GERIATRICS, GERONTOLOGY AND ELDERLY ISSUES

NEW HORIZONS IN GERIATRIC MEDICINE

VOLUME 1

GERIATRICS, GERONTOLOGY AND ELDERLY ISSUES

Additional books in this series can be found on Nova's website under the Series tab.

Additional e-books in this series can be found on Nova's website under the e-book tab.

GERIATRICS, GERONTOLOGY AND ELDERLY ISSUES

NEW HORIZONS IN GERIATRIC MEDICINE

VOLUME 1

AHMET TURAN ISIK, M.D.,
M. REFIK MAS, M.D.,
M. AKIF KARAN, M.D.,
AND
GEORGE T. GROSSBERG, M.D.
EDITORS

New York

Library of Congress Cataloging-in-Publication Data

ISBN: 978-1-62808-972-1

ISSN: 2330-5134

Published by Nova Science Publishers, Inc. † New York

CONTENTS

PREFACE

Old age is associated with a number of medico-social problems such as: hypertension, diabetes mellitus, thyroid disorders, osteoarthritis, tremor, pain, gait and balance impairment, incontinence, urinary tract infection, sarcopenia, osteoporosis, polypharmacy, pressure ulcers, sleeping problems, cardiocerebrovascular disorders, fluid and electrolyte disturbance, nutritional disorders, immunization and disease prevention rehabilitation and care. The management of these problems differs significantly between younger and older adults. All of these problems are evaluated in this book in two parts with the contributions of experienced clinicians and researchers. In addition, cellular aging, comprehensive geriatric assessments, and medicolegal and ethical principles in geriatric medicine are also evaluated. This book will be a valuable tool for all clinicians involved in the management of elderly people.

Chapter 1 - Many authors have searched oxidative stress and apoptosis on cellular aging process in literature. The chapter principally relate with cellular aging theories and also apoptotic process. According to the free radical theory of aging, free oxygen radicals accumulate over time leading to molecular damage, which causes aging. Investigators have also been evaluated in relating telomeres and aging. Aging is driven by the accumulation of damaged macromolecules, which appear as oxidized, cross-linked macromolecules that cause cells to function incorrectly. As a defensive mechanism, autophagy plays major catabolic role in all eukaryotic cells that degrades accumulated damaged macromolecules and also organelles. Programmed cell death which is called as apoptosis, is an active cell biochemical mechanism and causes cell death in tissues as the outcome of injury and degeneration. Shortly; relation between the cellular aging and the mitochondrial free radical theory of aging, telomeres, autophagy and apoptosis and their relation between some diseases are evaluated in detailed.

Chapter 2 - The term geriatrics comes from the Greek “geron” meaning "old man" and “iatros” meaning "healer”. According to World Health Organization (WHO), aim of geriatrics described as promoting health by preventing and treating diseases and disabilities in older adults. The geriatric population increased by achieving improvements in science, medicine and finance, especially in developed countries. As a result of that, each passing day doctors encounter more and more geriatric patients, thus the medical, social, psychological, cognitive and functional assessments of a geriatric patient have become essential. Here authors explain the important aspects of geriatric assessments.

Chapter 3 - Prevention through the life-course is a key to maintaining good health and a good quality of life in old age. Prevention in the elderly is more important than ever before, as this rapidly growing segment consumes a disproportionately high amount of health resources. Knowledge and consideration of unique aspects of preventive care in elderly can help better utilize limited resources and prevent hazards that may unintendedly be associated with health service utilization in this population.

In addition to targeting the universal causes of premature death, namely (1) heart disease and stroke, (2) cancer, (3) lung disease and (4) diabetes; health care providers will need to address factors such as limited life expectancy, multiple comorbidity, frailty and geriatric syndromes such as falls and inappropriate medication use in the preventive health care for the elderly. This chapter is intended to provide a framework for utilization of preventive services including counseling on lifestyle, immunization, cardiovascular disease prevention, cancer screening and other services relevant to the elderly by emphasizing unique aspects of prevention in this group.

Chapter 4 - The International Association for the Study of Pain (IASP) defines pain in terms of both actual or potential tissue damage and the emotional experiences associated with pain.

Pain is one of the most common complaints that remains poorly treated in the elderly. As we become older, different changes occur in the body and effect how it works.

Pain that is under-recognized and undertreated can result in significant physical and social disability in the elderly long-term care population. An aging adult may not respond to pain in the way that a younger person would. Their ability to recognize and report the pain often change according their illnesses, social conditions and dementia. The elderly need to detail the history of the pain, drugs and other complementaries that they have. They also need a good individual pain management plan. Most pain problems can be improved by proper assessment and careful use of analgesic drugs and nondrug strategies.

Chapter 5 - Anemia is defined as hemoglobin levels <13 g/dl in men and <12 g/dl in women according to World Health Organization criteria. Anemia incidence is reported 11.0% in men and 10.2% in women above 65 years of age in the "National Health and Nutrition Examination Survey (NHANES) III" in United States of America. There are three major causes of anemia in the elderly: nutritional anemia, mostly iron deficiency anemia, anemia of chronic disease or anemia of chronic inflammation and unexplained anemia. NHANES III data reveals that nutritional deficiency which is the mostly iron deficiency, vitamin B_{12} and/or folate deficiency is the major cause of anemia (34% in the elderly people). Iron deficiency alone or with folate and vitamin B_{12} deficiency compromise the 20% of the anemia in the elderly. Anemia of chronic disease is common and an important cause like iron deficiency anemia. Chronic renal disease is an important cause of anemia which is commonly seen in the elderly population. Unexplained anemia is present in the 20-30% of the elderly patients according to variety of epidemiological studies. Some theories that support the high incidence of anemia in the elderly are decrease in hematopoietic stem cells, decrease in the production of hematopoietic growth factors, decrease of the sensitivity of stem cells and progenitors to growth factors, bone marrow microenvironment abnormalities, androgen deficiency, age-related decrease in renal functions and/or erythropoietin release, undiagnosed chronic renal disease or myelodysplasia or early period of anemia of chronic disease. Some of the elderly patients with unexplained anemia have myelodysplastic syndrome which is defined as ineffective hematopoiesis, cytopenias, and an increased incidence of transformation into acute myeloid leukemia. Anemia increases the risk of mortality, cardiovascular diseases, fractures, and decreases the cognitive functions and physical performance. It should be implied that these symptoms appear not only in major reduction in hemoglobin levels also in slight fluctuations from the normal values. In the management of anemia, etiology should be investigated and treated if possible in the elderly population. Management is limited to transfusion of erythrocyte suspensions and erythropoiesis stimulating agents in patients with symptomatic anemia.

Chapter 6 - Vertigo is a term used for the complaint of disorientation in space mostly caused by an inner ear problem. It is a sense of unsteadiness or feeling of movement within the head such as giddiness or a swimming sensation. Equilibrium is affected by vision, vestibular sensation, proprioception, muscle strength and reaction time. There are many factors which may affect balance. Causes and treatment approaches of disequilibrium in elderly are discussed in this chapter.

Chapter 7 - As the population of seniors grows astoundingly, medical professionals will more frequently face to challenges in management of elderly patients with altered mental status. The general term "mental status change" has numerous synonyms. These terms are applied to a broad spectrum of conditions. Dementia, delirium, sepsis, hypoxia, hypoglycemia, depression and iatrogenic causes are common in the elderly and must be considered in differential diagnosis of altered mental status. Misdiagnosis and lack of recognition of underlying cause of altered mental status is costly to society and the family and is immeasurable in personal tragedy. Adopting an organized approach to the evaluation of mental status is therefore important for the evaluation of all older patients.

This chapter reviews the significance of altered mental status in the elderly. Specific diagnoses, including delirium, dementia, common medical conditions as a cause of altered mental status, depression and polypharmacy are discussed.

Chapter 8 - Presbystasis and falling are major disasters in geriatric patients. The proportion of geriatric population is increasing and so are their medical expenditures. The causes of dizziness and falling in elderly patients are different than other age groups, and are mainly non-vestibular disorders. The main vestibular cause of dizziness and vertigo in elderly patients is benign paroxysmal pozisyonel vertigo. Dizziness accounted for one third of all visits to the primary care physician in patients over the age of 65 years. More than half of all elderly falls occur in the home. The ideal testing modality in evaluating age-related balance loss and risk factors is Computer Dynamic Posturography. There are many exercise protocols for vestibular balance rehabilitation therapy.

Chapter 9 - A tremor is a rhytmic, oscillatory movement produced by alternating or synchronous contractions of antagonist muscles. It is the most common form of involuntary movements and is common in the elderly population. The cause of the tremor in old age ranges from a benign physiological tremor to a more serious tremor of neurodegenerative disorders like Parkinson's disease (PD). We can classify tremors according to their phenomenology (rest or action tremors), distribution (hand, head, jaw, tongue, leg, trunk), frequency (slow, medium or fast) or etiology (physiologic, semptomatic, degenerative). The prevelance of tremors in people aged 50-85 was found to be 15 % where the most common type of tremor was physiological tremor or Essential Tremor (ET) and tremor related to parkinsonism was only 2.75%. The prevelance of the postural tremor increases with age. Beta blockers and antiepileptic drugs can be used for ET or physiological tremor, while dopaminergic drugs are used for the tremor of patients in PD. It is important to be aware of the side effects of these drugs in the elderly. Semptomatic tremors, like the serebellar tremor, can also be seen in the elderly and are mostly the result of a stroke or a tumor. Neuropathic and ortostatic tremors are less frequent tremors which may also be seen in old age.

Chapter 10 - The prevention and management of systemic arterial hypertension (HT) remains a major public health challenge worldwide due to its high prevalance and importance as a cardiovascular disease (CVD) risk factor.

Chapter 11 - When considering changes in endocrine function of the elderly, it is important to distinguish between the effects of aging per se on the physiology of the endocrine system and those caused by age-related diseases, given the high prevalence of disorders both symptomatic and asymptomatic in the elderly. Moreover, the distinction between age and disease related to the change does not necessarily determine the therapeutic intervention.

The action of certain hormones decrease with age, the secretion of growth hormone may or may not offset these reductions in the responsiveness of the tissue.

The appropriate goal for hemoglobin A1C (HbA1c) in elderly patients who have a life expectancy of more than ten years should be similar to those developed for younger adults (<7.0 percent). The aim should be slightly higher (≤ 8.0 percent) in frail elderly with multiple medical comorbidities and functional and those whose life expectancy is less than ten years. Individual goals for the very elderly may be even greater and should include efforts to preserve the quality of life and prevent hypoglycemia and complications.

The risk of hypoglycemia, which can lead to a deterioration of cognitive functions and is significantly higher in the elderly. Therefore, avoiding hypoglycemia is an important consideration in the choice of therapeutic agents in the elderly.

Elderly patients with diabetes should receive individualized advice on lifestyle changes, including medical nutrition assessment. The prescription of nutrition for the elderly with diabetes based on medical, lifestyle and personal factors.

In the absence of specific indications-cons, suggested metformin as initial therapy for elderly patients with diabetes (Grade 2B). In patients with against-indications and/or intolerance to metformin, a sulfonylurea short-acting (e.g., glipizide) is an alternative option.

In patients who can not tolerate or are not candidates for metformin or sulfonylureas, repaglinide is a reasonable alternative, especially in a patient with chronic renal failure with risk of hypoglycemia.

If glycemic targets are not met a single agent, the elderly patient should be evaluated by the contributing causes, such as difficulty adhering to medication side effects, or a misunderstanding of the terms of nutrition.

Indications for a second officer and the treatment options for patients who fail initial treatment with a lifestyle intervention and metformin or a sulfonylurea were similar in elderly and younger.

Chapter 12 - This chapter will give insights for the diagnosis and treatment of thyroid disorders in the elderly. Thyroid disorders may cause significant morbidity if left untreated in the geriatric population. The diagnosis of the thyroid dysfunction in older patients is challenging since the presenting symptoms are sometimes atypical. Also the comorbidities and the confounders, common in this age group, may obscure the diagnosis. Therefore, it is always important to consider the possibility of thyroid disease in the elderly population. Serum TSH measurement should be performed as a screening test in the elderly. As the gland is often shrunken, the physical examination gives almost nothing in the elderly patient. The prudent physician should be patient while treating overt hypothyroidism. Low-dose levothyroxine should be implemented while starting the treatment and gradually increased within months. In treating hyperthyroidism, radioactive iodine rather than antithyroid medication seem to be definitive, well tolerated and effective. Surgical thyroid ablation is rarely necessary when the radioactive iodine therapy is not successful or in patients with multinodular goiter. Fine needle aspiration for cytology should be considered if the ultrasound findings are suspicious for malignancy.

Chapter 13 - Osteoarthritis (OA) is one of the most common causes of chronic disability in elderly and is related with a reduced quality of life. OA is clearly associated with aging, but there are additional factors that contribute to the development of OA like systemic (genetics, diet, estrogen use, and bone density) and local factors (muscle weakness, obesity, injury, malalignment). OA occurs as a result of various biochemical, biomechanical, inflammatory, and immunologic factors, not solely from the wearing down of the joints.

Aging-related changes of joint tissues that occur at the cellular level are cell senescence, decreased anabolic response to growth factors, accumulation of oxidative damage to DNA and telomere shortening. Changes within the extracellular matrix are increased collagen crosslinking by advanced glycation end products (AGEs), accumulation of modified and degraded extracellular matrix components and increased calcification. Age-related changes also occur in muscle, bone, fat, and the nervous system in elderly people that suggests OA to be a complex disease. How these aging changes interact with etiological factors to cause OA is unknown. Advanced imaging methods, evidence from genetic and biomarker studies has led to better understanding of the natural course of OA, provides information for early diagnosis and understanding the basic mechanisms by which aging affects joint tissues.

Although OA is most common in the hands, involvement of the knees and hips is usually much more disabling. OA management should consist of a combination of nonpharmacologic and pharmacologic treatment options. Usually all OA guidelines agree on shared recommendations for treatment. A wide array of agents have been studied for disease modification in OA, but the existing pharmacologic agents have not been shown to have convincing disease- modifying efficacy. More research is needed to provide new targets for slowing or preventing the development of OA. In the elderly, the management of OA has to be individualized for each patient according to the severity of symptoms and joint damage, joints affected, comorbidities, drug interactions, prior treatments, patient wishes and illness perceptions. Difficulties for patients to access health professional services also has to be considered in the treatment plan.

There is a rapid increase in the prevalence of OA because of aging population. This places a tremendous burden on health care system and causes great impact on elderly people and society. Further studies are needed to provide the early diagnosis and interventions that can help reduce the impact of OA on health care.

Chapter 14 - An elder patient with a urinary tract infection (UTI) is not an infrequent applicant in the emergency department and poor outcome in this patient population admitted to emergency room with UTI has been known. UTIs have been classified as complicated or uncomplicated to emphasize the underlying urinary comorbid conditions, upper or lower to point anatomic localization, catheter-associated symptomatic or asymptomatic to delineate the catheterization status of a given patient. Contributing factors specific to gender include prostate enlargement in men, the increase of vaginal pH, vaginal atrophy due to postmenopausal estrogen depletion, and incomplete emptying of the bladder in elder women. Since classic clinical manifestations of UTIs such as dysuria, fever, urinary frequency and suprapubic tenderness may be absent or masked in the elderly, treating these infections in this group of patients is a special challenge for physicians. Vague symptoms such as nausea, vomiting and decreased urinary output must be distinguished from symptoms of other common illnesses. Thus, infections often present in subtle fashion in the elderly. Physicians must be aware of unique predispositions to infection among elder adults and must seek early recognition and diagnosis of disease and early initiation of therapy.

SECTION 1: CELLULAR AGING

In: New Horizons in Geriatric Medicine. Volume 1
Editors: Ahmet Turan Isik, M. Refik Mas et al.
ISBN: 978-1-62808-972-1

Chapter 1

CELLULAR AGING

Yasemin Soysal[1], Murat Tosun[2] and Nuket Gocmen Mas[3]

[1]Afyon Kocatepe University, Medical Faculty, Department of Medical Genetics, Afyonkarahisar, Turkey

[2]Afyon Kocatepe University, Medical Faculty, Department of Histology and Embryology, Afyonkarahisar, Turkey

[3]Dokuz Eylul University, Medical Faculty, Department of Anatomy, Izmir, Turkey

ABSTRACT

Many authors have searched oxidative stress and apoptosis on cellular aging process in literature. The chapter principally relate with cellular aging theories and also apoptotic process. According to the free radical theory of aging, free oxygen radicals accumulate over time leading to molecular damage, which causes aging. Investigators have also been evaluated in relating telomeres and aging. Aging is driven by the accumulation of damaged macromolecules, which appear as oxidized, cross-linked macromolecules that cause cells to function incorrectly. As a defensive mechanism, autophagy plays major catabolic role in all eukaryotic cells that degrades accumulated damaged macromolecules and also organelles. Programmed cell death which is called as apoptosis, is an active cell biochemical mechanism and causes cell death in tissues as the outcome of injury and degeneration. Shortly; relation between the cellular aging and the mitochondrial free radical theory of aging, telomeres, autophagy and apoptosis and their relation between some diseases are evaluated in detailed.

Keywords: Cellular aging, free radicals, telomeres, autophagy, disease

Aging is a multifactorial degenerative process and can be defined as the steady increase with time of the probability of dying because of a gradual loss of the metabolic and genetic substances that maintain cellular function [1]. Many theories of aging have been proposed and can be divided into two main categories: the stochastic and the genetic theories [2].

The biological theory of why we age and the question of what exactly is happening inside our cells still leave one question unanswered. That is, how does aging take place at the cellular level? This is a difficult question demanding detailed molecular mechanisms. It is straightforward to assume that organism aging is caused by the accumulation of cellular changes that lead to cell aging. However, there is difficulty in conducting human *in vivo* studies because of the duration of aging. Alternatively, cellular cultures have been used, because aging is in part of a cellular origin.

Biogerontology studies the biological basis of aging. Age-related changes are characterized by the accumulation of worn-out organelles and cellular substructures over time, reducing the molecular efficiency of biological processes, which in turn decreases the ability of the organism to survive and increases the risk of death [2]. In 1965, The Cellular Senescence Theory of aging was formulated after *in vitro* experimental studies demonstrated a limited number of cell divisions in normal human cell cultures [3, 4].

This chapter mainly deals with cellular aging theories and also apoptotic process. Briefly; causal connection of aging process with the mitochondrial free radical theory of aging, telomeres, autophagy and apoptosis are discussed.

THE MITOCHONDRIAL FREE RADICAL THEORY OF AGING

The mitochondrion (Greek *Mito*, thread; *chondrion*, granule) is believed to be a once free-living bacteria that our ancient eukaryotic ancestors absorbed within their organisms [5, 6]. This view can explain why this organelle contains its own genome as well as its own biosynthetic machinery to make organelle proteins and RNA. The biosynthesis of mitochondria relies on special genes in nuclear DNA for its replication as well as transcription and translation. The structure of mitochondrial DNA resembles that of bacteria, which is a likely relation; even through mitochondria contain no histones. In 1981, researchers published the human mitochondrial genome complete sequence of 16,569 nucleotides in a simple circular structure. The primary function of mitochondria is to generate ATP via several protein complexes in ezymatic machinery for oxidative phosphorylation or the electron transport chain system [5]. Mitochondria consist of three structures, outer and inner membranes and the matrix, into which cristae protrude [7].

Free radicals or reactive oxygen species are any atoms or molecules that contain an unpaired electron in the outer shell, which makes them unstable. This unstable structure makes them highly reactive and inclined to pick up an electron to add to their last orbital to balance themselves; in this way, the attacked molecule is transformed into a free radical. Major free radicals are the superoxide radical ($O_2^{\bullet -}$) and hydroxyl radical ($OH^{\bullet}$). Cells protect themselves from oxidative damage by free radical scavengers, which are called antioxidants and include the flavonoids, carotenoids, glutathione, uric acid, and vitamins A, C, and E and the superoxide dismutase and catalase and glutathione peroxidase enzymes [2]. The balance between the level of pro-oxidant and antioxidant factors determines the outcome of age-causing oxidative damage. As a natural byproduct of oxidative phosphorylation, reactive oxygen species (ROS) are thought to damage proteins, lipids, and DNA as well as mitochondrial DNA [5].

In 1956, D. Harman first proposed the association between free radicals at the level of the electron transport chain and aging, and, over the years, other reactive species such as hydrogen peroxide (H_2O_2) and singlet oxygen also have been included in this association [8]. Damage to the mitochondrial DNA has been proposed as being responsible for the increased production of ROS and thus, the subsequent dysfunction of mitochondria has been hypothesized as being responsible for aging [8,9]. According to the mitochondrial free radical theory of aging (MFRTA), the core statement is that ROS arise from normal mitochondrial metabolism and damage mitochondrial and cytosolic constituents and this accumulated damage causes aging. In addition to this main statement, associated hypotheses include the deterioration of mitochondrial function over time because of more ROS production from malfunctioned mitochondria and the progressive accumulation of non-mitochondrial oxidative damage [1].

Since the MFRTA was proposed, numerous papers have provided evidence both for and against its core statement and satellite hypotheses [1, 9-14]. To date, the findings have revealed that the core statement of the theory is wrong but the associated hypotheses are correct [1]. Accordingly, the theory is now under challenge [15-17]. Dietary administration of antioxidant compounds, which decreases the incidence of free radicals, did not extend the lifespan in experimental studies in mammals, but the results are inconsistent in Drosophila [18-20]. Howes reviewed the papers about antioxidants, which were conducted on more than 550,000 humans and concluded that "not only have antioxidants failed to stop disease and aging but also they may cause harm and mortality" [9, 18]. Even resveratrol, a potential antioxidant compound, has been shown to extend lifespan in invertebrates, but not in mice. Also, feeding mice with the well-known mitochondrial antioxidant coenzyme Q_{10} has had no effect on extending lifespan [1]. It has been demonstrated that the deletion of mitochondrial superoxide dismutase (Sod-2) extended lifespan in *C.elegans* [17, 21]. However, in a study, the overexpression of the mitochondrial superoxide dismutase did not extend lifespan in single transgenic mice, while normally it is expected to show a defense against mitochondrial superoxide [13]. In an experimental study in young MCLK1+/- (MCLK1; a mitochondrial enzyme necessary for ubiquinone (coenzyme Q) biosynthesis) mice, the reduced energy metabolism and increased oxidative stress in the mitochondria resulted in protection against mitochondrial dysfunction, which is increased by age [17, 22]. This study demonstrates mitochondrial oxidative stress does not cause aging [22]. However, the only experimental data that supports the mitochondrial oxidative theory is the high degree of expression in mice of human peroxisomal catalase targeted to mitochondria, resulting in a longer life of 17–21% in mutant mice than in wild types [22, 23].

The free radical theory of aging allows for a wide spectrum of both ROS sources and molecular targets of ROS, including mtDNA. In 2003, Jacobs pointed out this theory had been neither proven nor disproven [9, 24]. Today, most experimental evidence does not support the mitochondrial theory of aging but it is likely to be recognized that damage to mitochondrial components plays an important but not essential role in aging. Mitochondrial dysfunction which is clinically important, intimately associated to the production of reactive oxygen species (ROS) and mitochondrial related apoptosis. It also appears to be aggravated in some brain disorder patients like Alzheimer Disease [25].

TELOMERES IN CELLULAR AGING

Telomeres are special repetitive DNA sequences and associated proteins that cap both ends of linear chromosomes, which were first discovered by Barbara McClintock and

Hermann Müller in 1930. Müller first termed these structures telomeres, from the Greek for "end" (telos) and "part" (meros) [26]. Telomeres are essential for chromosome integrity and represent the cellular biological clock. Forty years later, Alexey Olovnikov realized that there is a problem in the semiconservative replication of DNA. As conventional DNA polymerases needed a primer to start DNA synthesis, the space occupied at the end by these RNA primers is not filled with new DNA synthesis, so with every cell division, some genetic information from the leading DNA strand end part would be lost [27]. This problem was known as the "end replication problem" [28]. Cellular senescence (p53 tumor-induced suppressor protein) or death occurs when telomeres become critically short and the nucleus signals the cell to stop proliferation [27]. The prediction that somatic cells would have a finite lifespan was proven in 1961 by Hayflick and Moorhead. These researchers discovered that embryo-derived fibroblasts could only divide around 50 times in culture; this is known as replicative senescence (RS). Also, the potential number of divisions a cell is capable of is known as the "Hayflick limit" [8].

Elizabeth Blackburn and Joe Gall were the first to sequence *Tetrahymena thermophila*, and showed the tandem G-rich continues (TTAGGG in humans) expanding until the chromosome ends [Finkel, 2007]. Later, it was realized that some cells could elongate pre-existing telomeres either by recombination events between telomeres or by enzymatic activity that could synthesize telomere nucleotides *de novo* [28]. Elizabeth Blackburn and Carol Greider discovered an enzyme that repairs the loss of telomeres, which was then named as telomerase (TERT), a ribonucleoprotein with reverse transcriptase activity [29]. Telomerase is present in male and female germinal cells and hematopoietic stem cells but not in somatic cells. However, most tumor cells express telomerase at high levels [30]. Following this discovery, an alternative lengthening of the telomeres (ALT) pathway by recombination mechanisms was demonstrated in tumor cells [27, 31].

Most studies have shown that telomere lengths decrease with age in nucleated mammalian cells, particularly in the highly proliferative leukocytes [30]. In adulthood, a telomere shortens 60 base pairs at 20 years of age, but at age 80, the attrition rate decreases to 20 base pairs and, older than this age, the decrease is nondeductible [30, 32]. In a study, it was found that individuals around 60 years with shorter telomeres live less long lives than the individuals who had longer telomeres [33]. Cardiovascular (CV) disease in elderly men as the cause of death was also common in subjects with short peripheral leukocytes telomere length (TL) [34]. Furthermore, psychological stressors might influence immune cell proliferation and be associated with a decrease in blood telomere lengths [35]. Telomeres that shortened till the threshold level resemble damaged DNA and activate the p53-dependent pathway, which causes cellular senescence [36]. Treatments that inactivate the tumor suppressor protein p53 in senescent cells were found to trigger reentry into the replication cycle and cell proliferation [4]. Telomerase overexpression can improve wound healing by cell proliferation; on the other hand, it can also induce cancer cells to proliferate indefinitely in mice [37]. There is some evidence that telomeres may contribute to human aging. It has been demonstrated that, characteristically, vascular cells have a finite lifespan and the telomere shortening that occurs in human vessels might be related to atherogenesis [36]. In vascular endothelial cells from the abdominal aorta and the iliac arteries, telomere length decreases with age [36, 38]. Also, CV disease and stress-induced damage override the telomere shortening in endothelial cells.

Leukocyte TL always measure cellular aging. It is related with age connected disease onset, psychosocial stress, and health caused functional decline [39]. Several endogenous factors causing telomere shortening are present such as aging, oxidative stress and inflammation. Leukocyte TL shortening is inhibited by estrogen and endogenous antioxidants. Accelerated telomere attrition is also linked by CV risk factors such as age, gender, sedentary life-style, obesity, smoking, excess alcohol intake, and even mental stress. CV diseases and CV aging are generally but not invariably correlated with shorter telomeres than in healthy people. Psychosocial stress has been related with the onset of chronic pain and chronic pain is experienced as a physical and psychosocial stress factors [39, 40]. In an animal study, an atherosclerotic mouse model was used and, perhaps because of the reduced proliferation of macrophages, telomere shortening has been shown to decrease the area of atherosclerotic lesions [41]. In another study, mice lacking telomerase activity developed hypertension as a result of the overexpression of endothelin-converting enzyme [36]. Telomere dysfunction was first implicated in dyskeratosis congenita (DC), which is present in a variety of inheritance patterns, with the mutations in the dyskerin gene (DKC1) [4, 26]. The mutation in nucleolar protein dyskerin affects an enzyme that is involved in the telomerase RNA subunit (hTR) metabolism [42]. The telomerase levels of dyskeratosis congenita patients may be reduced by one-half to one-fifth, but not be completely absent. However, individuals develop pathologies at an earlier age when the telomerase deficiency degree is high [4]. More recently, a number of polymorphisms and mutations that cause telomerase deficiencies have been described [43, 44]. For progeroid syndromes patients who were suffering from accelerated aging, neither the direct nor the indirect effects of telomere length have been proven [26]. The indirect effect could be the increased cell death resulting from defective DNA repair, which in turn causes telomere shortening by increased stem cell turn over. For example, the cells of Werner syndrome patients divide slower than normal while Hutchinson-Gilford syndrome patients' cells divide faster than normal [45]. In addition, these progeroid disease cells tend towards apoptosis and stress [46]. Fanconi anemia and ataxia telangiectasia, segmental aging disorders, are associated with accelerated telomere shortening [26]. These observations suggest that alterations at a cellular level may explain the aging phenotype.

A number of clinical trials and interventions have been conducted to rescue human cells *in vitro* from senescence by targeting the activity of telomeres or telomerase [26, 47]. Also, the inhibition of telomerase activity is an interesting research area for cancer treatment. Today, in spite of accumulated data that telomere shortening mediates human aging, the effects of the organism's environment on telomere degradation are poorly understood.

Autophagy in Cellular Aging

Autophagy, from the Greek "to eat oneself," is the major catabolic process present in all eukaryotic cells that degrades damaged macromolecules and organelles, through a lysosomal pathway [48]. For cells to operate properly, these waste molecules must be eliminated. Although the autophagy process was described over 40 years ago, its role in longevity and healthy aging is only now largely accepted. Autophagy is characterized by the engulfment of part of the cytoplasm inside double-membrane vesicles, fusion with lysosomes, and degradation of cytoplasmic macromolecules. Newly formed vesicles called autophagosomes and the products of degradation are recycled for the synthesis of new molecules. The types of autophagy depend on the mechanism by which the cytosolic materials are transported into the lysosomes and the type of waste [49]. There are three main types of autophagy: macroautophagy, microautophagy, and chaperone-mediated autophagy [2]. Macroautophagy can be induced by stress conditions like nutrient deprivation, infections, and toxins. Transmission electron microscopic (TEM) evaluation may show autophagy in detailed. In macroautophagy, a *de novo*-synthesized membrane, which is encased into an autophagosome (Figure: 1), disunites the entire regions of the cytosol [50]. This form of autophagy is the most important form that has been implicated in lifespan control [2, 49]. Cellular damage is an important contributory factor. Molecular chaperones and cellular self-degradative systems and lysosome-mediated autophagy maintain cellular homeostasis and play an essence role in the aging process [51]. Autophagic degradation components of amino acids and fatty acids are used as alternative energy sources for cells during starvation and the elimination of damaged organelles' macromolecules contributes to cellular clearance. Also, when rapid reorganization of the cellular functions is necessary, autophagy becomes part of the cellular response. In rat liver, the degradation rate of long-lived proteins were measured and it was shown that there was an age-dependent reduction in autophagic activity because of the progressive accumulation of damaged proteins in aged cells. Further, it was proposed that calorie restriction can prevent a decline in autophagic activity [49]. Autophagy activation during cellular senescence was correlated with negative feedback in the PI3K-m TOR pathway. In the sub group of autophagy-related genes, when the ULK3 gene was overexpressed, autophagy and senescence were induced [17].

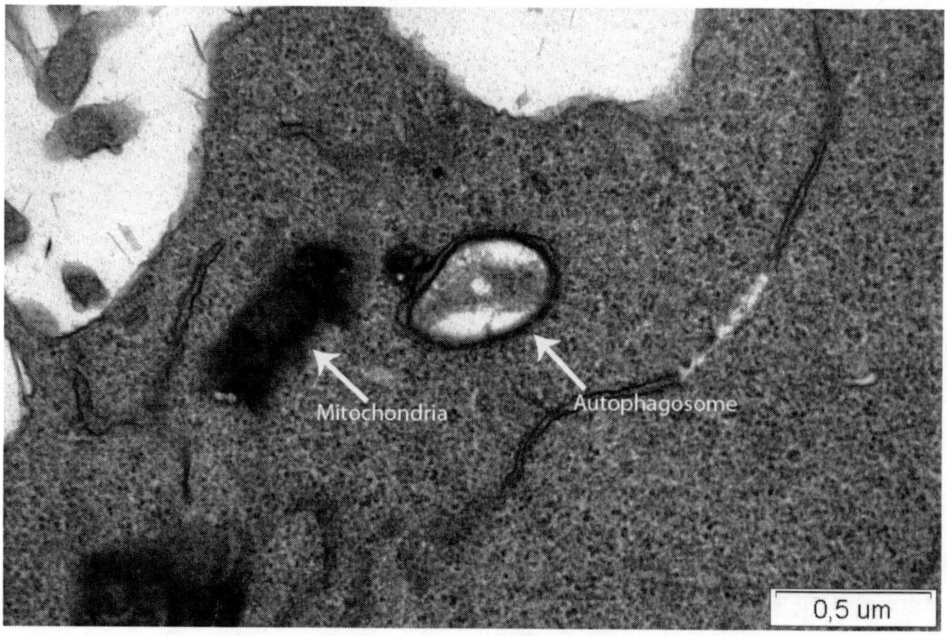

Figure:1. Autophogosome formation after macroautophagy (TEM).

Apoptosis in Cellular Aging

All the cells are born, live, sometimes differentiate to other cells, age, and always die, like everything in the universe. Although sometimes the cell dies from different intrinsic causes such as autoimmune diseases, cancer etc. or extrinsic agents such as bacterium or infection, generally most of the cells in the body die physiologically during all stages of life by programmed cell death, which is also known as apoptosis. Recently, several authors have searched oxidative stress and apoptotic process in developmental brain disorders like hereditary DNA repair disorders, congenital metabolic errors and childhood-onset neurodegenerative disorders; CV events, infections, autoimmune, colon and renal diseases [52-55].

The apoptosis concept was first described by Kerr, Wyllie, and Currie in 1972. Nowadays, this concept has been much improved and many mechanisms that regulate this process in cell have been discovered [56,57].

Programmed cell death can also be described as the suicide of normal cells by intrinsic and/or extrinsic pathways' activation. This mechanism may occur during different times of life from conception to death. Because apoptosis controls the number of cells in tissues, it can be accepted as one of the most important regulatory mechanisms in tissue reparation, regeneration, remodeling, and resurrection. In the embryonic and fetal periods, different tissue remodeling such as neural canal formation, the disappearance of interdigital mesenchymal tissue to form fingers, and formation of all the tubular organs' lumens is managed by apoptotic cell death [56]. Also, after birth, billions of cells in the body, especially in bone marrow, intestines, skin etc. die and are eliminated from the body without the retention of any harmful waste. At the same time, apoptosis is a fundamental mechanism in tissue homeostasis, immune response, metamorphosis, and development. Contrary to apoptosis, in necrosis, a kind of cell death, the cell is destroyed and many harmful agents such as enzymes, cytokines etc. are released in the cells' environment and damage the nearest cells and activate immunological responses. This activation is rapidly augmented by the other cells nearest to the damage and inflammation occurs [58]. All these reactions have an effect on the cells' lifetime. Even though the cells do not die, because of many biochemical reactions during the inflammatory process, the cells' organelles are aged and the lifetimes of the cells are shortened.

Apoptosis is activated by different stimuli from the intrinsic or extrinsic environment. Although toxins, nitric oxide, and the activation of different signal transduction pathways, such as by hormones, cytokines, and growth factors are extrinsic apoptotic factors, the factors such as heat, malnutrition, hypoxia, glucocorticoids, and high intracellular calcium levels are some of the intrinsic factors [58,59]. However, it should be noticed that these factors can either activate or suppress apoptotic cell death. Occasionally, the same factor can work as both stimulant and suppressant on apoptosis in different milieu interiors. For example, although under normal conditions p53 is a guardian of the genome, and has an antiapoptotic effect on cells, if cell damage cannot be repaired well; it stimulates the intrinsic apoptotic pathways and triggers apoptosis [60].

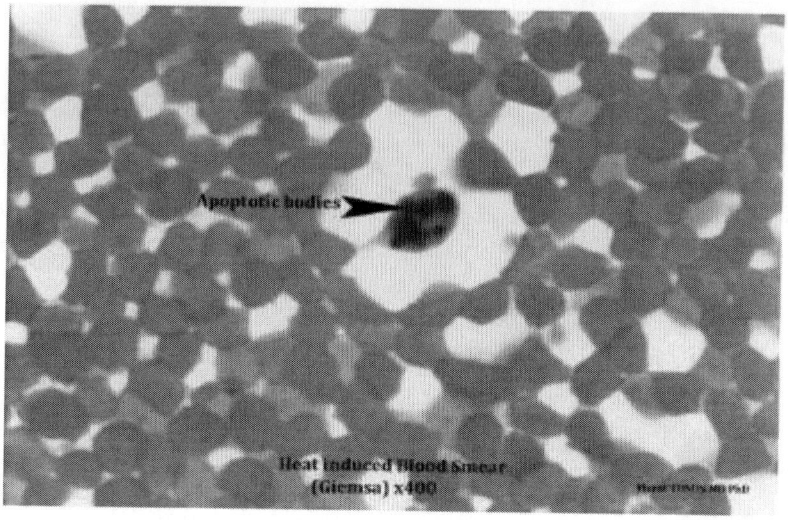

Figure 2. Apoptotic bodies in an apoptotic Neutrophil in heat-induced blood smear. Giemsa.

Apoptosis has the main morphological features such as membrane blebbing, nuclear condensation due to degradation of DNA also known as pyknosis, shrinkage by breakdown of cell cytoskeleton by the induction of caspases, and formation of apoptotic bodies (Figure:2) in the cytoplasm. On the other hand, nucleosomal 180-200 bp DNA laddering after endonuclease activation is another feature of apoptosis [58]. However, different studies have revealed that morphological and biochemical changes in apoptotic cell death can be different for each cell. On the other hand, in a molecular aspect, different markers have been defined to detect apoptosis in the cell. These markers include caspases, mainly caspase 3 and Annexin V, changes in mitochondrial membrane potential, and the detection of different signal transduction pathways members such as TRAIL R2, Apaf-1, p53, Bax family, Fas, and associated pathways [61]. However, the presence of these markers in the cell does not mean mainly that that cell is apoptotic. If the cell stress that is activating these pathways interrupts, the suicide of the cell stops their suicide and the cell returned to a healthy state. In this case, a change in mitochondrial membrane potential is the most critical landmark for the cell life. If this potential changes, the cell will certainly go into apoptosis. As known, because mitochondria are very essential organelle for multicellular organisms, and any damage to them results in the cessation of aerobic respiration of the cell and the cell dies. For example, nitric oxide triggers to cell into apoptosis via dissipation of mitochondrial membrane potential, which causes an increase of the membrane's permeability [58]. Then, under the influence of SMACs (small mitochondria-derived activator of caspases), the mitochondrial proteins are released into the cytoplasm and bind and deactivate the IAPs (inhibitor of apoptosis proteins). Accordingly, apoptotic activity of the caspases, which is normally blocked by the IAPs, activates apoptotic cell death [62]. On the other hand, Cytochrome C, which is released from the mitochondria, generates the mitochondrial apoptosis-induced channel formation (MAC) in the outer mitochondrial membrane. These channels serve a regulatory function for the morphological change associated with apoptosis. [58,63,64]. After Cytochrome C is released into the cytosol, it binds to Apaf-1 (Apoptotic protease activating factor – 1) and ATP and builds the apoptosome complex, which cleaves pro-caspase to caspase 9 and then to caspase 3. Besides these intrinsic apoptotic factors, different extrinsic factors activate apoptotic cell death in tissue. The direct signal transduction induced by Fas-Fas ligand and TNF family-induced pathways can also result in apoptosis. TNF is mainly activated by macrophages and is a major extrinsic mediator of apoptosis. When the TNF is released, it binds to the TNF receptor-associated death domain (TRADD) and Fas-associated death domain protein (FADD) and cleaves into caspases [58,61]. This mechanism is very useful for understanding the mechanisms of different diseases and also senescence. Because recurrent infections cause TNF-related apoptotic cell death, the number of cells in tissues decreases faster via apoptosis and organ dysfunction may occur [56,57]. On the other hand, the Fas receptor, also known as Apo-1, binds to the Fas ligand as a transmembrane protein and activates the formation of DISC (death-inducing signaling complex) and causes the activation of apoptotic pathways [65].

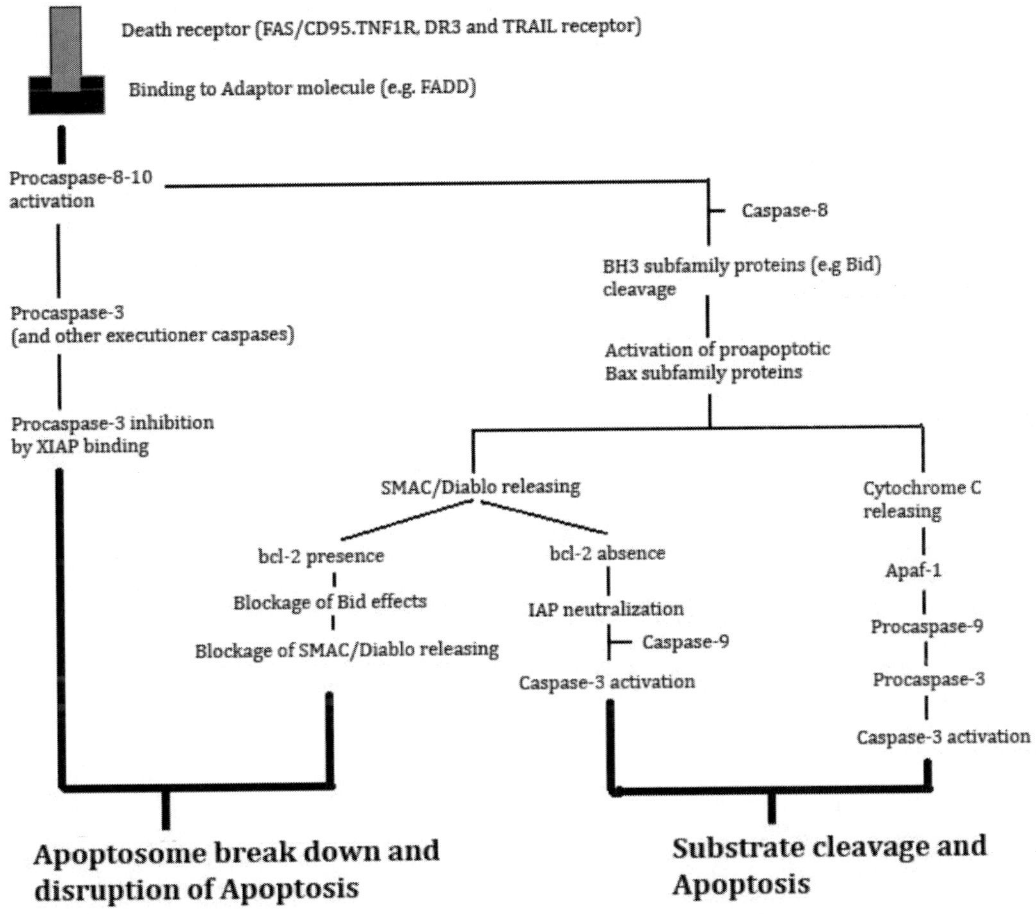

Figure:3. Intrinsic apoptotic pathways.

Caspases are proteins that are highly conserved, cysteine-dependent aspartate-specific proteases and play a very important role in apoptotic cell death. There are two types of caspases: initiator caspases (caspase 2, 8, 9, 10) and effector caspases (caspase 3, 6, 7). In the execution of apoptosis after initiator caspases bind to a specific oligomeric adaptor protein, effector caspases are activated and these trigger apoptotic cell death cascades. In the tissues, different molecules and factors control apoptotic cell death and establish a balance between living and apoptotic cells. Although some of these factors, such as p53, Bax, Bid, Bak, and Bad are proapoptotic, some of them, such as bcl-2 and bcl-Xl, are antiapoptotic [58]. Maintaining a balance between these factors is important to healthy body functions. For example, if proapoptotic factors are more effective than antiapoptotic factors, the cells in tissues die faster and the body ages. On the other hand, if antiapoptotic factors are more active, the cells cannot be dying and senile and damaged cells cannot be removed from the body and different diseases, including autoimmune deficiencies, chronic conditions, and even malignancies can occur. All the removal of the apoptotic cells in the body that takes place by neighboring phagocytic cells is termed as efferocytosis [66]. The importance of this mechanism is independent of the inflammatory response contrary to necrosis.

In summary, apoptosis is one of the most important mechanisms in the body during life. Manifestation of initial definition of programmed cell death has appeared as a basic biological circumstance fundamental for development and alignment of homeostasis whose alteration has significant implications in pathologies. Dysregulation of apoptotic cell death results in the dysfunction of tissue, organs, and even systems and may predispose the organism toward diseases as well as preaging. Over 65 years of survey in the territory of cell death and its relation with clinical manifestations are still tried to explain by many mechanism and theories. We thought that in the foreseeable future more circumstances based on control of the variant forms of cell deathor apoptosis may enter the clinical applications. Many troubles need to be analyzed such as activation of alternative cellular death cascades when one is averted via gene or drug therapy, in diseases as well as unexpected death when trying to eliminate pathological cells such as in anti-cancer treatments.

REFERENCES

[1] Lapointe J and Hekimi S. 2010. When a theory of aging ages badly. *Cell Mol Life Sci.,* 67; 1-8.

[2] Rajawat YS, Hilioti Z, Bossis I. 2009. Aging: central role for autophagy and the lysosomal degradative system. *Ageing Research Reviews,* 8; 199-213.

[3] Hayflick L. 1985. Theories of biological aging. *Exp Gerontol.,* 20; 145-159.

[4] Weinert BT and Timiras PS. 2003. Invited review: theories of aging. *J Appl Physiol,* 95; 1706-1716.

[5] Reeve AK, Krishnan KJ, Turnbull D. 2008. Age related mitochondrial degenerative disorders in humans. *Biotechnology J.,* 3; 750-756.

[6] Kierszenbaum AL. 2007. *Epithelial glands: mitochondria in 2nd Ed, Histology and cell biology: an introduction to pathology,* Mosby Elsevier, Philadelphia, pp.77.ISBN 0-323-04527-8.

[7] Frey TG, Renken CW, Perkins GA. 2002. Insight into mitochondrial structure and function from electron tomography. *Biochim Biophys Acta.,* 1555; 196-203.

[8] Passos JF and von Zglinicki T. 2005. Mitochondria, telomeres and cell senescence. *Experimental Gerontology.* 40; 466-472.

[9] Alexeyev MF. 2009. Is there more to aging than mitochondrial DNA and reactive oxygen species? *FEBS Journal,* 276; 5768-5787.

[10] Martin GM. 2011. The biology of aging: 1985-2010 and beyond. *FASEB J.,* 25;3756-3762.

[11] Pérez VI, Bokov A, Van Remmen H, Mele J, Ran QT, Ikeno Y, Richardson A. 2009. Is the oxidative stress theory of aging dead? *Biochim Biophys Acta.,* 1790; 1005-1014.

[12] Gruber J, Schaffer S, Halliwell B. 2008. The mitochondrial free radical theory of ageing –where do we stand? *Front Biosci.,* 13; 6554-6579.

[13] Muller FL, Lustgarten MS, Jang Y, Richardson A, Van Remmen H. 2007. Trends in oxidative aging theories. *Free Radic Biol Med.,* 43; 477-503.

[14] Miquel J, Economos AC, Fleming J, Johnson JE Jr. 1980. Mitochondrial role in cell aging. *Exp Gerontol.,* 15; 575-591.

[15] De Magalhaes JP, Church GM. 2006. Cell discover fire: employing reactive oxygen species in development and consequences for aging. *Exp Gerontol.,* 41; 1-10.

[16] Fukui H, Moraes CT. 2008. The mitochondrial impairment, oxidative stres and neurodegeneration connection: reality or just an attractive hypothesis? *Trends Neurosci.,* 31; 251-256.

[17] Mikhail VB, Blagosklonny MV, Campisi J, Sinclair DA, Bartke A, Blasco MA, Bonner WM, Bohr VA, Brosh RM Jr, Brunet A, Depinho RA, Donehower LA, Finch CE, Finkel T, Gorospe M, Gudkov AV, Hall MN, Hekimi S, Helfand SL, Karlseder J, Kenyon C, Kroemer G, Longo V, Nussenzweig A, Osiewacz HD, Peeper DS, Rando TA, Rudolph KL, Sassone-Corsi P, Serrano M, Sharpless NE, Skulachev VP, Tilly JL, Tower J, Verdin E, Vijg J. 2010. *Impact papers on aging in 2009.* Aging, 2(3), 111-121.

[18] Howes RM. 2006. The free radical fantasy: a panoply of paradoxes. *Ann AY Acad Sci.,* 1067, 22-26.

[19] Magwere T, West M, Riyahi K, Murphy MP, Smith RA, Partridge L. 2006. The effects of exogenous antioxidants on lifespan and oxidative stres resistance in Drosophila melanogaster. *Mech Ageing Dev.,* 127; 356-370.

[20] Pérez VI, Van Remmen H, Bokov A, Epstein CJ, Vijg J, Richardson A. 2009. The overexpression of major antioxidant enzymes does not extend the lifespan of mice. *Aging Cell,* 8; 73-75.

[21] Van Raamsdonk JM, Hekimi S. 2009. Deletion of the mitochondrial superoxide dismutase sod-2 extends lifespan in Caenorhabditis elegans. *PLoS Genet.,* 5; e1000361.

[22] Lapointe J, Stepanyan Z, Bigras E, Hekimi S. 2009. Reversal of the mitochondrial phenotype and slow development of oxidative biomarkers of aging in long-lived Mclk1+/- mice. *J Biol Chem.,* 284; 20364-20374.

[23] Schriner SE, Linford NJ, Martin GM, Treuting P, Ogburn CE, Emond M, Coskun PE, Ladiges W, Wolf N, Van Remmen H, Wallace DC, Rabinovitch PS. 2005. Extension of murine life span by overexpression of catalase targeted to mitochondria. *Science,* 308; 1909-1911.

[24] Jacobs HT. 2003. The mitochondrial theory of aging: dead or alive? *Aging Cell,* 2; 11-17.

[25] Ferreiro E, Baldeiras I, Ferreira IL, Costa RO, Rego AC, Pereira CF, Oliveira CR. 2012. Mitochondrial- and endoplasmic reticulum-associated oxidative stress in Alzheimer's disease: from pathogenesis to biomarkers. *Int J Cell Biol,* 735206. Epub 2012 Jun 4.

[26] Aubert G, Lansdorp PM. 2008. Telomeres and aging. *Physiol Rev.,* 88; 557-579.

[27] Calado R, Young N. 2012. *Telomeres in disease.* F1000 Medicine Reports, 4; 8.

[28] Finkel T, Serrano M, Blasco MA. 2007. The common biology of cancer and ageing. *Nature,* 448;767-774.

[29] Greider CW, Blackburn EH. 1985. Identification of a specific telomere terminal transferase activity in Tetrahymena extracts. *Cell,* 43; 405-413.

[30] Eisenberg DTA. 2011. An evolutionary review of human telomere biology: the thrifty telomere hypothesis and notes on potential adaptive paternal effects. *American Journal of Human Biology,* 23; 149-167.

[31] Lundblad V, Blackburn EH. 1993. An alternative pathway for yeast telomere maintenance rescues est1-senescence. *Cell,* 73; 347-360.

[32] Valdes AM, Andrew T, Gardner JP, Kimura M, Oelsner E, Cherkas LF, Aviv A, Spector TD. 2005. Obesity, cigarette smoking, and telomere length in women. *Lancet,* 366; 662-664.

[33] Cawthon RM, Smith KR, O'Brien E, Sivatchenko A, Kerber RA. 2003. Association between telomere lenght in blood and mortality in people aged 60 years or older. *Lancet,* 361; 393-395.

[34] Epel ES, Merkin SS, Cawthon R, Blackburn EH, Adler NE, M.J.P, Seeman TE. 2009. The rate of leukocyte telomere shortening predicts mortality from cardiovascular disease in elderly men. *Aging,* 1; 81-88.

[35] Tryka AR, Price LH, Kao H-T, Porton B, Marsella SA, Carpenter LL. 2010. Childhood maltreatment and telomere shortening: Preliminary support for an effect of early stres on cellular aging. *Biol Psychiatry,* 67; 531-534.

[36] Minamino T. 2010. Role of cellular senescence in lifestyle-related disease. *Circ J.,* 74; 2527-2533.

[37] Campisi J, Yaswen P. 2009. Aging and cancer cell biology, 2009. *Aging Cell,* 8; 221-225.

[38] Chang E, Harley CB. 1995. Telomere length and replicative aging in human vascular tissues. *Proc Natl Acad Sci USA,* 92; 11190-11194.

[39] Sibille KT, Langaee T, Burkley B, Gong Y, Glover TL, King C, Riley JL 3rd, Leeuwenburgh C, Staud R, Bradley LA, Fillingim RB. 2012Chronic pain, perceived stress, and cellular aging: an exploratory study. *Mol Pain,* 12;8:12.

[40] Fyhrquist F, Saijonmaa O. 2012. Telomere length and cardiovascular aging. *Ann Med,* 44: 138-142.

[41] Poch E, Carbonell P, Franco S, Diez-Juan A, Blasco MA, Andres V. 2004. Short telomeres protect from diet-induced atherosclerosis in apolipoprotein E-null mice. *Faseb J.,* 18; 418-420.

[42] Mitchell JR, Wood E, Collins K. 1999. A telomerase component is defective in the human disease dyskeratosis congenita. *Nature,* 402; 551-555.

[43] Savage SA, Stewart BJ, Weksler BB, Baerlocher GM, Lansdorp PM, Chanock SJ, Alter BP. 2006. Mutations in the reverse transcriptase component of telomerase (TERT) in patients with bone marrow failure. *Blood Cell Mol Dis.,* 37; 134-136.

[44] Vulliamy TJ, Walne A, Baskaradas A, Mason PJ, Marrone A, Dokal I. 2005. Mutations in the reverse transcriptase component of telomerase (TERT) in patients with bone marrow failure. *Blood Cells Mol Dis.,* 34; 257-263.

[45] De Magalhães JP. 2004. From cell to ageing: a review of models and mechanisms of cellular senescence and their impact on human ageing. *Experimental Cell Research,* 300; 1-10.

[46] Bridger JM, Kill IR. 2004. Aging of Hutchinson-Gilford progeria syndrome fibroblasts is characterised by hyperproliferation and increased apoptosis. *Exp Gerontol.,* 39; 717-724.

[47] Vaziri H, Benchimol S. 1998. Reconstitution of telomerase activity in normal human cells leads to elongation of telomeres and extended replicative life span. *Curr Biol.,* 8; 279-282.

[48] Rajawat YS, Hilioti Z, Bossis I. 2009. Aging: central role for autophagy and the lysosomal degradative system. *Ageing Research Reviews,* 8; 199-213.

[49] Vellai T, Takacs-Vellai K, Sass M, Klionsky DJ. 2009. The regulation of aging: does autophagy underlie longevity. *Trends in Cell Biology,* 19(10); 487-494.

[50] Yorimitsu T, Klionsky DJ. 2005Autophagy: molecular machinery for self-eating. *Cell Death Differ,* 12: 1542-1552. Review.

[51] Levine B, Kroemer G. 2008. Autophagy in the pathogenesis of disease. *Cell,* 132; 27-42.

[52] Hayashi M, Miyata R, Tanuma N. 2012. Oxidative stress in developmental brain disorders. *Adv Exp Med Biol,* 724:278-290.

[53] Erkan G, Gonul II, Kandilci U, Dursun A. 2012. Evaluation of apoptosis along with BCL-2 and Ki-67 expression in patients with intestinal metaplasia. *Pathol Res Pract,* 208: 89-93. Epub Jan 25.

[54] Grönwall C, Akhter E, Oh C, Burlingame RW, Petri M, Silverman GJ. 2012. IgM autoantibodies to distinct apoptosis-associated antigens correlate with protection from cardiovascular events and renal disease in patients with SLE. *Clin Immunol,* 142(3):390-398.

[55] Favaloro B, Allocati N, Graziano V, Di Ilio C, De Laurenzi V. 2012. Role of Apoptosis in disease. *Aging,* 4:330-349.

[56] Warner HR. 2004. Cell death, aging phenotypes, and models of premature aging. In: *When cells die II* (Ed: Lockshin RA, Zakeri Z), John Wiley & Sons, Inc. pp241-253.

[57] Jordan LB. and Harrison DJ. 2003. Apoptosis and Cell Senescence In: *Molecular Biology in Cellular Pathology* Murray PG, Crocker J 2nd ed, John Wiley & Sons, Inc. pp153-193.

[58] Cotran, Kumar, Collins. 1998. *Robbins Pathologic Basis of Disease*. Philadelphia: W.B Saunders Company.

[59] Brüne B. 2003. Nitric oxide: NO apoptosis or turning it ON?. *Cell Death Differ.* 10(8); 864–869.

[60] Levine AJ. 1997. p53, the cellular gatekeeper for growth and division. *Cell,* 88; 323–331.

[61] Pagliari LJ, Pinkoski MJ, and Green DR Bradshaw RA, Dennis EA. 2003. Apoptosis Signaling: A Means to an End In: *Handbook of Cell Signaling* (Ed: Bradshaw RA, Dennis EA), Elsevier Science (USA). pp 431-441.

[62] Fesik SW, Shi Y. 2001. Controlling the caspases. *Science,* 294(5546); 1477–1478.

[63] Laurent P, Chevalier C, Wood CM. 2006. Appearance of cuboidal cells in relation to salinity in gills of Fundulus heteroclitus, a species exhibiting branchial Na+ but not Cl- uptake in freshwater. *Cell Tissue Res,* 325:481-492.

[64] Dejean LM, Martinez-Caballero S, Kinnally KW. (2006). Is MAC the knife that cuts cytochrome c from mitochondria during apoptosis?. *Cell Death and Differentiation,* 13(8); 1387–1395.

[65] Wajant H. 2002. The Fas signaling pathway: more than a paradigm. *Science,* 296(5573); 1635–1636.

[66] Vandivier RW, Henson PM, Douglas IS. 2006. Burying the dead: the impact of failed apoptotic cell removal (efferocytosis) on chronic inflammatory lung disease. *Chest* 129(6); 1673–1682.

SECTION 2: APPROACH TO THE ELDERLY PATIENT

In: New Horizons in Geriatric Medicine. Volume 1
Editors: Ahmet Turan Isik, M. Refik Mas et al.
ISBN: 978-1-62808-972-1

Chapter 2

COMPREHENSIVE GERIATRIC ASSESSMENT

***Bilgin Bahadır Başgöz*[1]*, Birol Yildiz*[1] *and M. Refik Mas*[2]**
[1]Gulhane School of Medicine, Department of Internal Medicine, Ankara, Turkey
[2]Dokuz Eylul University, School of Medicine, Department of Geriatric Medicine, Izmir, Turkey

ABSTRACT

The term geriatrics comes from the Greek "geron" meaning "old man" and "iatros" meaning "healer". According to World Health Organization (WHO), aim of geriatrics described as promoting health by preventing and treating diseases and disabilities in older adults. The geriatric population increased by achieving improvements in science, medicine and finance, especially in developed countries. As a result of that, each passing day doctors encounter more and more geriatric patients, thus the medical, social, psychological, cognitive and functional assessments of a geriatric patient have become essential. Here we explain the important aspects of geriatric assessments.

INTRODUCTION

As a result of achieved developments in science, medicine, finance and technology, human life is extended. Nowadays, it is estimated that the number of people aged 65 years and over in the developed countries is 146 million and it is expected to increase approximately 232 million in 2020, and will reach 1,4 billion in 2030. It is explain that in USA one of each five people will be 65 years and over old ages in 2030 [1-4].

The geriatric period is like the childhood period which has its own specialties. Some factors such as diseases, traumas, socio-economic factors, way of life and education make a contribution to the changes on the body which is physiologically getting older. Generally, the problems of the geriatric periods don't occur as expected, and the management could be different for the reasons why metabolic or multiple diseases occur at the same time on the same body. That's why the management of elder patient should be different than other patients. For that reason, to know the differences of elderly patients' assessments is very important for the daily practice.

DESCRIPTION

For the elder patient's assessment, there are some differences regarding history and physical examination. Under the situations which seem like the natural results of the getting older, there could silently lay some disease which poses a serious threat, but also the common diseases could show atypical symptoms(5). These show that the knowledge of the physiology of aging and its risks and diseases is necessary. Because of the elder's complicated and interacting problems, a geriatric assessment needs intense interdisciplinary and multidisciplinary management, after that large amount of data is gathered and finalizes the future lifestyle of the patient that may be the healthiest way.

Geriatric patients require a holistic and multidisciplinary management which includes medical, social, psychological and ethic items. Comprehensive geriatric assessment (CGA) is a multidimensional, interdisciplinary diagnostic process to determine the medical, psychological, and functional capabilities of a frail elderly person in order to develop a coordinated and integrated plan for treatment and long-term follow-up [6-8].

While integrating standard medical diagnostic evaluation, CGA emphasizes quality of life and functional status, prognosis, and outcome that entails a workup of more depth and breadth. Thus, the hallmarks of CGA are the employment of interdisciplinary teams [9] and the use of any number of standardized instruments to evaluate aspects of patient functioning, impairments and social supports [10, 11]. The roots of modern CGA practice go back approximately 70 years and are conventionally traced to the work of Marjory Warren in the United Kingdom [12, 13]. Warren created a specialized geriatric assessment unit in a large chronic disease hospital (a "workhouse infirmary").

The hospital had been filled with elderly patients who were neglected and bedridden. By systematically evaluating these patients, Warren was able to determine who might benefit from medical and rehabilitation efforts. She remobilized a majority of these patients, and in many cases discharged them to their homes. These experiences led her to become a leading proponent of comprehensive assessment of the elderly prior to their placement in a chronic hospital or a nursing home facility. Since then, the concepts and practice of CGA have evolved to include a medical history, a physical examination, a functional assessment, rehabilitation, a social work assessment, and other aspects of psychometric measurements. CGA is now applied internationally and has a central position in the systems of geriatric care rather than at the point of entry into institutional long term care alone [14, 15].

CGA is a planning process which starts after a geriatric history and a physical examination of the patient. In the process of CGA, patients should be evaluated mainly according to basic items as listed below and the data such as monthly income and social insurance should be recorded [16]. Cultural factors such as support of their family, nursing and other issues should not be ignored.

Components of CGA consist of the basic items below:

- Medical assessment,
- Functional assessment,
- Psychological assessment,
- Cognitive assessment,
- Social assessment,
- Environmental assessment,
- Assessment of comorbidities,
- Regulation of drugs, polypharmacy, the prevention of drug interactions,
- Nutrition assessment and planning,
- Walking, balance and mobility assessment,
- Needs which requires support and necessary equipment,
- Care facilities / financial status,
- Home security/transport,
- Tele-health systems are made used in the future [17-20]

The patient should be re-assessed in each visit about the positive and negative changes. All patients' problems should be listed as medical, social, functional, psychiatric and cognitive processes. Each problem should be evaluated with an identifier, as well as a therapeutic and educational solution plan [18, 21].

Therefore, the interdisciplinary team members could be listed as;

- Doctor (geriatrist, internal medicine specialist, internal medicine assistant, family physician, medical practitioner),
- Geriatrics nurse,
- Patient, relatives of patient and care members,
- The social worker,
- Psychologist,
- Nutrition expert,
- Physiotherapist,
- Occupational therapist,
- Pharmacologist [18, 22, 23]

Now, we are going to assess the basic components which take the major role of increasing the quality of life and relief of health problems, individually.

MEDICAL ASSESSMENT

The assessment of a geriatric patient begins like the other patients, such as taking medical history and performing a physical examination. Because of distractibility and the current cognitive statement of the patient, taking a medical history could be difficult. The patient should be questioned carefully and answers should be recorded in detail in his medical history [17, 18, 24].

The medical exam starts the moment the patient is met (his sight, speech, awareness of his environment, the ability of movement) and continues until the exam is completed and the patient leaves the hospital. (e.g., difficulty in wearing himself and finding the exit). All symptoms should be recorded in the part of general examination. If a well-rounded physical examination couldn't be completed at the first visit, the deficiency should be eliminated at the later controls.

Functional Assessments

The functional assessments, the ability of performing the activity which is required in the daily life, should be evaluated. The information could be obtained by observing the patient directly, or from the nurse and the patient's family. Geriatric patients ability of perform the daily life activities classified in three different levels. These are gathered under three headings as basic, medium (tools) and high level daily life activities guides the clinicians [25].

Basic daily life activities are the evaluation of the whether the geriatric patients are able to care for themselves. Medium level [with tools] daily life activities are the evaluation of the whether the geriatric patient takes care of their house without anyone's help. High level daily life activities should be evaluated individually instead of gathering under the general headings, which could be described as the fulfillment of the social roles, in both the community and their family [25].

For each level, some scales that provide the patients' functional assessments are developed and had been made useful. Individuals who are expressed as The Vulnerable Elders and had five properties observed in them (*involuntary weight loss, feeling of exhaustion, muscle weakness, slow walking and decrease of physical activity)* are the group that will benefit the most from CGA. The Vulnerable Elders Scale -13/ VES-13 is the scale which is developed for the purpose of evaluating patients based on their age and health situations, and measures their abilities of functional and physical activities. The evaluation includes 13 questions and presents the risks of functional decline or death in the following 5 years for the elderly people who live in society [26-28] (Table 1).

Psychological Assessment

Although depression is observed frequently in old age, symptoms of depression are perceived as if the requirement of the old age brings on the diagnostic difficulties [29].

Depression is one of the common psychiatric disorders. If it didn't cure, some negative results such as deterioration in general health status, early death occurs. When it is diagnosed correctly and cured properly, it is possible to raise the quality of life of the old people. During assessment of the geriatric patients, as the depression scan tool two questions test could be apply, easily and it is the guide to identify to the patient who is under the risk if each two question answered positively [30].

These Questions:

1) Did you ever feel yourself addicted, depressed or hopeless, in the last month?
2) Did you ever feel your interest and happiness is less while you are doing something?

Table 1. The Vulnerable Elders Scale -13/ VES-13

The Vulnerable Elders Scale -13/ VES-13	
Assessment Questions	***POINT***
Age	
75-85	*1*
>85	*3*
Personal Self Evaluation	
Good, Very Good, Excellent	*0*
Breakdown or Bad	*1*
Daily Life Activities – The Situation which Need Help	
Bath or Shower	*1*
Shopping	*1*
Budget Management	*1*
Ability of Moving in the House	*1*
Slight Housework	*1*
Difficulty in Specific Cases	
Knell, Bend, Fold	*1*
Performance while Making Housework (e.g., Brushing the floor)	*1*
Reaching the Top or Arms Up to Shoulder Level	*1*
Lifting Approximately 5 kg Weight and Carry	*1*
Walking 400 meters	*1*
Writing or Holding the Small Items	*1*

**Result≥3 :Vulnerable Elder*

Although a two-question-test is sensitivity as the depression scan test, its specificity is low (Sensitivity 97%, Specificity 67%), so it can be used simultaneously with the *Patient Health Questionnare-9/ PHQ-9 [31]. The use of the Patient Health Questionnare-9 for the older patients is gradually increased in order to detect and clarify the symptoms of depression [32]. This test offers reliable and valid measurements for determining the severity of depression.*

COGNITIVE ASSESSMENT

In the process of getting older, the neurological changes and dysfunction which appears in the other systems affects the cognitive and physical functions. Nero-psychiatric disorders that affect memory, especially, and various cognitive disorders, personality changes and various behavioral symptoms which are seen together are frequently found in the elderly [33].

Assessments of cognitive functions, behavioral and emotional states are the most important elements of CGA in the elderly. The scanning tests consisting of "3 words and remind 5 minutes later test", "drawing a clock test", etc. could be used, but also the "Mini Mental Situation Test" could be used most frequently. A score of 24 or less over thirty shows the cognitive disorders. But it is necessary to know that this test is just a scanning test and it doesn't run out the requirement to do advanced cognitive assessment.

ASSESSMENT OF MEDICINE

Due to the comorbidity, the geriatric patients have to be evaluated by different branch doctors and as a result they are exposed to polypharmacy, frequently. As a result of the toxic effect of polypharmacy, the interactions of drugs cause a decrease in expected benefits or an aggravation of the toxic table. Thus, in each visit, the patient's drugs should be evaluated one by one and the medicine the patient will use should be noted.

REFERENCES

[1] The World Health Report. World Health Organization 1999.

[2] Özcan S, Güzel R, Koç F, et al. "Yasli Bireye Multidisipliner Yaklasim Modülü'nün Degerlendirilmesi. Turkish Journal of Geriatrics 2008;11:1-6.

[3] Clark GS, Siebens HC. Geriatric Rehabilitation. In: De Lisa J, editor. Physical Medicine and Rehabilitation. Philadelphia: Lippincott Williams Wilkins; 2005. p. 1531-60.

[4] Meyer KC. Aging. Proc Am Thorac Soc 2005; 2: 433-439.

[5] Gallo JJ, Fulmer T, Paveza GJ, Reichel W. Handbook of Geriatric Assessment. 3rd ed. Gaithersburg, MD: Aspen Publishers, 2000: 52-7.

[6] Rubenstein LZ. An overview of comprehensive geriatric assessment: rationale, history, program models, basic components. In: Rubenstein LZ, Wieland D, Bernabei R, eds. Geriatric Assessment Technology: The State of the Art. New York, NY: Springer; 1995.

[7] Osterweil D, Brummel-Smith K, Beck JC, eds. Comprehensive Geriatric Assessment. New York, NY: McGraw Hill; 2000.

[8] Bernbei R,Venturiero V,Tarsitani P, et al. The comprehensive geriatric assessment: when, where, how. Crit Rev Oncol Hematol. 2000;33:45-56.

[9] Wieland D, Kramer BJ, Waite MS, et al. The interdisciplinary team in geriatrics. Am Behav Sci. 1996;39:655-664.

[10] Kane RL, Kane RA, eds. Assessing Older Persons: Measures. Meaning, and Practical Application. New York, NY: Oxford University Press; 2000.

[11] Gallo JJ, Fulmer T, Paveza GJ, eds. Handbook of Geriatric Assessment. 3rd ed. Gaithersburg, Md: Aspen; 2000.

[12] Warren MW. Care of the chronic aged sick. Lancet. 1946;841-843.

[13] Matthews DA. Dr. Marjory Warren and the origins of British geriatrics. J Am Geriatr Soc. 1984;32:253-258.

[14] Beers MH, Berkow R. Section 1. Basics of geriatric care. Chapter4. Comprehensive geriatric assessment. The Merck Manual of Geriatrics. 3rd ed. New Jersey: Merck Research Laboratories, 2000: 40-6.

[15] Williams ME. Assessment of the geriatric patient initial impressions. Medscape CME/CE activity. June 16, 2005.

[16] A. Döventas; Çok Yönlü Geriatrik Degerlendirme: Pratik Yaklasimlar Akad Geriatri 2009; 1: 125-131.

[17] Isik AT, Doruk H, Mas MR. Çok yönlü geriatrik degerlendirme:Geriatrik olguya yaklasim.

[18] A. Döventas;Çok Yönlü Geriatrik Degerlendirme: Pratik Yaklasimlar Akad Geriatri 2009; 1: 125-131.

[19] Landefeld CS, Palmer RM, Johnson MA, Johnston CB, Lyons WL. Chapter 4. Geriatric assessment. Current Geriatric Diagnosis & Treatment. New York, Toronto: Lange Medical Books/McGraw-Hill, 2004: 16-20.

[20] Wieland D, Ferrucci L. Multidimensional geriatric assessment: Back to the future. J Gerontol A Biol Sci Med Sci 2008; 63: 272-4.

[21] Stott DJ, Langhorne P, Knight PV. Multidisciplinary care for elderly people in the community. Lancet 2008; 371: 699] 700.

[22] Miller KE, Zylstra RG, Standridge JB. The geriatric patient: A systematic approach to maintaining health. AFP 2000; 61:1089-104.

[23] Cankurtaran M. Çok yönlü geriatrik degerlendirme (ÇYGD).

[24] Ellis G, Langhorne P. Comprehensive geriatric assessment for older hospital patients. Br Med Bull 2005; 71: 45-59.

[25] Comprehensive geriatric assessment: Up to date:19.1.

[26] Saliba D, Elliot M, Rubenstein LZ, et al. The vulnerable Elders Survey:a tool for identifying vulnerable older people in the community. J Am Geriatr Soc 2001; 49:1691.

[27] Min L, Yoon W, Mariano J, et al. The vulnerable elders-13 survey predicts 5-year functional decline and mortality outcomes in older ambulatory care patients. J Am Geriatr Soc 2009; 57:2070.,

[28] Min LC, Elliot MN, Wenger NS, Saliba D. Higher vulnarable elders survey scores predict death and functional decline in vulnerable older people. L Am Geriar Soc 2006; 54:507.

[29] Yüksel N. Yaslilik çagi depresyonlari. Türk Geriatri Dergisi 1998; 1: 19-23.

[30] Arroll B, Khin N, Kerse N. Screening for depression in primary care with two verbally asked questions:cross sectional study BMJ 2003; 327:1144.

[31] Rinaldi P, Mecocci P, Benedetti , et al. Validation of the five-item geraitric depression scale in elderly subjects in three different settings. J Am Geriatr Soc 2003; 51:694.

[32] Kroenke K, Spitzer RL, Williams JB. The PHQ-9: validity of brief depression severity measure. J Gen Intern Med 2001; 16:606.

[33] Çuhadar D, Sertbas G, Tutkun H. Huzurevinde yasayan yaslilarin bilissel islev ve günlük yasam etkinligi düzeyleri arasindaki iliski. Anatolian J Psychiatry 2006; 7: 232-9.

In: New Horizons in Geriatric Medicine. Volume 1
Editors: Ahmet Turan Isik, M. Refik Mas et al.

ISBN: 978-1-62808-972-1

Chapter 3

IMMUNIZATION AND DISEASE PREVENTION

Zeynep Dilek Aydın
Süleyman Demirel University Medical School, Department of Internal Medicine, Division of Geriatrics, Turkey

ABSTRACT

Prevention through the life-course is a key to maintaining good health and a good quality of life in old age. Prevention in the elderly is more important than ever before, as this rapidly growing segment consumes a disproportionately high amount of health resources. Knowledge and consideration of unique aspects of preventive care in elderly can help better utilize limited resources and prevent hazards that may unintendedly be associated with health service utilization in this population.

In addition to targeting the universal causes of premature death, namely (1) heart disease and stroke, (2) cancer, (3) lung disease and (4) diabetes; health care providers will need to address factors such as limited life expectancy, multiple comorbidity, frailty and geriatric syndromes such as falls and inappropriate medication use in the preventive health care for the elderly. This chapter is intended to provide a framework for utilization of preventive services including counseling on lifestyle, immunization, cardiovascular disease prevention, cancer screening and other services relevant to the elderly by emphasizing unique aspects of prevention in this group.

INTRODUCTION

The number of persons aged 60 years or older in the world is estimated to be 605 million in 2000. This number is projected to grow to nearly 2 billion by 2050. Persons aged 60 or older currently comprise 10 per cent of the world population with a much higher percentage in the more developed regions (20 per cent) compared to less developed (8 per cent) and the least developed countries (5 per cent). By 2050, the older ages will make up a projected 22 per cent of the world population—33 per cent in the more developed regions, 21 per cent in the less developed regions and 12 per cent in the least developed countries [1]. Given the absolute and proportional growth in the elderly population, preventive health care in the elderly deserves much more emphasis today than ever before in almost every country in the world. The aim in preventive health care is to promote healthy aging which can be defined as "being free of any chronic disabling conditions and the prevalent conditions of older age; having the ability to be content or enjoy life; and being able to perform desired physical, mental and social activities without any limitations." [2]

Prevention can be categorized as primary, secondary or tertiary prevention [3, 4]. In general, primary prevention refers to activities that aim to avert the development of disease. Immunizations, lifestyle modifications and chemoprophylaxis (i.e., aspirin) before disease development fall under the category of primary prevention. Secondary prevention refers to activities that focus on early detection and treatment of asymptomatic disease. Screening for cancer, hearing or vision impairment, osteoporosis, hypertension, and abdominal aortic aneurysm are examples of secondary prevention. Tertiary prevention targets established conditions to prevent further morbidity or functional decline. Targeting cognitive problems, disorders of gait and balance, malnutrition, and urinary incontinence are examples.

Table 1. United States Preventive Services Task Force (USPSTF) grades of recommendation

Grade	Definition	Suggestions for Practice
A	USPSTF recommends the service. There is high certainty that the net benefit is substantial.	Offer or provide this service.
B	USPSTF recommends the service. There is high certainty that the net benefit is moderate or moderate certainty that the net benefit is moderate to substantial.	Offer or provide this service.
C	USPSTF recommends against routinely providing the service. There may be considerations that support providing the service in an individual patient. There is at least moderate certainty that the net benefit is small.	Offer or provide this service only if other considerations support the offering or providing the service in an individual patient.
D	USPSTF recommends against the service. There is moderate or high certainty that the service has no net benefit or that the harms outweigh the benefits.	Discourage the use of this service.
I	USPSTF concludes that the current evidence is insufficient to assess the balance of benefits and harms of the service. Evidence is lacking, of poor quality, or conflicting, and the balance of benefits and harms cannot be determined.	Read the clinical considerations section of USPSTF Recommendation Statement. If the service is offered, patients should understand the uncertainty about the balance of benefits and harms.

Evidence-based recommendations are useful in order to assist the physician in the practice of preventive medicine. Such recommendations include those of the United States Preventive Services Task Force (USPSTF) and the Canadian Task Force on the Periodic Health Examination. The task force is an independent panel of experts in primary care and prevention that systematically reviews the evidence of effectiveness and develops recommendations for clinical preventive services. Since May 2007, USPSTF has been grading its level of recommendation as shown in table 1. However, not infrequently, the evidence base guiding the management of conditions affecting older persons is insufficient, especially for those aged 80 years or older. Older individuals and those with comorbidities are often excluded from clinical trials, and some conditions are difficult to study or have not received priority for research [5]. Consequently, some of the preventive recommendations must extrapolate beyond the evidence base.

Cost Effectiveness

An ageing population, population growth, technological advances and increasing expectations of the health system necessitates ensuring that scarce health resources are utilized in the most effective way for improving the health and quality of life. For this purpose cost-effectiveness or cost-utility analysis [when the benefit is measured in quality adjusted life years (QALY)] is frequently used.

Effectiveness analysis assesses net health benefit which usually consists of extended survival, reduced morbidity, and enhanced quality of life. Effectiveness is generally expressed in terms of years of life gained or, preferably, quality adjusted years of life (QALY) gained by which length of survival is weighted by the quality of survival [6]. Aspects of quality of life may include improvements in functional status and reductions in the anxiety and disutility that accompany diseases. Cost refers to net cost of health care resources consumed such as the costs of physician services, counseling, tests, case finding and monitoring, treatments, and treatment of complications and side effects. Subtracted from these costs are savings from reductions in medical care resources utilized and savings from decreased economic losses.

There are no explicit criteria for what is or is not cost-effective. Acceptable thresholds for cost effectiveness are a reflection of available resources and cultural, social, political and individual values. World Health Organization recommends that interventions with cost-effectiveness ratios less than gross domestic product (GDP) per capita are highly cost-effective, between one and three times GDP per capita are cost-effective and more than three times GDP per capita are not cost-effective [7]. In US generally, interventions are considered highly cost-effective when the cost per QALY gained is below $20,000–$25,000, moderately high in cost-effectiveness when the cost per QALY is between $25,000–$50,000, borderline cost-effective when the cost per QALY is between $50,000–$100,000, and generally not cost-effective as the cost per QALY further increases [6]. In Turkey, interventions with a cost below 10.000 $ per QALY have been considered cost effective [8].

An Outline for Preventive Health Services in the Elderly

Preventive health services can be categorized as 1. Screening, 2. Counseling, 3. İmmunization and Chemoprophylaxis. Another useful categorization is based on whether preventive health services can be applied irrespective of age or not [9]. Some types of preventive care (i.e., flu vaccine, counseling about physical activity and nutrition) are helpful at all ages, whereas others (i.e., screening for many types of cancer) have been found to be helpful only if life expectancy is more than 5 years when the screening is done. Determining which preventive care to undergo depends on weighing the likelihood that the person will benefit from the preventive measure against the likelihood that the person will experience harm.

Estimating life expectancy may not be an easy task. Risk of mortality is based on functional status (an individual's ability to perform normal daily activities required to meet basic needs, fulfill usual roles, and maintain health and well-being) and number and severity of medical conditions [5, 9, 10, 11].

In 2003 American Geriatrics Society made 6 recommendations about screening decisions for the elderly in a position paper [12]. These are as follows:

1. *For patients who have a short life expectancy, clinical care should focus on conditions whose treatment is likely to be of immediate benefit rather than on screening for asymptomatic disease.*
2. *Older patients with multiple medical problems, life shortening conditions, or dementia may find routine screening tests to be more burdensome than younger patients. This potential increased burden needs to be taken into account in screening decisions.*
3. *Screening decisions for older adults should be individualized rather than set strictly by age. The expected benefit of the screening test should be considered for each patient, with consideration of such factors as the expected time until anticipated benefit of the test, the patient's life expectancy, and the patient's preferences.*
4. *Healthcare systems and insurance policies that allow coverage for screening procedures should not restrict coverage for older adults on the basis of age alone.*
5. *Quality assessment and quality improvement systems that use rates of screening tests in defined subpopulations as a performance indicator should allow for patients to be excluded from the denominator if the screening test is unlikely to be of benefit to the patient.* (Indeed given the recent findings on the uncertain risk-benefit balance for screening of some cancers, whether an opportunity for shared decision making is provided would be a better quality indicator. See cancer screening.)
6. *Older patients should have access to screening tests for prognostic information and planning if that is their wish, even if they do not plan to pursue active treatment of a condition if it is found.*

There is much enthusiasm for increasing life expectancy and quality of life through screening for asymptomatic conditions. However the balance between the aims of prolonging life and reducing suffering through screening versus behavioral approaches needs to be thought twice. This is particularly true for the elderly. Instead of screening, practicing a few simple behavioral measures such as exercising, drinking in moderation, eating enough fruits and vegetables, and not smoking may more efficiently increase the likelihood of enjoying a long and reasonably healthy life [13]. Prevention through successful behavior modification would therefore be much more cost effective.

Table 2 provides a list of preventive services for the elderly based on recommendations of USPSTF. However, this list may not be readily applicable to other nations as discussed in specific sections. For the frail elderly with more complex multisystem problems, this list gets longer to include the components of a comprehensive geriatric assessment which has been shown to reduce the decline in functional status, prevent nursing home admission and decrease mortality [14, 15]. The components of comprehensive geriatric assessment are shown in table 3 [10].

Table 2. Recommended preventive care for adults 65 years and older based on us preventive services task force (modified from Chang et al. 2010 [9])

Vaccinations
Influenza vaccine (annual) Pneumococcal vaccine (one time) Tetanus vaccine (every 10 years) Zoster (shingles) vaccine (one time)
Screening
Alcohol use screening and counseling Breast cancer screening (biennial mammography for women aged 50 to 74 years) Blood pressure screening Colon cancer screening (up to age 75) Depression screening (When staff-assisted depression care and support is in place) Diabetes screening (in those with blood pressure over 135/80 mm Hg) Lipid disorder screening (men aged 35 and older and women aged 45 and older) Obesity screening (with counseling intervention for those who are obese) Osteoporosis screening (in women at risk and aged 65 and over) Ultrasound to screen for abdominal aortic aneurysm (one-time screen for men aged 65-75 who have ever smoked)
Preventive Actions
Aspirin to prevent cardiovascular disease (to age 79, if benefit outweighs the possible harm) Exercise and healthy diet Limit alcohol consumption (no more than 1 drink/day for women and 2 drinks/ day for men) Don't smoke; smoking cessation counseling (for anyone who smokes)

Table 3. Components of comprehensive geriatric assessment for frail elderly patients (Reuben 2009 [5])

Functional status (Activities of daily living and independent activities of daily living) Visual and hearing impairment Urinary incontinence Malnutrition Gait, balance, falls Depression Cognitive problems Inappropriate medication use Environmental Problems

COUNSELING ON LIFESTYLE

A healthy lifestyle is key to primary prevention and it ought to be implemented from the earlier stages of life to be most effective. However, even if implemented later in life, it is invaluable for attaining a better quality of life and health outcomes.

Even though the value of lifestyle practices are indisputable, the evidence base regarding the value of physician counseling on lifestyle practices is scarce, such that USPSTF concluded that evidence is insufficient to recommend for or against behavioral counseling in primary care settings to promote neither physical activity (2002) [16] nor healthy diet in unselected patients (2003) [16]. This statement does not mean that the benefits of exercise or a healthy diet are uncertain but uncertainty is whether advice from a doctor or nurse causes patients to change behavior. Indeed primary prevention through lifestyle is not a medical problem but is instead a societal, cultural, and environmental problem [18, 19]. Nevertheless others have concluded that physical activity counseling in clinical settings provides "exceptional value for money" [20].

In this section, we will touch upon some useful guidelines for counseling patients on how to safely be physically active and consume a healthy diet [21, 22]. We will also review recommendations on prevention of smoking, alcohol and illicit drug related problems as well as recommendations on ultraviolet radiation (UVR) exposure and how to achieve optimal vitamin D levels.

Physical Activity

The benefits of regular exercise and cardiorespiratory and general physical fitness are numerous and contribute significantly to health impact and cost savings, including lower risk for cardiovascular disease and diabetes mellitus, improved musculoskeletal health, better weight management, reduced risk for hypertension, less dyslipidemia, preserved cognitive function, reduced symptoms of depression, and improved overall quality of life [19].

A recent British physical activity guideline made specific recommendations for adults younger and older than age 65 [23]. Based on a series of recent systematic reviews, the guideline recommends 150 minutes of moderate intensity physical activity per week for both younger and older adults as providing substantial benefits for the prevention of chronic diseases. The recommendations are to undertake this exercise as 30 minutes of moderate intensity physical activity on five days of the week. However, overall volume of activity appears to be key to the beneficial effects rather than specific types of activity or combinations of intensity or frequency. Brisk walking which can be done either as leisure walking or as part of shopping and social routines is probably best way of achieving this. Strength and balance training are also recommended with physical activity to improve muscle strength on at least two days a week and activity to improve balance and co-ordination on at least two days a week for those at risk of falls. Another recommendation is to minimize the amount of time spent being sedentary (sitting) for extended periods for all older adults. It is also critical to consider the level of physical and cognitive function, recent physical activity levels and health status, as well as age itself and individualize the prescription for exercise [23].

Another useful resource for prescribing physical activity is the Swedish book "Physical Activity in the Prevention and Treatment of Disease" which categorizes the prescription according to levels of patient frailty and provides exercise recommendations for 33 specific conditions such as diabetes, hypertension, coronary artery disease, chronic obstructive pulmonary disease and osteoarthritis [24].

Unfortunately physical activity is a complex behavior which is discouraged by modern physical and social environments. Therefore not only individual efforts but also a coordinated approach involving multiple societal, institutional, and departmental collaborations is needed to counter these influences [21]. Nevertheless clinicians are in the best suited position for promoting physical activity. A systematic approach which considers physical activity as a modifiable vital sign incorporates its assessment, counseling and follow-up into routine care may help clinicians provide this service to a greater proportion of their both older and younger patients.

Nutrition

Diet is a powerful common determinant of cardiovascular disease, obesity, diabetes, and several cancers [25]. Evidence suggests that dietary improvements at the population level can result in improved health outcomes [26, 27]. However it has been difficult for nutrition researchers to pinpoint to the best dietary patterns for decades. As nicely stated by Willett "A focus on foods, rather than individual nutrients, is particularly important because the relationship between diet and chronic disease cannot be adequately predicted from the effects of individual nutrients, and because people choose foods, not nutrients, when deciding what to eat" [28, 29].

The latest (2010) US dietary guidelines (USDG), intend to summarize and synthesize knowledge about individual nutrients and food components into an interrelated set of recommendations for healthy eating [22]. The Guidelines' recommendations emphasize two concepts: 1. maintaining calorie balance over time to achieve and sustain a healthy weight and, 2. focusing on consuming nutrient-dense foods and beverages. Accordingly USDG recommend limiting the intake of sodium, solid fats, particularly trans fats, added sugars, and refined grains and emphasizes nutrient-dense foods and beverages—vegetables, fruits, whole grains, fat-free or low-fat milk and milk products, seafood, lean meats and poultry, eggs, beans and peas, and nuts and seeds. Specific recommendations about salt is to reduce daily sodium intake to less than 2,300 mg and further reduce intake to 1,500 mg among persons who are 51 and older and those of any age who are African American or have hypertension, diabetes, or chronic kidney disease. Another recommendation is to increase the amount and variety of seafood consumed by choosing seafood in place of some meat and poultry.

USDG make a specific recommendation for individuals ages 50 years and older to consume foods fortified with vitamin B12, such as fortified cereals, or dietary supplements given that individuals ages 50 years and older may have reduced ability to absorb naturally occurring vitamin B12 [22]. This recommendation may be approached with caution given the fact that vitamin B12 supplementation has not been proven as safe and may even be associated with adverse outcomes [30]. According to USDG review, moderate evidence suggests an association between the increased intake of processed meats and increased risk of colorectal cancer and cardiovascular disease [22]. Therefore it would be wise to reduce the consumption of processed meat products [31, 32, 33]. Also olives and olive oil is mentioned as part of a Mediterranean diet and a source of mono-unsaturated fats. Given the evidence on benefits of olive oil in cancer and cardiovascular protection and longevity [34, 35, 36], it is prudent to recommend the consumption of mono-unsaturated fats through olive oil as part of a healthy diet.

As for physical activity, promoting healthy diets to reduce the global burden of noncommunicable diseases requires a multisectoral approach involving the various relevant sectors in societies including agriculture and food sector [37]. For instance, there have been encouraging examples of change in regulations in some countries such as the ban of trans fats in Denmark [38] and reduced sodium intake in Finland [27].

Even though it makes sense to continue to adhere to dietary guidelines with advancing age, there is also a concern for loss of appetite and malnutrition with very restricted diets in the frail elderly with comorbidities. It is the position of the American Dietetic Association that the quality of life and nutritional status of older adults residing in health care communities can be enhanced by individualization to less-restrictive diets [39].

As a nutritional issue, a final comment deserves to be made on the role of multivitamins and other dietary supplements as aids to healthy aging. Growing evidence suggests that there does not appear to be much role for dietary supplements for this aim. Dating back to 2003, USPSTF concluded that the evidence is insufficient to recommend for or against the use of supplements of vitamins A, C, or E; multivitamins with folic acid; or antioxidant combinations for the prevention of cancer or cardiovascular disease. Concurrently USPSTF recommended against the use of beta-carotene supplements, either alone or in combination, for the prevention of cancer or cardiovascular disease [40]. Accumulating evidence since then suggests that some other supplements such as vitamin E [41], vitamin A [42], vitamin B(6), folic acid, iron, magnesium, zinc, and copper [43] may not also be safe at all. Some recent findings raise concern even about safety of very widely used supplements such as calcium [43], vitamin D [44] and vitamin B12 [30]. Therefore unless a deficiency state exists, a balanced diet and lifestyle instead of supplements may be in the best interest of most adults.

Smoking, Alcohol and Illicit Drugs

Smoking, alcohol and illicit drug use share the common feature that they have harms at both individual and society levels and they can apparently best be controlled by measures at population level through effective policies [45, 46, 47].

Based on data for the year 2004, tobacco use ranks second and alcohol use ranks 8th among global deaths whereas alcohol use ranks third and tobacco use ranks 6th among global DALYs attributed to 19 leading risk factors [48]. Although alcohol use declines with age and illicit drug use is uncommon in the over-65 age group, substance misuse/abuse may still occur in the elderly. A significant number of older people may consume alcohol at dangerous levels. Also high rates of mental health problems in older people are accompanied by complex patterns and combinations of substance use (e.g., alcohol plus inappropriate use of prescribed medications) and high rates of misuse (both intentional and inadvertent) particularly in older women [49].

The USPSTF (2009) recommends that clinicians ask all adults about tobacco use and provide tobacco cessation interventions for those who use tobacco products (Grade A recommendation) [50] USPSTF (2004) also recommends screening and behavioral counseling interventions to reduce alcohol misuse by adults in primary care settings (Grade B recommendation) [51]. On the other hand, USPSTF (2008) concludes that the current evidence is insufficient to assess the balance of benefits and harms of screening for illicit drug use (Grade I recommendation) [52].

For tobacco control effective policies to reduce tobacco use at population level exist. These include: raising tobacco taxes, extending laws regarding clean indoor air to additional sites, running counter-marketing campaigns, and banning cigarette advertising and promotion [47]. However cessation is the only intervention with the potential to reduce tobacco-related mortality in the short- and medium-term. Treatment of tobacco dependence refers to a range of techniques including motivation, advice and guidance, counseling, telephone and internet support, and appropriate pharmaceutical aids, all of which aim to encourage and help tobacco users to stop using tobacco and to avoid subsequent relapse. The success of these interventions depends on their synergistic use in a broader context of a comprehensive tobacco-control strategy [48].

Tobacco cessation treatments in general are accepted highly cost effective in developed countries [19]. For less developed regions, there is no single approach that should be emphasized to the exclusion of others because the therapies vary widely in their efficacy, acceptability, cost-effectiveness, and cost on an individual and population basis [48]. Although there are no randomized studies of smoking cessation at higher ages, all available observational data suggest that smoking cessation is beneficial at higher age and the absolute benefit in life years gained remains substantial [53].

Although harms of tobacco use are very well known, the case for alcohol has been perceived differently as it may have some health benefits when used in moderation. Alcohol contributes to more than 60 types of disease (including alcohol-use disorders, cancer, cardiovascular disease, liver cirrhosis) and injury, although it can also decrease the risk of coronary heart disease (CHD), stroke and diabetes [49]. However, the net effect of alcohol consumption on health is detrimental, with an estimated 3·8% of all global deaths and 4·6% of global DALYs attributable to alcohol. Globally, the effect of alcohol on burden of disease is about the same size as that of smoking in 2000, and it is greatest in developing countries [54]. Therefore consumption of alcohol should never be encouraged on health grounds [55]. Moreover studies evaluating the alcohol-cancer association suggest that there is no level of consumption that is risk-free for the individual [56, 57, 58].

With regard to use of alcohol and illicit drugs, the clinician needs to be aware of subtle signs and symptoms of hazardous use. Recently, in the first report on "Older Persons' Substance Misuse", Royal College of Psychiatrists in Britain emphasize that signs and symptoms of substance misuse may be mistakenly attributed to other physical or mental health conditions, or may be masked by the presence of other illnesses. Thus, an underlying substance use disorder may be missed unless a high degree of clinical suspicion is maintained. The working committee recommended that the following physical symptoms should trigger screening [50]: sleep complaints, cognitive impairment, memory or concentration disturbance, seizures, malnutrition, muscle wasting, liver-function abnormalities, persistent irritability without obvious cause, unexplained chronic pain or other somatic symptoms, incontinence, urinary retention, poor hygiene and self-neglect, unusual restlessness and agitation, complaints of blurred vision or dry mouth, unexplained nausea and vomiting, changes in eating habits, slurred speech, tremor, poor motor coordination, shuffling gait, frequent falls and unexplained bruising.

Elderly are more sensitive to alcohol's negative health effects compared to younger adults and are more prone to fall injuries. Research also suggests that alcohol use disorders among the elderly are frequently misdiagnosed or overlooked [59, 60]. Clinicians need to screen for alcohol use, drinking consequences, and possible interactions of alcohol and medications. Screening should be updated annually, before the older adult begins taking any new medications, or in response to problems that may be related to alcohol or medication [61]. One of the most simply implemented screening tools is the AUDIT-C test [61], which has the advantage of identifying heavy drinking as well as more severe drinking patterns. The CAGE questionnaire [63] is perhaps the most widely known alcohol screening test, but it mostly identifies patients with probable alcohol dependence, rather than the broader public health problems of at-risk drinking and binge drinking [62].

It is recommended that if alcohol is consumed, it should be consumed in moderation—up to one drink per day for women and two drinks per day for men [22]. However current recommended 'safe limits' for alcohol consumption are based on work in younger adults. Because of physiological and metabolic changes associated with ageing, these 'safe limits' may be too high for older people. [50]

Ultraviolet Radiation (UVR) Exposure and Vitamin D

UVR exposure may be beneficial not only for skeletal health but also for cardiovascular, neuromuscular, cognitive health and prevention of certain cancers. On the other hand it is well known to cause skin cancers, cataracts and other eye diseases [64, 65, 66]. However, the optimal UV exposure practices to gain benefits while avoiding harms is not well known. This dilemma represents a serious problem, for which the best solution for the time being appears to be supplementation with vitamin D. However it is not yet known whether naturally attained and exogenously maintained levels of vitamin D produce the same health effects or whether vitamin D can account for all potential benefits associated with UVR exposure [66].

On the other hand, UVR exposure increases the risk for skin cancer among people with all skin types, but especially fair-skinned people. Basal cell carcinoma is the most common skin cancer, with squamous cell carcinoma coming in second. However melanoma remains the most deadly [67]. Although primary prevention efforts have focused on young people, the elderly (especially elderly men) bear a disproportionate burden of morbidity and mortality from melanoma and non-melanoma skin cancer [68]. Using sunscreen, particularly those that block both ultraviolet A and ultraviolet B, has been shown to prevent squamous cell skin cancer. However, the evidence for the effect of sunscreen use in preventing melanoma is mixed [69]. Other measures for preventing skin cancer include avoiding direct exposure to midday sun (between the hours of 10:00 AM and 4:00 PM) and covering skin exposed to the sun (by wearing protective clothing such as broad-brimmed hats, long-sleeved shirts, long pants, and sunglasses). However USPSTF found insufficient evidence to recommend for or against routine counseling by primary care clinicians to prevent skin cancer (I Recommendation). At the time of the USPSTF review, the effects of sunlamps and tanning beds on the risk for melanoma were unclear. However The World Health Organization's International Agency for Research on Cancer has later reported a significantly increased risk of melanoma with sunbed use and labeled tanning devices as carcinogenic to humans [69]. Others have also reported an increased risk of melanoma and non-melanoma skin cancer and eye melanoma as well as increased overall mortality risk for women associated with solarium use [70, 71].

Vitamin D deficiency is highly prevalent both in young and the elderly [72]. Recent evidence implicates optimum levels of vitamin D not only as an essential contributor to musculoskeletal health but also as a correlate of lower prevalence of chronic disease such as diabetes, hypertension, cardiovascular disease, colorectal, breast and prostate cancers, and autoimmune disease [67, 73]. An optimum level of vitamin D is particularly important for muscle strength and balance in the elderly [67]. Many intervention studies of supplementation with vitamin D have shown a reduction in fractures and falls [74]. However the Institute of Medicine suggested that the evidence for vitamin D on fall prevention is inconsistent [75] whereas the benefit of vitamin D in fracture prevention is evidenced for institutionalized individuals but inconsistent in community-dwelling individuals [76].

Of note, supplementation with vitamin D has not been shown to consistently improve non-skeletal health outcomes. For instance it was not found to reduce the risk of cardiovascular disease [75] and no large-scale randomized clinical trial of vitamin D has been completed with cancer as the primary prespecified outcome [77]. On the contrary, a large randomized controlled study of annual oral high dose (500 000 IU) cholecalciferol was found to result in greater number of falls and fractures particularly in the several months following the dose [78].

Vitamin D deficiency is defined as a 25-hydroxyvitamin D level below 20 ng/ml (50 nmol/liter) and vitamin D insufficiency as a 25-hydroxyvitamin D level of 21–29 ng/ml (52.5–72.5) nmol/liter [75]. Frank or severe vitamin D deficiency is observed with serum level of 25-hydroxyvitamin D below 10 ng/ml (25 nmol/liter) [74]. Unfortunately, there is no widely accepted recipe for the optimal duration of sun exposure to attain the optimal levels of vitamin D. Vitamin D synthesis is influenced by many factors including time of day, season of the year, latitude, aging, sunscreen use, and degree of skin pigmentation [67]. Therefore supplementation with 25-hdroxy vitamin D is recommended to maintain the desired levels of vitamin D. The recent Institute of Medicine and Endocrine Society clinical guideline recommends 600 IU per day for persons 1 to 70 years of age and 800 IU per day for persons over 70 or — intakes corresponding to a serum 25-hydroxyvitamin D level of at least 20 ng/ml (50 nmol/ liter) [75,76,78]. The Endocrine Society clinical guideline also suggests that doses as high as 1500-2000 IU/day may be needed to obtain 25-hydroxyvitamin D concentration above 30 ng/ml (75 nmol/liter) in order to achieve potential non-skeletal health benefits associated with vitamin D [75]. The Institute of Medicine has a more cautious approach with regard to higher doses given that the evidence that vitamin D reduces cancer incidence and related mortality is yet inconsistent and inconclusive as to causality [75,78].

IMMUNIZATION

Vaccination of the adult population can have an important impact on morbidity, mortality and quality of life. Aging results in greater susceptibility to infection and increased severity as well as a reduced response to vaccination. The increased severity of infectious diseases in the older adult combined with increased number of co-morbidities leads to higher level of hospitalizations. There is also a strong relationship between infectious diseases and disability. Patients in long-term care facilities are particularly at higher risk from infectious diseases [79].

The Centers for Disease Control and Prevention's Advisory Committee on Immunization Practices (ACIP) publishes recommendations on immunizations for children and adults for effective control of vaccine-preventable diseases in US. World Health Organization also issues a series of regularly updated position papers on vaccines and vaccine combinations against diseases that have an international public health impact. In this section, the inactivated influenza, pneumococcal polysaccharide, tetanus and the zoster vaccines are going to be discussed.

Influenza

Worldwide estimates indicate that influenza infections cause 3–5 million of severe cases per year resulting in 250,000–350,000 deaths. The highest prevalence mainly occurs amongst older adults especially those with chronic medical conditions or immunological disorders, resulting in increased mortality in these high risk groups [80].

Influenza viruses undergo frequent changes in their surface antigens. Immunity resulting from infection by one influenza virus does not protect fully against antigenic or genetic variants of the same subtype (influenza A viruses) or type (influenza B viruses). As a consequence, influenza outbreaks occur every year. New influenza vaccines must be designed annually to match the circulating viruses which are expected to cause the next epidemic [81]. Trivalent inactivated influenza vaccine (TIV) prevents laboratory-confirmed influenza illness in approximately 70–90% of healthy adults below the age of 60 years in randomized controlled trials, whereas the picture for the aged individuals is not as clear. For obvious ethical reasons, it is not currently possible to resolve this issue by randomized placebo controlled trials. So the efficacy of the vaccine, especially in the elderly, has mainly been derived from observational studies [81, 82]. Although the vaccine is not highly effective in preventing clinical illness among the elderly, it is effective in preventing complications and death [82, 83]. Among elderly persons, the vaccine is 50%–60% effective in preventing hospitalization and 80% effective in preventing death [84].

There are two types of influenza vaccine: the TIV and live attenuated influenza vaccine (LAIV). LAIV is not approved for use in persons over 50 years of age. TIV is administered by the intramuscular route and contains three inactivated viruses: type A (H1N1), type A (H3N2), and type B. In 2009 the Food and Drug Administration approved a new formulation of inactivated influenza vaccine which contains 4 times as much hemagglutinin as the regular formulation only for persons 65 years of age or older. Among persons 65 years and older, the vaccine was found to result a higher rate of seroconversion and higher titer of influenza antibody against type A influenza, but not against type B influenza [84]. ACIP has not expressed a preference for the high dose formulation or any other inactivated vaccine for use in persons 65 years and older.

Influenza activity peaks in temperate areas between late December and early March. TIV should be offered each year as soon as it becomes available. Although most influenza vaccination activities should be completed by December, vaccine should be provided throughout influenza season. ACIP recommends annual influenza vaccination for all persons 6 months of age and older. The groups with a high priority for vaccination include persons 50 years and older, persons with chronic pulmonary (including asthma), cardiovascular (except hypertension), renal, hepatic, neurologic, hematologic, or metabolic disorders (including diabetes mellitus) and persons who are immunosuppressed [84]. Priority groups also include the residents of nursing homes and other chronic-care facilities and the health care personnel.

Pneumococcal Pneumonia

Streptococcus pneumoniae is the most commonly identified causative organism in cases of community-acquired pneumonia in both ambulatory and hospitalized patients. S. pneumoniae is a major source of morbidity and mortality, particularly in the very young and in the elderly [85]. There are 2 types of pneumococcal vaccine: 1. pneumococcal polysaccharide vaccine, 2. pneumococcal conjugate vaccine. The 23-valent polysaccharide vaccine contains polysaccharide antigen from 23 types of pneumococcal bacteria that cause 88% of bacteremic pneumococcal disease. Conjugate vaccines, have superior immune-genicity, but are not yet offered for adult vaccination. There is reasonable skepticism about the effectiveness and efficacy of the 23-valent polysaccharide vaccine, especially in the elderly and in immunocompromised adults. Data suggest that polysaccharide vaccine raises inadequate protection against non-bacteremic pneumonia, while the benefit against invasive pneumococcal disease in high-risk population is uncertain [86].

Current recommendations for pneumococcal polysaccharide vaccine from ACIP is to administer it routinely to all adults 65 years of age and older. In addition vaccine is recommended for persons 2 years of age or older with chronic illness, anatomic or functional asplenia, depressed immunity, Human Immunodeficiency Virus (HIV) infection, environments or settings with increased risk and cochlear implant. In 2008 ACIP added two new indications for pneumococcal polysaccharide vaccine for adults 19 years of age and older. These new indications are asthma and cigarette smoking. Persons aged 65 years and older should be administered a second dose of pneumococcal vaccine if they received the vaccine more than 5 years previously, and were younger than 65 years of age at the time of the first dose [87].

Although many industrialized countries recommend immunization with 23-valent pneumococcal polysaccharide vaccine for their elderly and other high-risk groups, in 2008 the World Health Organization concluded that in resource-limited settings where there are many competing health priorities, the evidence does not support routine immunization of the elderly and high-risk populations with this vaccine [86].

Tetanus-Diphteria-Pertussis

Tetanus is readily preventable through immunization and tetanus toxoid-containing vaccines, which are included in childhood immunization programs all over the world. To obtain long-lasting immunity, however, booster doses are required. Where national immunization programs have maintained high coverage with tetanus toxoid containing vaccines for several decades, tetanus has become very rare, but occurs occasionally in the elderly and other non-

or insufficiently immunized people [87]. Cases most likely to be fatal are those occurring in persons 60 years of age and older (18%) and unvaccinated persons (22%) [88].

In subjects who have completed a primary vaccination series, routine boosters with Td (adult tetanus-diphteria toxoid) are recommended every 10 years. Tdap (adult tetanus diphtheria toxoid and acellular pertussis) vaccines are approved by the Food and Drug Administration for a single (booster) dose for persons who have completed the recommended childhood vaccination series [89]. Though not previously approved for persons ≥65, in 2011 ACIP recommended Tdap for persons ≥65 who are close contacts of infants younger than 12 months of age and who have not received Tdap previously. Either Td or Tdap can be used if there is no infant contact. Also persons who sustain a wound that is other than clean and minor should receive a tetanus booster if more than 5 years have elapsed since their last booster. Persons with wounds that are neither clean nor minor, and who have had 0–2 prior doses of tetanus toxoid or have an uncertain history of prior doses should receive tetanus immune globulin as well as Td or Tdap [90].

For unvaccinated persons 7 years and older (including persons who cannot document prior vaccination), the primary series is three doses of Td. The first two doses should be separated by at least 4 weeks, and the third dose given 6 to 12 months after the second. ACIP recommends that one of these doses (preferably the first) be administered as Tdap. Again, booster dose of Td should be given every 10 years. Tdap is approved for a single dose at this time (i.e., it should not be used for all the doses of Td in a previously unvaccinated person 7 years or older) [90].

Herpes Zoster

Herpes zoster (HZ) or shingles results from reactivation of the varicella-zoster virus. The lifetime risk of zoster is estimated to be at least 32%. Increasing age and cellular immunosuppression are the most important risk factors; 50% of persons living until age 85 years will develop zoster '[90].

Postherpetic neuralgia is the most common and serious complication of zoster. The incidence of PHN after HZ is directly related to age, with 50% of affected individuals older than 60 years experiencing persistent and unrelieved pain [91]. Postherpetic neuralgia may last a year or longer after the episode of zoster. Ocular nerve and other organ involvement with zoster can occur, often with severe sequelae [92].

The zoster vaccine has been licensed in the US for the prevention of herpes zoster and post herpetic neuralgia in immuncompetent adults 60 years of age and older. ACIP recommends a single dose of zoster vaccine for adults 60 years of age and older whether or not they report a prior episode of herpes zoster [92]. The live virus HZ vaccine reduces the incidence of HZ by about 50% and the occurrence of postherpetic neuralgia by two-thirds, with vaccinated individuals experiencing attenuated or shortened symptoms. The vaccine is contraindicated in immunocompromised patients and might not be effective in patients taking antiviral medications active against the HZ virus [93]. Even though the vaccine is considered cost effective for developed countries [93], cost effectiveness of this vaccine needs to be established in country-specific circumstances.

Cardiovascular Disease Prevention

In 2004, ischemic heart disease and cerebrovascular disease (stroke) were the leading causes of death in both middle- and high-income countries, and also in the top five causes for low-income countries. These two causes were together responsible for 22% of all deaths worldwide [92]. Given the scope of the problem, cardiovascular disease prevention is a major public health goal that should focus on all life stages. Even though the long time frames involved in evaluating preventive interventions make cost-effectiveness analysis difficult and necessarily flawed, public policy, community efforts, and specific pharmacological interventions for cardiovascular prevention are thought to be cost-effective and cost saving [19].

Numerous studies have shown the efficacy of controlling individual cardiovascular risk factors in preventing or slowing cardiovascular disease. Elderly people are more likely to have multiple risk factors or clinical cardiovascular disease and large benefits are seen when multiple risk factors are addressed globally [93, 94]. However the presence of greater comorbidity makes cardiovascular prevention in the elderly more complicated. For instance "the lesser the better" approach may not hold true for the elderly, at least for blood pressure and blood glucose control [95]. Given a limited focus of most intervention studies on the elderly, there are still large evidence gaps as to best approaches in prevention of cardiovascular disease in this population.

Another problem with cardiovascular prevention strategies on a global scale, albeit not only for the elderly, is the limited applicability of risk prediction tools such as the Framingham risk score to population of less developed countries. The World Health Organization/ International Society of Hypertension risk prediction charts are a valuable effort to fill in this gap until more data is available to develop necessary tools for these regions [96, 97].

Type 2 Diabetes

The incidence and prevalence of diabetes mellitus markedly increase with age and people with diabetes mellitus have cardiovascular disease mortality rates that are 2 to 4 times higher than those for people without diabetes mellitus [19].

The USPSTF (2008) [98] recommends screening for type 2 diabetes in asymptomatic adults with sustained blood pressure (either treated or untreated) greater than 135/80 mm Hg (Grade: B Recommendation). On the other hand American Diabetes Association (2012) recommends universal screening for type 2 diabetes after 45 years of age at least every 3 years. Testing is also recommended for adults of any age who are overweight or obese [body mass index (BMI) ≥25 kg/m2] and who have one or more additional risk factors for diabetes including physical inactivity, first-degree relative with diabetes, high-risk race/ethnicity, hypertension (blood pressure ≥140/90 mmHg or on therapy for hypertension), HDL cholesterol level <35 mg/dL and/or a triglyceride level >250 mg/dL, A1C≥5.7%, IGT, or IFG on previous testing, other clinical conditions associated with insulin resistance (e.g., acanthosis nigricans) and history of cardiovascular disease. To test for diabetes or to assess risk of future diabetes, the A1C, fasting plasma glucose, or 2 hour 75-g oral glucose tolerance test are recommended [95].

Lifestyle modification can reduce the risk of developing diabetes. For individuals at high risk for developing type 2 diabetes, American Diabetes Association recommends structured programs that emphasize lifestyle changes that include moderate weight loss (7% body weight) and regular physical activity (150 min/week), with dietary strategies including reduced calories and reduced intake of dietary fat [95]. A dietary pattern which is recommended for general health promotion such as the USDA Food Patterns and the DASH Eating Plan are also beneficial for the prevention of diabetes [22].

The 2012 American Diabetes Association guidelines recommend an individualized approach for diabetes treatment goals in the elderly. Even though older adults who are functional, cognitively intact, and have significant life expectancy should receive diabetes care using goals developed for younger adults, glycemic goals for older adults not meeting the above criteria may be relaxed using individual criteria, but hyperglycemia leading to symptoms or risk of acute hyperglycemic complications should be avoided in all patients [95].

Lipid Disorders

Dyslipidemia has consistently been linked with cardiovascular disease and the association between dyslipidemia and coronary artery disease holds true for patients older than 65 years of age [99]. Statins are the most well studied and widely used medications for the management of patients with dyslipidemia. There is strong evidence that statins reduce major vascular evens and mortality in people with atherosclerotic cardiovascular disease. Although there is some debate [100, 101, 102], evidence is thought to support the use of statins in primary prevention for adults with increased risk of cardiovascular disease [6, 103, 104, 105, 106]. However, the evidence on the use of statins in older adults is mostly derived from post hoc and subgroup analysis of major trials [101] and data is even more limited for those over 80 [103] resulting in concern over unknown risk-benefit relationship. This concern could best be resolved with RCTs in the elderly [109] given the side effects of statins including increased occurrence of diabetes [103, 108].

Nevertheless USPSTF recommends screening for lipid disorders with no upper age limit, endorsing the National Cholesterol Education Program (NCEP) Adult Treatment Panel (ATP III) recommendations [6, 107]. USPSTF (2008) strongly recommends screening men aged 35 and older and women aged 45 and older for lipid disorders (Grade A recommendation) [108] whereas in UK the National Collaborating Centre for Primary Care and Royal College of General Practitioners recommends a systematic strategy to identify people aged 40–74 who are likely to be at high risk for the primary prevention of cardiovascular disease in primary care [106].

The NCEP ATP III recommends that fasting lipid panel should be measured at least once every 5 years in all adults 20 years of age and older without a history of CHD or other atherosclerotic diseases [6]. The first line of prevention in patients with lipid disorders should include therapeutic lifestyle change, including physical activity, diet and weight control, and statin therapy should be used in patients with established cardiovascular disease and patients at high risk. In ATP III, the risk assessment is based on Framingham risk score which is available to estimate the 10-year risk of CHD (hp2010.nhlbihin.net/atpiii/calculator.asp).

In ATP-III guidelines, the high risk group with priority for treatment includes the CHD or CHD equivalents [6]. The CHD group includes persons with coronary disease and persons with an absolute 10-year risk of myocardial infarction and coronary death >20%. CHD risk equivalent refers to diabetes, peripheral arterial disease, abdominal aortic aneurysm, and symptomatic carotid artery disease. In high risk group, the LDL cholesterol cutpoint to initiate drug therapy is 100 mg/dL with a goal of <100 mg/dL and an optional goal of <70 mg/dL. Only high risk diabetic patients are recommended statins in more recent guidelines, i.e., diabetics with overt cardiovascular disease and without cardiovascular disease who are over the age of 40 and who have one or more other cardiovascular disease risk factors [95]. Risk factors include age (men 45 years or older and women 55 years or older), smoking, hypertension (>140/90mmHg or use of antihypertensive medication), family history of premature CHD (CHD in first-degree male relatives before the age of 55 years and in a first-degree female relative before the age of 65 years), and low HDL cholesterol levels (<40 mg/dl).The low risk group includes persons with 0–1 risk factor. The LDL cutpoint to initiate drug therapy for this group is ≥190 mg/dL with a goal of <160 mg/dL. For the intermediate risk group LDL cutpoint to initiate drug therapy is either ≥160 mg/dL (if 10 year risk is <10%) or ≥130 mg/dL (if 10 year risk is 10% to 20%). The LDL goal is <130 mg/dL in both categories of intermediate risk [6, 107].

Because the decision for statin treatment in primary prevention relies on estimate of future cardiovascular disease risk, accurate risk prediction is vital for different regions of the world. For regions where charts to predict the risk of cardiovascular disease do not exist (low- and middle-income countries), the World Health Organization/ International Society of Hypertension risk prediction charts have been developed from best available mortality and risk factor data of these populations [98, 99]. The World Health Organization recommendations for statins based on risk estimates are as follows: In secondary prevention, World Health Organization recommends statins for everyone. In persons with a 10-year cardiovascular disease risk between 20-30 %, WHO recommends statins for adults >40 years with persistently high serum cholesterol (>5.0 mmol/l or 193.4 mg/dL) and/or LDL cholesterol >3.0 mmol/l (116 mg/dL) despite a lipid-lowering diet and in all adults with a risk ≥30%. The Turkish Society of Cardiology issued guidelines on the prevention and treatment of cardiovascular disease in 2002 which incorporates metabolic syndromeand total cholesterol/HDL cholesterol into the cardiovascular disease risk assessment in addition to classical risk factors for cardiovascular disease [8].

High Blood Pressure

Hypertension is a major risk factor for coronary artery disease, stroke, heart failure, and renal failure [19]. Until recently treatment of high blood pressure was of proven benefit only in younger adult population and elderly younger than 80 [109]. The Hypertension in the Very Elderly Trial (HYVET) showed that the use of antihypertensive drugs to reduce high blood pressure in patients aged 80 years or more is associated with a significant and marked reduction in the incidence of stroke and heart failure as well as all-cause mortality [110, 111]. The HYVET study suggested that a goal of 150/90 mmHg can be reasonable in patients aged

80 years or more [112]. With regard to the target blood pressure to be reached in the elderly, several lines of evidence suggest a J curve with lower blood pressures increasing the risk of adverse events such as myocardial infarction and mortality [112, 113].

Nevertheless most recent guidelines recommend lowering BP in elderly hypertensives to below 140/90mmHg [114, 115, 116, 117]. However the more recent British guidelines relaxes treatment thresholds and goals by limiting the antihypertensive drug recommendation for people with stage 1 hypertension (clinic blood pressure ≥140/90 mmHg but <160/100 mmHg) to those aged under 80 years who have one or more of the following (target organ damage, established cardiovascular disease, renal disease, diabetes or a 10-year cardiovascular risk equivalent ≥ 20%) with a treatment goal of <140/90 mmHg. For people with stage 2 hypertension (Clinic blood pressure ≥ 160/100 mmHg) drug treatment is recommended irrespective of age to a goal blood pressure of <140/90 mmHg in people aged under 80 years and to a goal blood pressure of <150/90 mmHg in people aged over 80 years [118]. Also the 2011 American College of Cardiology Foundation/American Heart Association 2011 Expert Consensus Report on Hypertension in the Elderly distinguishes the over 80 year age group and recommends SBP values of 140 to 145 mm Hg, if tolerated, as acceptable in contrast to the goal of <140 mm Hg for patients ≤79 years of age [119].

USPSTF (2007) recommends screening for high blood pressure in adults aged 18 and older (Grade A recommendation) with no recommendation for an optimal interval for screening due to lack of evidence [120]. The seventh report of the Joint National Committee on Prevention, Detection, Evaluation, and Treatment of High Blood Pressure (JNC 7) recommends screening every 2 years in persons with blood pressure less than 120/80 mm Hg and every year with systolic blood pressure of 120 to 139 mm Hg or diastolic blood pressure of 80 to 89 mm Hg [116].

Obesity

Overweight and obesity are major risk factors for a number of chronic diseases, including diabetes, cardiovascular diseases and cancer. Once considered a problem only in high income countries, overweight and obesity are now dramatically on the rise in low- and middle-income countries, particularly in urban settings [121].

Even though the prevalence of obesity (defined as BMI ≥30 kg/m2) increases into old age, the prevalence in the over 80-year group is about half of that in the 50–59-year group [122]. In addition the body weight associated with maximal survival increases with increasing age [123, 124] resulting in some hesitation when recommending weight loss in the elderly. Even though evidence suggests that obesity in the elderly increases cardio-metabolic risk, physical disability, impaired quality of life and sexual dysfunction, lower urinary tract symptoms as well as impaired cognition and dementia, there are mixed reports over the effects of weight loss on mortality in the elderly and it may have slightly negative effects on bone mineral density (BMD) and lean body mass. Nevertheless, evidence is more clearly positive in the reduction of morbidity from arthritis, diabetes and cardiovascular risk factors with weight loss [125].

The USPSTF (2003) recommends that clinicians screen all adult patients for obesity and offer intensive counseling and behavioral interventions to promote sustained weight loss for obese adults irrespective of age (Grade B Recommendation) [125]. USPSTF recommends

BMI as a reliable and valid tool for identifying adults with overweight and obesity. However in the elderly, BMI may not reliably identify central obesity in the face of decreasing lean mass. Also height loss in older ages may positively bias BMI values. Waist circumference may be a better predictor of health risks, particularly CHD, than BMI [125].

The recent USDG make an emphasis on obesity in elderly. USDG recommend that adults ages 65 years and older who are overweight should be encouraged not to gain additional weight. USDG also suggest that among older adults who are obese, particularly those with cardiovascular disease risk factors, intentional weight loss can be beneficial and result in improved quality of life and reduced risk of chronic diseases and associated disabilities [22]. Therapeutic lifestyle changes should be the key elements for promoting weight loss. There is limited evidence on the effectiveness of anti-obesity medications and bariatric surgery in the elderly [126].

Aspirin

Although aspirin reduces mortality in treatment of acute coronary syndromes and in secondary prevention of cardiovascular disease, recent evidence introduced some debate as to its effectiveness in primary prevention [126, 127, 128]. In primary prevention aspirin appears to reduce the risk of the composite of cardiovascular events primarily by reducing the risk of ischemic stroke with no significant effect on the risk of myocardial infarction in women and predominantly by reducing the risk of myocardial infarction with no significant effect on the risk of stroke in men. Aspirin has no significant influence in overall mortality in either sex [128] and the benefits are observed at the price of increased adverse effects, mainly upper-gastrointestinal toxicity, extra-cranial and intracranial haemorrhage.

Findings of a very recent meta-analysis which looked at approximately 102,000 people with an average of more than 6 years of follow-up suggest that for every nonfatal myocardial infarction prevented, there were about 2.5 extra bleeds during 6 years of aspirin use [129]. Given the uncertainties in the risk-benefit balance, it is best to convey such information to the patient in a shared decision making process and future guidelines are expected to take the recent findings into account. Some recent issues that may contribute to a more refined risk-benefit balance for aspirin are reduced cancer incidence [131] and possible increased risk of age related macular degeneration [130]. However it may take longer time periods than has been possible in most trials to observe these long term effects. It is also wise to keep in mind that the risk-benefit relationship for aspirin may be different for non-Caucasian populations necessitating the evaluation of its use in population specific settings. For instance based on a higher risk of hemorrhagic complications in the Japanese population, Morimoto et al. concluded that the coronary artery disease risk threshold to initiate antiplatelet therapy for Asian populations should be two to five times higher than those for the U.S. population [132].

As of 2009 USPSTF recommends the use of aspirin for men age 45 to 79 years and women age 55 to 79 years when the potential benefit due to a reduction in myocardial infarctions outweighs the potential harm due to an increase in gastrointestinal hemorrhage (Grade A recommendation). The USPSTF concludes that the current evidence is insufficient to assess the balance of benefits and harms of aspirin for cardiovascular disease prevention in men and women 80 years or older (Grade I statement). The USPSTF recommends against the use of aspirin for stroke prevention in women younger than 55 years and for myocardial infarction prevention in men younger than 45 years (Grade D recommendation) [132]. The risk level cardiovascular disease events prevented exceeds gastrointestinal harms varies for different age groups and gender. For diabetic men and women, the risk is deemed to justify the use of aspirin for most men >50 years of age or women >60 years of age who have at least one additional major risk factor (family history of cardiovascular disease, hypertension, smoking, dyslipidemia, or albuminuria)[95].

The aspirin regimens shown to be effective in primary prevention trials include dosages of 75 and 100 mg/day and 100 and 325 mg every other day. A dosage of approximately 75 mg/day seems as effective as higher dosages. The risk for gastrointestinal bleeding may increase with dose [134]. The recent meta-analysis by Seshasai et al. suggests that taking aspirin on alternate days may significantly diminish bleeding risk, so that there is a 48% increase in bleeding risk if aspirin is taken daily versus a 16% increased risk when it is taken on alternate days [131].

Anticoagulation in Atrial Fibrillation

Atrial fibrillation is the most common clinically significant arrhythmia in the elderly and it confers a 5 fold increased risk of stroke [133]. The guidelines recommend antiplatelet agents for people at low risk of stroke and anticoagulants for those at higher risk. Oral anticoagulant therapy with Vitamin K antagonists has been the cornerstone therapy in atrial fibrillation patients at high risk of stroke. Both aspirin monotherapy and the combination of aspirin and clopidogrel are inferior to vitamin K antagonists with increased risk of complications in the face of modest benefit [134, 135, 136].

Two risk assessment schemes on which to base treatment decisions to reduce the risk of stroke and systemic thromboembolism are recommended in the 2010 guidelines of the European Society of Cardiology [137]. CHADS2 score (an acronym for Congestive heart failure, Hypertension, Age >75, Diabetes Mellitus, and prior Stroke or transient ischemic attack) is recommended as an initial, rapid, and easy-to-remember means of assessing stroke risk. This scoring system assigns 2 points for a history of stroke or transient ischemic attack and 1 point each for age 75 years, a history of hypertension, diabetes, or recent cardiac failure. In patients with a CHADS2 score ≥2, chronic oral anticoagulant therapy with a vitamin K antagonist is recommended in a dose-adjusted approach to achieve an international normalized ratio (INR) target of 2.5. A more refined risk stratification scheme is the CHA2DS2-VASc score [congestive heart failure, hypertension, age ≥75 (doubled), diabetes, stroke (doubled), vascular disease, age 65–74, and sex category (female)]. This scheme is based on a point system in which 2 points are assigned for a history of stroke or transient ischemic attack, or age ≥75; and 1 point each is assigned for age 65–74 years, a history of hypertension, diabetes, recent cardiac failure, vascular disease [myocardial infarction, complex aortic plaque, and peripheral artery disease (PAD), including prior revascularization, amputation due to PAD, or angiographic evidence of PAD, etc.], and female sex. A greater number of persons are estimated to be at elevated risk by this scoring system.

Despite a better appreciation of benefits of treatment with oral anticoagulants, under-treatment is common particularly due to fear of hemorrhage [137]. Unfortunately factors that increase risk of stroke are also associated with increased risk of hemorrhage. A scoring system such as HAS-BLED (acronym for (Hypertension, Abnormal renal/liver function,

Stroke, Bleeding history or predisposition, labile INR, elderly (>65), Drugs/alcohol concomitantly) may be helpful in treatment decisions [137]. With the introduction of newer oral anticoagulant agents such as the direct thrombin inhibitor dabigatran, proportion of people at high risk of stroke who can safely be treated with an anticoagulant is likely to increase.

Abdominal Aortic Aneurysm

By definition, an abdominal aortic aneurysm is present when the infrarenal aortic diameter exceeds 3.0 cm. The prevalence of abdominal aortic aneurysms found in population-based ultrasonography screening studies from various countries is about 4 percent to 9 percent in men and 1 percent in women. The prevalence of an abdominal aortic aneurysm greater than 5.0 cm in men aged 50 to 79 is estimated to be 0.5 percent. The major risk factors include age (being 65 or older), male sex, and a history of ever smoking (at least 100 cigarettes in a person's lifetime) [138]. Abdominal aortic aneurysm is the tenth most common cause of death in individuals aged >55 years and the mortality rate associated with rupture of a previously unknown aneurysm is 50-80% [139].

The USPSTF (2005) recommends one-time screening for abdominal aortic aneurysm by ultrasonography in men aged 65 to 75 who have ever smoked (Grade B recommendation). The USPSTF makes no recommendation for or against screening in men aged 65 to 75 who have never smoked (Grade C recommendation). The USPSTF recommends against routine screening in women (Grade D recommendation) [140].

Open surgical repair for an abdominal aortic aneurysms of at least 5.5 cm leads to an estimated 43-percent reduction in abdominal aortic aneurysms -specific mortality in older men even though screening does not reduce all-cause mortality in this population [138]. When utilized in the appropriate indication screening is found to be a cost-effective strategy in developed countries [141, 142].

Cancer Screening

Cancer is a leading cause of death worldwide, accounting for 7.6 million deaths (around 13% of all deaths) in 2008 [143]. In all age groups, lung, stomach, liver, colon and breast cancer cause the most cancer deaths each year. About 70% of all cancer deaths in 2008 occurred in low- and middle-income countries [145]. With increased age, there is an increased risk for the development of cancer with most new cancers and cancer deaths occurring in persons older than 65 years [144]. However older adults with cancer are likely to be living with additional comorbidities which makes the prevention and treatment efforts more complicated.

According to World Health Organization, more than 30% of cancer deaths could be prevented by modifying or avoiding key risk factors, including: tobacco use, being overweight or obese, unhealthy diet with low fruit and vegetable intake, lack of physical activity, alcohol use, sexually transmitted Human Papilloma Virus (HPV) infection, urban air pollution, indoor smoke from household use of solid fuels [145].

Although prevention by avoidance of risk factors can apply to all ages, secondary prevention through early detection may have somewhat decreased utility in the elderly. The reader is referred to the section on "outline for preventive health services in the elderly" for a discussion of the limitations and principles of screening in the elderly. It should also be emphasized that it is no longer wise to routinely order cancer screening without first informing the patient of his/her cancer risk, educating about the natural history of the screened cancer, the accuracy of screening and diagnostic tests, and the potential benefits and harms of screening [145], a process called shared decision making. This section will provide an overview on the value of screening for lung, breast, prostate, colorectal and cervical cancers.

Lung Cancer

Lung cancer is the third leading cause of death in high-income countries, and the fifth leading cause in middle-income countries [94]. Cigarette smoking is the major risk factor for lung cancer. Other risk factors include family history, chronic obstructive pulmonary disease, idiopathic pulmonary fibrosis, environmental radon exposure, passive smoking, asbestos exposure, and certain occupational exposures [146].

In 2004 the USPSTF concluded that the evidence is insufficient to recommend for or against screening asymptomatic persons for lung cancer with either low dose computerized tomography, chest x-ray, sputum cytology, or a combination of these tests [148]. Although no randomized controlled trials up to that date have shown benefits in terms of mortality, the national lung screening trial (NLST) study of over 53,000 smokers and ex-smokers age 55-74 showed a 20% mortality reduction in lung cancer among those who underwent low dose helical computed tomography (CT) screening as compared to the control group imaged with a chest radiograph. In addition an all-cause mortality reduction of 6.7% was also found in the study group [147]. The study participants were required to have a smoking history of at least 30 pack-years and were either current or former smokers without signs, symptoms, or history of lung cancer. Participants received their screening tests at enrollment and at the end of their first and second years on the trial and were then followed for up to another five years.

For contemplating future lung-cancer screening programs, the NLST authors suggest that the cost-effectiveness of low-dose CT screening must be rigorously analyzed and the reduction in lung-cancer mortality must be weighed against the harms from positive screening results and overdiagnosis, as well as the costs. The authors also thoughtfully suggest that cost-effectiveness of low-dose CT screening must also be considered in the context of competing interventions, particularly smoking cessation [149].

Breast Cancer

Breast cancer is the most common cancer in women worldwide, comprising 16% of all female cancers [148]. As of 2004 it is among the top 10 causes of death for women in middle and high income countries, killing more women than any other cancer [149] and only second to lung cancer in some countries including US [150] and Turkey [151].

Even though several risk factors for breast cancer have been well documented, risk factors are not clear for the majority of women presenting with breast cancer [150, 512]. The risk for breast cancer increases with age, with 80% of all new breast cancer diagnoses occurring in women over the age of 50 [153]. A positive family history, genetic factors, reproductive factors including early menarche, late menopause, late age at first childbirth, use of oral contraceptives and hormone replacement therapy are associated with increased risk whereas breastfeeding has a protective effect [154]. It has been estimated that modifiable risk factors (alcohol use, overweight and obesity, and physical inactivity) account for 21% of all breast cancer deaths worldwide [155].

Although some risk reduction might be achieved with prevention, these strategies cannot yet eliminate the majority of breast cancers [150, 156]. Moreover neither clinical breast examination nor teaching breast self-examination has been shown to benefit women, whereas evidence suggests that teaching BSE is associated with harms that are at least small [152]. Mammography screening is the only screening method that has proven to be effective. It is reported to reduce breast cancer mortality in high-income countries when the screening coverage is over 70% [156]. Mammography screening is very complex and resource intensive and it is important to keep in mind that no research of its effectiveness has been conducted in low resource settings [150].

Nevertheless, according to USPSTF 2009 review, screening with film mammography is found to reduce breast cancer mortality, with a greater absolute reduction for women aged 50 to 74 years than for women aged 40 to 49 years. The strongest evidence for the greatest benefit is among women aged 60 to 69 years. Among women 75 years or older, evidence of benefits of mammography is lacking [152]. Even though mammography screening decreases breast cancer specific mortality, evidence for a beneficial effect on all-cause mortality is also lacking [152, 155].

The harms associated with breast cancer screening include psychological harms, unnecessary imaging tests and biopsies in women without cancer, inconvenience due to false-positive screening results, overdiagnosis (diagnosis of cancer that would not become clinically apparent during a woman's lifetime), harms of unnecessary earlier treatment of breast cancer that would have become clinically apparent but would not have shortened a woman's life and radiation exposure (from radiologic tests). Components of the harms shift over time with false-positive results being more common for women aged 40 to 49 years, whereas overdiagnosis being a greater concern for women in the older age groups [152]. There are conflicting estimates about the magnitude of the harm caused by overdiagnosis [156]. Also the financial cost diverting limited resources from other preventive services is another issue that should be well-evaluated particularly in low resource settings.

Based on the reported risks and benefits, USPSTF recommended biennial screening mammography for women aged 50 to 74 years [152]. USPSTF recommended that the decision to start regular, biennial screening mammography before the age of 50 years should be an individual one and take patient context into account, including the patient's values regarding specific benefits and harms. The USPSTF concluded that the current evidence is insufficient to assess the additional benefits and harms of screening mammography in women 75 years or older. The USPSTF recommended against teaching breast self-examination and concluded that the current evidence is insufficient to assess the additional benefits and harms of clinical breast examination beyond screening mammography in women 40 years or older.

Although these recommendations created lots of controversy, particularly part of the recommendations pertaining to 40-49 year old women, Canadian Task Force on Preventive Health Care have also reached similar conclusions [155]. According to USPSTF's analysis number needed to invite to screening to prevent 1 breast cancer death is 1904 among 39-49 year old women, 1339 among 50-59 year old women and 377 among 60-69 year old women. The relative risk of mortality for women assigned to screening is 0.85, 0.86 and 0.68 for 39-49, 50-59 and 60-69 year old women respectively. However, the relative risk of mortality for the 70-74 year age group is 1.12 and not significant [152]. Therefore the recommendation to screen women in the over 70 year age group is based on lower quality of evidence [155]. For the frail elderly women who have serious coexisting illnesses and a life expectancy of less than 5 to 10 years, there is agreement that screening is not indicated [157].

Prostate Cancer

Urological cancers comprise approximately one third of all cancers diagnosed in men worldwide, and prostate cancer is the commonest of these [158]. Older age, African-American ancestry, and a family history of prostate cancer are risk factors for diagnosis of and death from prostate cancer [159]. However, very little is known about modifiable risk factors [160].

The Prostate Specific Antigen (PSA) test is more sensitive than the digital rectal examination for detecting prostate cancer and has been widely used for screening despite uncertainty about its risks and benefits. The 2008 USPSTF guidelines recommended against screening for prostate cancer in men age 75 years or older and also concluded that the evidence is insufficient to assess the balance of benefits and harms in men younger than age 75 years. After the completion of two major trials, USPSTF issued a draft recommendation and advised against routine screening with the PSA test. In their current analysis, USPSTF found that after about 10 years, PSA-based screening is associated with the detection of additional cases of prostate cancer, but small to no reduction in prostate cancer-specific mortality and no reduction in overall mortality [161].

On the other hand there are considerable potential harms associated with prostate cancer screening. Men undergoing regular PSA screening are much more likely than unscreened men to receive a diagnosis of prostate cancer. However, 23 to 42% of PSA-detected prostate cancers are estimated to be overdiagnosed [160]. Such cancers would not be expected to cause clinical problems during the patient's lifetime, but the diagnosis exposes these men to adverse effects of treatment such as of urinary, sexual, and bowel dysfunction and decreased quality of life. Complications from biopsies include stress and anxiety and, the infrequent occurrence of bleeding, pain, or infection [161].

Nevertheless, current American Cancer Society guidelines deviate from the USPSTF draft recommendations in that American Cancer Society recommends that asymptomatic men who have at least a 10-year life expectancy have an opportunity to make an informed decision with their health care provider about screening for prostate cancer after they receive information about the uncertainties, risks, and potential benefits associated with prostate cancer screening [162]. American Cancer Society recommends that this information should be conveyed to men at average risk beginning at age 50 years and to higher risk groups before age 50 years (40 or 45 depending on risk).

Colorectal Cancer

Colon and rectal cancers (CRC) account for approximately 9.4% of total worldwide cancer cases. Worldwide, there is at least a 25-fold variation in occurrence of CRC, with high incidence rates in affluent societies [163]. Differences in diet and lifestyle, particularly alcohol intake and physical inactivity, are believed to account for a large proportion of this variation. Nevertheless, major risk factors for CRC incidence and mortality include older age, black race, personal history of polyps, inflammatory bowel disease, or CRC, and family history of CRC [164]. The majority (~75%) of CRC are sporadic whereas the remainder are comprised of hereditary syndromes (i.e., familial adenomatous polyposis and hereditary nonpolyposis colorectal cancer), family/personal history of the disease or adenomatous polyps, or other high-risk conditions (inflammatory bowel diseases, previous diagnoses for cancers of the ovary, endometrium, breast, bile duct, pancreas, stomach). [165]

Several methods are currently available for CRC screening. These include stool-based tests, including guaiac-based fecal occult blood test, immunochemical-based fecal occult blood test, and stool DNA panel; and endoscopic and radiologic tests, including flexible sigmoidoscopy, optical colonoscopy, double-contrast barium enema, and computed tomography colonography (virtual colonoscopy). Of these screening methods, only guaiac-based fecal occult blood test and flexible sigmoidoscopy were found to be associated with decreased CRC–related mortality in randomized, controlled trials [166]. Of note, although screening for CRC apparently reduces disease specific mortality, it was not found to reduce all-cause mortality [165, 166].

USPSTF recommendations target the general adult population excluding those with specific inherited syndromes and inflammatory bowel disease. USPSTF in 2008 recommended screening for CRC using fecal occult blood testing, sigmoidoscopy, or colonoscopy in adults, beginning at age 50 years and continuing until age 75 years. USPSTF recommended against routine screening for CRC in adults aged 76 to 85 years though there may be exceptions to this on an individual basis and USPSTF recommended against screening in adults older than age 85 years. In addition USPSTF concluded that the evidence is insufficient to assess the benefits and harms of computed tomographic colonography and fecal DNA testing as screening modalities for CRC. Using any of the following 3 regimens for screening is thought to be equally effective 1) annual high-sensitivity fecal occult blood testing, 2) sigmoidoscopy every 5 years combined with high-sensitivity fecal occult blood testing every 3 years, and 3) screening colonoscopy at intervals of 10 years [167].

Based on a critical review of the existing guidelines developed by other US organizations, the American College of Physicians recently recommended starting CRC screening at the age of 50 years for people at average risk, and at 40 years (or 10 years before the age of the youngest case of CRC in a family) for people at high risk. Though stool-based tests, flexible sigmoidoscopy, and optical colonoscopy are all acceptable for people at average risk, optical colonoscopy is prioritized for people at high risk [166].

There are potential harms associated with CRC screening. These include perforation, bleeding, false-negative results as well as discomfort and embarrassment for many. Therefore, choice of tests should also take into account people's personal and cultural preferences. In addition, there are substantial international variations among screening recommendations. For instance, UK recommends once-only screening for people aged 55–60 years using flexible sigmoidoscopy and the faecal occult blood test for those aged 60 years and older. [168, 169].

Cervical Cancer

Cervical cancer is the second most common cancer among women worldwide and more than 80% of the global burden of cervical cancer is found in developing countries [170]. The incidence of cervical cancer begins to rise at ages 30–39, and then increases rapidly to reach a peak in the fifth or sixth decade of life [172]. Human papillomavirus (HPV) infection is associated with nearly all cases of cervical cancer. Other factors that increase the risk of cervical cancer include HIV infection, a compromised immune system, in utero exposure to diethylstilbestrol, and previous treatment of a high-grade precancerous lesion or cervical cancer [171]. In addition sexual intercourse at an early age, multiple sexual partners, multiparity, long-term oral contraceptive use, tobacco smoking, low socioeconomic status, infection with Chlamydia trachomatis, and micronutrient deficiency in vegetables and fruits are associated with increased risk [172].

Population-based screening, leading to early detection of cervical precancerous lesions and their treatment, has led to greatly reduced cervical cancer incidence and mortality in developed countries. In addition primary prevention through HPV vaccination offers a promising option for cervical cancer prevention [172].

As of 2012 the USPSTF issued new recommendations which applies to all women who have a cervix, regardless of sexual history but not to women who have received a diagnosis of a high-grade precancerous cervical lesion or cervical cancer, women with in utero exposure to diethylstilbestrol, or women who are immunocompromised (such as those who are HIV positive). In the new guidance, USPSTF recommends screening for cervical cancer in women ages 21 to 65 years with cytology (Pap smear) every 3 years or, for women ages 30 to 65 years who want to lengthen the screening interval, screening with a combination of cytology and human HPV testing every 5 years (Grade A recommendation) [173].

The USPSTF recommends against screening for cervical cancer in women older than age 65 years who have had adequate prior screening and are not otherwise at high risk for cervical cancer (Grade D recommendation). Most guidelines from other organizations agree on the upper age limit [173]. The USPSTF definition of adequate prior screening is based on ACS/ASCCP/ASCP (American Cancer Society, American Society for Colposcopy and Cervical Pathology, and American Society for Clinical Pathology) guidelines [172], which is "3 consecutive negative cytology results or 2 consecutive negative HPV results within 10 years before cessation of screening, with the most recent test occurring within 5 years". Routine screening should continue for at least 20 years after spontaneous regression or appropriate management of a high-grade precancerous lesion, even if this extends screening past age 65 years. Screening should not resume after cessation in women older than age 65 years, even if a woman reports having a new sexual partner [173, 174]. Screening is also not recommended for women who have had a hysterectomy with removal of the cervix and who do not have a history of a high-grade precancerous lesion (i.e., cervical intraepithelial neoplasia grade 2 or 3) or cervical cancer (Grade D recommendation) [173].

OTHER PREVENTIVE SERVICES

Several other problems that may be amenable to screening and prevention in the elderly include depression, osteoporosis, falls and fractures, vision and hearing impairment, and dementia. Comprehensive geriatric assessment is also briefly reviewed as a preventive service particularly targeting the frail elderly.

Depression

Depression makes a large contribution to the burden of disease, being at third place worldwide and eighth place in low-income countries, but at first place in middle- and high-income countries among causes of disability in adults [173]. Depression in later life is associated with disability, increased mortality, and poorer outcomes from physical illness [174].

In their 2009 review the USPSTF found good evidence that treating depressed adults and older adults identified through screening in primary care settings with antidepressants, psychotherapy, or both decreases clinical morbidity but also concluded that screening programs without staff-assisted depression care supports are unlikely to improve depression outcomes. Based on this evaluation, the USPSTF recommended screening adults for depression when staff-assisted depression care supports are in place to assure accurate diagnosis, effective treatment, and follow-up (Grade B recommendation) and recommended against routine screening when such supports are not in place though there may be considerations that support screening for depression in individual patients (Grade C recommendation) [175].

The emphasis on "staff-assisted depression care supports" is important and refers to clinical staff that assists the primary care clinician by providing some direct depression care, such as care support or coordination, case management, or mental health treatment. In the available evidence, the lowest effective level of staff-assisted depression care supports consisted of a screening nurse who advised resident physicians of positive screening results and provided a protocol that facilitated referral to behavioral treatment [176, 177]. The USPSTF found no evidence of harms of screening for depression in adults or older adults, but found at least fair-quality evidence that second-generation antidepressants (mostly selective serotonin reuptake inhibitors) increase suicidal behaviors in adults aged 18 to 29 years, especially those with major depressive disorder and those who receive paroxetine. Also USPSTF found at least fair-quality evidence that SSRI use is associated with an increased risk for upper gastrointestinal bleeding in adults older than 70 years, with risk increasing with age.

The USPSTF suggested that asking 2 simple questions about mood and anhedonia ("Over the past 2 weeks, have you felt down, depressed, or hopeless?" and "Over the past 2 weeks, have you felt little interest or pleasure in doing things?") may be as effective as using more formal instruments and did not recommend one screening method over another. Therefore, clinicians may choose the method most consistent with their personal preference, the patient population being served, and the practice setting; and all positive screening tests should trigger full diagnostic interviews [177].

On the other hand UK National Screening Committee (NSC) (2009) concluded that screening alone can improve the detection of depression, but not the management or outcome of depression. This result is thought to be due to inadequate systems for managing depression in primary care. The UK NSC also emphasizes that the ratio of costs to benefits is unacceptable for screening. The UK NSC states that depression is a life-long and relapsing condition for many people and population strategies aimed at reducing morbidity are more efficient when targeted at minimizing the chronic effects of existing depression, rather than identifying more minor psychiatric morbidity [176].

Osteoporosis, Falls and Fractures

Osteoporosis – an excessive decrease in bone mass – is more common in women than in men. It is a particularly common condition among elderly women in affluent countries. Osteoporosis and the fractures associated with it are a major public health concern, because of related morbidity and disability, diminished quality of life, and mortality [177].

For all demographic groups, the rates of osteoporosis increase with age. Additional risk factors for fractures include poor bone quality, tendency to fall, previous fractures, low bone density, inadequate physical activity, impaired vision, smoking, alcohol use and the use of corticosteroids [178, 179]. The USPSTF used the FRAX (Fracture Risk Assessment) tool (World Health Organization Collaborating Centre for Metabolic Bone Diseases, Sheffield, United Kingdom), available at www.shef.ac.uk/FRAX/, to estimate 10-year risks for fractures (clinical spine, hip, forearm, proximal humerus and hip), because this tool relies on easily obtainable clinical information (with or without femoral neck BMD). The FRAX tool was derived from data on 9 different cohorts in Europe, Canada, the United States, and Japan. Seven of these cohorts included men. The FRAX tool was validated in 11 different cohorts, but only 1 of these cohorts included men [178, 180]. The clinical risk factors used for the assessment of fracture probability are shown in table 4 [179].

USPSTF states that bone measurement tests such as dual-energy x-ray absorptiometry (DXA) of the hip and lumbar spine and quantitative ultrasonography of the calcaneus predict short-term risk for osteoporotic fractures in women and men whereas clinical risk assessment instruments have only modest predictive value for low bone density or fractures [180]. Even though USPSTF found no direct evidence that screening decreases fractures or fracture related morbidity and mortality, the task force found convincing evidence that drug therapies reduce the risk for fractures. The harms of treatment were found to range from no greater than small for bisphosphonates and parathyroid hormone too small to moderate for raloxifene and estrogen. Therefore USPSTF (2011) recommended screening for osteoporosis in women aged 65 years or older and in younger women whose fracture risk is equal to or greater than that of a 65-year-old white woman who has no additional risk factors (Grade B Recommendation).

The USPSTF concluded that the current evidence is insufficient to assess the balance of benefits and harms of screening for osteoporosis in men (Grade I Statement) [180]. The USPSTF did not define a specific upper age limit for screening in women. Clinicians should take into account the patient's remaining lifespan when deciding whether to screen patients with significant illness. Optimal screening intervals are unknown. However, a minimum of 2 years may be needed to reliably measure a change in BMD and repeated BMD measurement even after 8 years may not be more predictive of subsequent fracture risk than the original measurement [180, 180].

Although DXA screening of older women appears to be cost effective in US [180], widespread screening programs may not be feasible or cost-effective in many countries [179]. For instance, the UK NSC does not recommend screening for osteoporosis (this policy is currently being reviewed) [182]. In the UK, guidance for the identification of patients at high fracture risk has been provided by the Royal College of Physicians (RCP). In contrast to USPSTF guidelines, RCP guidelines, state that several of the risk factors used to trigger a BMD test is associated with a fracture risk greater than can be accounted for by BMD alone. Thus, the assessment of fracture risk should take account of those clinical risk factors that contribute to fracture risk in addition to BMD, since this increases the detection rate of individuals who would fracture [183].

Table 4. Clinical risk factors used for the assessment of fracture probability* (National Osteoporosis Guideline Group-2010 [182])

- Age
- Sex
- Low body mass index (≤19 kg/m2)
- Previous fragility fracture, particularly of the hip, wrist and spine including morphometric vertebral fracture
- Parental history of hip fracture
- Current glucocorticoid treatment (any dose, by mouth for 3 months or more)
- Current smoking
- Alcohol intake 3 or more units daily
- Secondary causes of osteoporosis including:
    - Rheumatoid arthritis
    - Untreated hypogonadism in men and women
    - Prolonged immobility
    - Organ transplantation
    - Type I diabetes
    - Hyperthyroidism
    - Gastrointestinal disease
    - Chronic liver disease
    - Chronic obstructive pulmonary disease

  Falls*

* Not presently accommodated in the FRAX® algorithm.

The UK National Osteoporosis Guideline Group (NOGG) recommends an opportunistic case finding strategy in which physicians are alerted to the possibility of osteoporosis and high fracture risk by the presence of clinical risk factors associated with fracture (table 4) [182, 184]. Briefly the guideline states that postmenopausal women with a prior fragility fracture should be considered for treatment without the need for further risk assessment, although BMD measurement may sometimes be appropriate. Assessment by the FRAX tool is recommended in men aged 50 years or more (with or without fracture) but with a clinical risk factor or a BMI < 19kg/m^2 and all postmenopausal women without fracture but with a clinical risk factor or a BMI < 19kg/m^2. The clinical risk factors are the same as those used in

FRAX® algorithm but also includes a history of falls which is not presently accommodated in FRAX® (table 4) [187].

Following the assessment of fracture risk using FRAX, the patient may be classified to be at low, intermediate or high risk. For the low risk group, the recommendation is to reassure and reassess in 5 years or less depending on the clinical context. For the intermediate risk group, the recommendation is to measure BMD and recalculate the fracture risk to determine whether an individual's risk lies above or below the intervention threshold. For the high risk group, treatment can be considered without the need for BMD, although BMD measurement may sometimes be appropriate [182, 187]. The recommended approach for decision making is based on fracture probabilities derived from FRAX® and can be applied to men and women. This approach is underpinned by cost-effectiveness analysis with generic alendronate as the intervention. The Guideline Group also comments on the view that treatment should not be undertaken in women without recourse to a BMD test except in women with prior fragility fractures. The Group thought that the strategy could be justified based on several studies which have shown little or no interaction of BMD on effectiveness of several agents, including bisphosphonates, raloxifene and teriparatide (evidence from at least one randomized controlled trial) [182].

The NOGG guidelines also list some potential approaches for decreasing fracture risk for the population such as increasing the level of physical activity at all ages, reducing the prevalence of smoking, and increasing dietary calcium intake, but makes no recommendations concerning such population-based strategies as the uptake and compliance of such strategies have not been adequately assessed, and value and feasibility of population programs in osteoporosis prevention or treatment cannot be evaluated [182]. The NOGG guidelines also recommend avoiding immobilization to prevent bone loss.

Fall-related risk factors add significantly to the risk of fracture and often overlap with risk factors for osteoporosis. Identification of elderly subjects at risk of fracture should therefore involve an integrated approach [182]. In 2010 American Geriatrics Society, British Geriatrics Society and American Academy of Orthopedic Surgeons issued a joint guideline on fall prevention [185]. The panel recommended that all older individuals should be asked whether they have fallen (in the past year), the frequency and circumstances of the fall(s) and if they experience difficulties with walking or balance. For those who report a single fall, gait and balance should be evaluated with tests such as "Get Up and Go Test" or "Timed Up and Go Test". A multifactorial fall risk assessment including a focused history, physical exam, functional assessment and environmental assessment is recommended for older persons with a history of single fall who cannot perform or perform poorly on a standardized gait and balance test and those who present with recurrent falls or difficulty walking.

The joint guideline on fall prevention [188] recommends that the multifactorial fall risk assessment should be followed by direct interventions tailored to the identified risk factors, coupled with an appropriate exercise program (good evidence benefits substantially outweigh harm). Of the components most commonly included in efficacious interventions, 2 were based on good evidence that benefits substantially outweigh harm (adaptation or modification of home environment and exercise, particularly balance, strength, and gait training), 1 was based on at least fair evidence that benefits outweigh harm (withdrawal or minimization of psychoactive medications) and 3 were based on at least fair evidence that the intervention can improve health outcomes, but the balance of benefits and harms is too close (withdrawal or minimization of other medications, management of postural hypotension, and management of foot problems and footwear).

In their draft recommendation statement, USPSTF also conclude that there is strong evidence that several types of primary care applicable falls interventions (i.e., comprehensive multifactorial assessment and management, exercise/physical therapy interventions, and vitamin D supplementation) reduce falls among those selected to be at higher risk for falling [186]. Of note, even though modification of such factors is important in preventing falls, randomized studies have not shown any significant decrease in fracture risk [182]. Some randomized trials but not a recent meta-analysis [187] have shown that wearing hip protectors can markedly reduce hip fracture risk, particularly in the elderly living in nursing homes [182].

NOGG (2010) found level level Ib evidence (evidence from at least one randomized controlled trial) that vitamin D supplements can reduce the risk of falling and level Ia evidence (evidence from meta-analysis of randomized controlled trials) that calcium and vitamin D supplements decrease secondary hyperparathyroidism and reduce the risk of proximal femur fracture in the elderly living in residential care homes. Therefore NOGG recommended that elderly living in residential care homes, the housebound elderly and those in nursing homes should be supplemented with 800 IU vitamin D and 1.0-1.2 g calcium daily. NOGG also recommended that daily intakes of 500-1000 mg/day of calcium and 800 IU of vitamin D can be adjuncts to other treatments in patients with osteoporosis [182]. However recent findings on the influence of calcium on cardiovascular events [44] may necessitate a reassessment of the risk-benefit balance of supplementing with calcium. The joint British-American Panel on Falls Prevention (2011) recommends vitamin D supplements of at least 800 IU/day to older persons with proven vitamin D deficiency (strong recommendation) and advised considering vitamin D supplements of at least 800 IU/day for people with suspected vitamin D deficiency or who are otherwise at increased risk for falls (a weaker recommendation) [188]. In contrast to NOGG and British-American Geriatrics Society joint guidelines, Institute of Medicine recently suggested that the evidence of vitamin D on fall prevention is inconsistent. With regard to fractures, Institute of Medicine concluded that the benefit of vitamin D supplementation was evidenced for institutionalized individuals but inconsistent in community-dwelling individuals [76]. The USPSTF is currently in the process of updating their statement on the preventive effects of vitamin D and calcium supplements on osteoporotic fractures [180].

Visual Impairment

Impairment of visual acuity is a serious public health problem in older adults. The prevalence in adults older than 60 years is approximately 9% [188]. About 90% of the world's visually impaired live in developing countries. Globally, uncorrected refractive errors are the main cause of visual impairment; cataracts remain the leading cause of blindness in middle- and low-income countries [189].

With regard to benefits of detection and early treatment USPSTF identified inadequate direct evidence that screening and early interventions for impairment of visual acuity by primary care physicians improve functional outcomes in older adults. The USPSTF found adequate evidence that early treatment of refractive error, cataracts, and age related macular degeneration improves or prevents loss of visual acuity. Although the USPSTF found adequate evidence that treatment of refractive error improves visual acuity, there was inadequate evidence that these improvements improve functional outcomes. Thus, USPSTF concluded that the current evidence is insufficient to assess the balance of benefits and harms of screening for visual acuity for the improvement of outcomes in older adults (Grade I statement) [191].

Nevertheless, in developing countries where % 50-90 of all blindness is caused by cataracts, programs to reduce the disease burden may be cost-effective [190, 191].However in developing countries, barriers may limit access to cataract surgery including, cost, distance, lack of awareness of the benefits of surgery, poor quality outcomes, and lack of adequate human resources for both case finding and surgery [192]. Among preventive strategies, reduction of cigarette smoking and ultraviolet light exposure may be of help [193].

Hearing Impairment

Hearing loss can affect quality of life and ability to function. The prevalence of hearing loss is 20% to 40% in adults aged 50 years or older and more than 80% for those aged 80 years or older. Other than age, factors contributing to hearing loss include genetic factors, exposure to loud noises, exposure to ototoxic agents, history of inner ear infections, and presence of systemic diseases (such as diabetes mellitus) [194].

Screening could identify people who could benefit from therapies for hearing loss. In 1996, the USPSTF issued a recommendation to screen adults aged 50 years or older for hearing loss (grade B recommendation). In a recently updated draft recommendation statement [197], USPSTF states that additional research is needed to understand effects of screening compared with no screening on health outcomes, and to confirm benefits of treatment under conditions likely to be encountered in most primary care settings. USPSTF also emphasizes that they did not find direct evidence on harms of screening or treatments with hearing aids, but harms are likely to be small based on the non-invasive nature of screening and treatment, with no known serious adverse events.

Dementia

Dementia is a significant public health problem. In 2003 the USPSTF concluded that the evidence is insufficient to recommend for or against routine screening for dementia in older adults [195].

The USPSTF found good evidence that some screening tests have good sensitivity but only fair specificity in detecting cognitive impairment and dementia. USPSTF found fair to good evidence that several drug therapies have a beneficial effect on cognitive function (equivalent to delaying the natural progression of Alzheimer's disease from 2 to 7 months), but the evidence of their beneficial effects on instrumental activities of daily living was rated as mixed, with the benefit being small, at best. USPSTF also found insufficient evidence to determine whether the benefits observed in drug trials are generalizable to patients whose disease would be detected by screening in primary care settings. The task force noted that accuracy of diagnosis, the feasibility of screening and treatment in routine clinical practice, and the potential harms of screening (e.g., labeling effects) are unknown. Therefore the task force concluded that the evidence is insufficient to recommend for or against routine screening for dementia in older adults (I Recommendation). Even though current evidence does not support routine screening of patients in whom cognitive impairment is not otherwise suspected, clinicians should assess cognitive function whenever cognitive impairment or deterioration is suspected, based on direct observation, patient report, or concerns raised by family members, friends, or caretakers [198].

Comprehensive Geriatric Assessment

The geriatric assessment is a multidimensional, multidisciplinary assessment designed to evaluate an older person's functional ability, physical health (including nutrition, vision, hearing, fecal and urinary continence, balance and medication use), cognition and mental health, and socio-environmental circumstances. The geriatric assessment differs from a standard medical evaluation by including nonmedical domains; by emphasizing functional capacity and quality of life; and, often, by incorporating a multidisciplinary team such that it aids in the diagnosis of medical conditions; development of treatment and follow-up plans; coordination of management of care; and evaluation of long-term care needs and optimal placement [196]. Comprehensive geriatric assessment has been shown to be of benefit in various settings particularly for frail elderly. Recent evidence suggests that in the setting of acute hospital care, comprehensive geriatric assessment improves outcomes not only for selected but for all elderly patients [197, 198]. This intervention appears to be particularly useful in the setting of wards designated for comprehensive geriatric assessment rather than its implementation by teams liaising with other specialties and appears to be associated with potential cost reductions compared with general medical care [201].

Also ambulatory older patients can apparently benefit from specific types of programs based on comprehensive geriatric assessment; with improved outcomes and a reduction in unnecessary hospital admissions in the subgroup of frail older patients. Preventive home visits in selected people above the age of 75 and programs based on comprehensive geriatric assessment for patients in need of palliative care were also found to be helpful. However widespread adoption of comprehensive geriatric assessment has not yet been possible even in developed countries [200]; this would require considerable resources particularly trained physicians and other health care personnel as well as system change.

Comprehensive geriatric assessment incorporates many tools for the evaluation of functional ability, physical health, cognition, mental health and socio-environmental circumstances [5, 199]. Readers are referred to specific chapters for details.

Miscellaneous Conditions and Interventions

The topic of preventive health care is broad and can be extended to include other specific screening and interventions in particular populations or settings such as screening for tuberculosis in risk groups [199] or screening for stomach cancer in some countries such as Japan [200].

In addition, physicians should be alert to subtle symptoms and risk factors for specific conditions in the elderly so as to provide targeted screening for problems such as thyroid dysfunction [201] or vitamin B12 deficiency [202, 203]

As a final comment, health care personnel and the public should be aware that there are no 'magic bullet' medicines to prevent or reverse the effects of aging [204] (See also section for lifestyle/nutrition). There is not sufficient evidence to support the promotion of most such products and it is unlikely that their multi-system effects will be tested in large randomized trials. Nevertheless, when it was possible to test the effects of some of these medicines in large randomized controlled trials, such as the once largely promoted hormone replacement therapy, the results were disappointing [205]. Therefore it may be to our best interest to keep a skeptical viewpoint on medicines claiming to be a panacea for aging and rather direct our efforts to try and achieve healthy lifestyles as the best anti-aging strategy [206]

CONCLUSION

Preventive healthcare in the elderly is rather complex and should take into account the multiple comorbidity and limited life expectancy at advanced age. Even though some preventive measures are applicable at certain ages, primordial prevention through lifestyle change can be applied at every stage of life and offers great value for money. These preventive services include counseling about physical activity, nutrition, smoking and alcohol use. Even though the clinician has a responsibility for counseling his/her patients on healthier lifestyle practices, prevention through lifestyle is not only a medical problem but instead a societal, cultural, and environmental problem.

Not infrequently, the evidence base guiding the management of conditions affecting older persons is insufficient, especially for those aged 80 years or older. Consequently, some of the preventive recommendations must extrapolate beyond the evidence base. There is also an evidence gap, albeit not only for the elderly, about the efficacy of many preventive interventions in non-caucasian populations.

Nevertheless, screening for and treating high blood pressure and influenza and tetanus vaccinations appear to be effective preventive strategies that can have an important impact on morbidity, mortality and quality of life in many countries. On the other hand some preventive measures including cancer screening and use of aspirin in primary prevention of cardiovascular disease requires a careful risk-benefit assessment for the individual and cost-benefit analysis for the society. Shared decision making which elicits the values and preferences of the patient for the potential consequences is invaluable before pursuing these preventive services. For many strategies, such as use of statins in primary prevention of cardiovascular disease or screening and treatment of depression in primary care, whether screening and intervening is cost-effective appears to depend on circumstances of the specific country.

Finally, comprehensive geriatric assessment including the assessment of functional ability, physical health, cognition and mental health, and socio-environmental circumstances is a resource-intensive process that is associated with improved outcomes and cost reductions in selected settings particularly for frail elderly. However its implementation would be a long-term goal for many countries which would necessitate investment in the education of health care personnel, creating infrastructure and mediating the system change.

REFERENCES

[1] Mirkin B, Weinberger MH. The demography of population ageing. Jan 14, 2002. http://www.un.org/esa/population/publications/bulletin42_43/weinbergermirkin.pdf (Accessed on April 20, 2012)

[2] Myint PK, Welch AA. Healthier ageing. *BMJ.* 2012 Mar 12;344:e1214. doi: 10.1136/bmj.e1214.

[3] Heflin, MT. Geriatric health maintenance. In: *Up To Date,* Basow, DS (Ed), Up To Date, Waltham, MA, 2012. (Accessed on April 22, 2012)

[4] Hensrud DD. Clinical preventive medicine in primary care: background and practice: 1. Rationale and current preventive practices. *Mayo Clin Proc.* 2000 Feb;75(2):165-72.

[5] Reuben DB. Medical care for the final years of life: "When you're 83, it's not going to be 20 years". *JAMA.* 2009 Dec 23;302(24):2686-94.

[6] *Third Report of the Expert Panel on Detection, Evaluation, and Treatment of High Blood Cholesterol in Adults* (ATP III Final Report). http://www.nhlbi.nih.gov/guidelines/cholesterol/atp3_rpt.htm (Accessed on April 20, 2012)

[7] WHO. *Choosing Interventions that are Cost Effective (WHO-CHOICE). Cost-effectiveness thresholds.* http://www.who.int/choice/costs/CER_thresholds/en/index.html

[8] *Türk Kardiyoloji Derneği Koroner Kalp Hastalığı Korunma ve Tedavi Kılavuzu 2002.* http://www.tkd.org.tr/kilavuz/k11/4e423.htm?wbnum=1604

[9] Chang HJ, Burke AE, Glass RM. JAMA patient page. Preventive care for older adults. *JAMA.* 2009 Dec 23;302(24):2722.

[10] Inouye SK, Peduzzi PN, Robison JT, Hughes JS, Horwitz RI, Concato J. Importance of functional measures in predicting mortality among older hospitalized patients. *JAMA.* 1998 Apr 15;279(15):1187-93.

[11] Lee SJ, Lindquist K, Segal MR, Covinsky KE. Development and validation of a prognostic index for 4-year mortality in older adults. JAMA. 2006 Feb 15;295(7):801-8. Erratum in: *JAMA.* 2006 Apr 26;295(16):1900.

[12] American Geriatrics Society Ethics Committee. Health screening decisions for older adults: AGS position paper. *J Am Geriatr Soc.* 2003 Feb;51(2):270-1.

[13] Clarfield AM. Screening in frail older people: an ounce of prevention or a pound of trouble? *J Am Geriatr Soc.* 2010 Oct;58(10):2016-21.

[14] Stuck AE, Iliffe S. Comprehensive geriatric assessment for older adults. *BMJ.* 2011 Oct 27;343:d6799.

[15] Ellis G, Whitehead MA, Robinson D, O'Neill D, Langhorne P. Comprehensive geriatric assessment for older adults admitted to hospital: meta-analysis of randomised controlled trials. *BMJ* 2011;343:d6553.

[16] USPSTF 2002. *Behavioral Counseling in Primary Care to Promote Physical Activity.* http://www.uspreventiveservicestaskforce.org/uspstf/uspsphys.htm (accessed on Mar 30, 2012)

[17] USPSTF 2003. *Behavioral Counseling in Primary Care to Promote a Healthy Diet.* http://www.uspreventiveservicestaskforce.org/uspstf/uspsdiet.htm (accessed on Mar 30, 2012)

[18] Tomaselli GF. Prevention of cardiovascular disease and stroke: meeting the challenge. *JAMA.* 2011 Nov 16;306(19):2147-8.

[19] Weintraub WS, Daniels SR, Burke LE, Franklin BA, Goff DC Jr, Hayman LL, Lloyd-Jones D, Pandey DK, Sanchez EJ, Schram AP, Whitsel LP; American Heart Association Advocacy Coordinating Committee; Council on Cardiovascular Disease in the Young; Council on the Kidney in Cardiovascular Disease; Council on Epidemiology and Prevention; Council on Cardiovascular Nursing; Council on Arteriosclerosis; Thrombosis and Vascular Biology; Council on Clinical Cardiology, and Stroke Council. Value of primordial and primary prevention for cardiovascular disease: a policy statement from the American Heart Association. *Circulation.* 2011 Aug 23;124(8):967-90.

[20] NHS 2009. *Let's Get Moving Commissioning Guidance A new physical activity care pathway for the NHS.* http://www.dh.gov.uk/prod_consum_dh/groups/dh_digitalassets/documents/digitalasset/dh_105944.pdf

[21] Khan KM. Prescribing exercise in primary care. *BMJ* 2011;343:d4141

[22] US Department of Health and Human Services 2010. *Dietary guidelines for Americans.* http://www.health.gov/dietaryguidelines/2010.asp Accessed April 1, 2012.

[23] Department of Health, Physical Activity, Health Improvement and Protection 2011. Start Active, Stay Active: A report on physical activity from the four home countries' Chief Medical Officers. http://www.dh.gov.uk/en/Publicationsandstatistics/Publications/PublicationsPolicyAndGuidance/DH_128209 (Accessed April 18, 2012).

[24] Swedish national institute of public health 2010. Physical Activity in the Prevention and Treatment of Disease: professional associations for physical activity (Sweden). http://www.fhi.se/PageFiles/10682/Physical-Activity-Prevention-Treatment-Disease-webb.pdf (Accessed April 18, 2012)

[25] Mozaffarian D. United Nations' dietary policies to prevent CVD. *BMJ* 2011;343:d5747.

[26] Capewell S, O'Flaherty M. Rapid mortality falls after risk-factor changes in populations. *Lancet.* 2011 Aug 27;378(9793):752-3.

[27] Karppanen H, Mervaala E. Sodium intake and hypertension. *Prog Cardiovasc Dis.* 2006 Sep-Oct;49(2):59-75.

[28] Willett WC, Ludwig DS. The 2010 Dietary Guidelines--the best recipe for health? *N Engl J Med.* 2011 Oct 27;365(17):1563-5.

[29] Mozaffarian D, Ludwig DS. Dietary guidelines in the 21st century—a time for food. *JAMA.* 2010 Aug 11;304(6):681-2.

[30] Ebbing M, Bønaa KH, Nygård O, Arnesen E, Ueland PM, Nordrehaug JE, Rasmussen K, Njølstad I, Refsum H, Nilsen DW, Tverdal A, Meyer K, Vollset SE. Cancer incidence and mortality after treatment with folic acid and vitamin B12. *JAMA.* 2009 Nov 18;302(19):2119-26.

[31] Micha R, Wallace SK, Mozaffarian D. Red and processed meat consumption and risk of incident coronary heart disease, stroke, and diabetes mellitus: a systematic review and meta-analysis. *Circulation.* 2010 Jun 1;121(21):2271-83.

[32] Kushi LH, Byers T, Doyle C, Bandera EV, McCullough M, McTiernan A, Gansler T, Andrews KS, Thun MJ; American Cancer Society 2006 Nutrition and Physical Activity Guidelines Advisory Committee. American Cancer Society Guidelines on Nutrition and Physical Activity for cancer prevention: reducing the risk of cancer with healthy food choices and physical activity. CA Cancer J Clin. 2006 Sep-Oct;56(5):254-81; quiz 313-4. Erratum in: CA *Cancer J Clin.* 2007 Jan-Feb;57(1):66. NcTiernan, Anne [added].

[33] Varraso R, Jiang R, Barr RG, Willett WC, Camargo CA Jr. Prospective study of cured meats consumption and risk of chronic obstructive pulmonary disease in men. *Am J Epidemiol.* 2007 Dec 15;166(12):1438-45.

[34] Psaltopoulou T, Kosti RI, Haidopoulos D, Dimopoulos M, Panagiotakos DB. Olive oil intake is inversely related to cancer prevalence: a systematic review and a meta-analysis of 13,800 patients and 23,340 controls in 19 observational studies. *Lipids Health Dis.* 2011 Jul 30;10:127.

[35] Ruiz-Canela M, Martínez-González MA. Olive oil in the primary prevention of cardiovascular disease. *Maturitas.* 2011 Mar;68(3):245-50.

[36] Trichopoulou A, Dilis V. Olive oil and longevity. *Mol Nutr Food Res.* 2007 Oct;51(10):1275-8.

[37] WHO Technical Report Series 916, Geneva 2003. Diet, Nutrition and the Prevention of Chronic Diseases. http://whqlibdoc.who.int/trs/who_trs_916.pdf

[38] Coombes R. Trans fats: chasing a global ban. *BMJ.* 2011 Sep 7;343:d5567.

[39] Dorner B, Friedrich EK, Posthauer ME; American Dietetic Association. Position of the American Dietetic Association: individualized nutrition approaches for older adults in health care communities. J Am Diet Assoc. 2010 Oct;110(10):1549-53. Erratum in: *J Am Diet Assoc.* 2010 Dec;110(12):1941.

[40] USPTF 2003. *Routine Vitamin Supplementation to Prevent Cancer and Cardiovascular Disease.* http://www.uspreventiveservicestaskforce.org/uspstf/uspsvita.htm (Accessed on Mar 30, 2012)

[41] Klein EA, Thompson IM Jr, Tangen CM, Crowley JJ, Lucia MS, Goodman PJ, Minasian LM, Ford LG, Parnes HL, Gaziano JM, Karp DD, Lieber MM, Walther PJ,Klotz L, Parsons JK, Chin JL, Darke AK, Lippman SM, Goodman GE, Meyskens FL Jr, Baker LH. Vitamin E and the risk of prostate cancer: the Selenium and Vitamin E Cancer Prevention Trial (SELECT). *JAMA.* 2011 Oct 12;306(14):1549-56.

[42] Bjelakovic G, Nikolova D, Gluud LL, Simonetti RG, Gluud C. Mortality in randomized trials of antioxidant supplements for primary and secondary prevention: systematic review and meta-analysis. JAMA. 2007 Feb 28;297(8):842-57.Review. Erratum in: *JAMA.* 2008 Feb 20;299(7):765-6.

[43] Bolland MJ, Avenell A, Baron JA, Grey A, MacLennan GS, Gamble GD, Reid IR. *Effect of calcium supplements on risk of myocardial infarction and cardiovascular events:* meta-analysis. BMJ. 2010 Jul 29;341:c3691. doi:10.1136/bmj.c3691.

[44] Sanders KM, Stuart AL, Williamson EJ, Simpson JA, Kotowicz MA, Young D, Nicholson GC. Annual high-dose oral vitamin D and falls and fractures in older women: a randomized controlled trial. *JAMA.* 2010 May 12;303(18):1815-22. Erratum in: JAMA. 2010 Jun 16;303(23):2357.

[45] Groves T. Preventing alcohol related harm to health. BMJ. 2010 Jan 20;340:c372. doi: 10.1136/bmj.c372. Erratum in: *BMJ.* 2010;340. doi: 10.1136/bmj.c694.

[46] Schroeder SA, Warner KE. Don't forget tobacco. N Engl J Med. 2010 Jul 15;363(3):201-4. Epub 2010 Jul 7. Erratum in: *N Engl J Med.* 2010 Aug 19;363(8):798.

[47] World Health organization 2003. Tools for Advancing Tobacco Control in the XXIst century. Policy Recommendations for Smoking Cessation and Treatment of Tobacco Dependence: Tools for public health. *WHO Library Cataloguing-in-Publication Data.* Edited by Dr Vera da Costa e Silva. http://www.who.int/tobacco/resources/ publications/en/intro_chapter3.pdf (Accessed on April 20, 2012)

[48] WHO. *Global health risks: mortality and burden of disease attributable to selected major risks.* 2009. www.who.int/healthinfo/global_burden_disease/GlobalHealth Risks_report_full.pdf. (Accessed on April 20, 2012)

[49] Royal College of Psychiatrists 2011. *Our Invisible Addicts* is at www.rcpsych.ac.uk /publications/collegereports/collegereports.aspx. (Accessed on April 20, 2012)

[50] USPSTF 2009. *Counseling and Interventions to Prevent Tobacco Use and Tobacco-Caused Disease in Adults and Pregnant Women.* http://www. uspreventiveservices taskforce .org/uspstf/uspstbac2.htm (Accessed on April 20, 2012)

[51] USPSTF 2004. *Screening and Behavioral Counseling Interventions in Primary Care to Reduce Alcohol Misuse.* http://www.uspreventiveservicestaskforce.org/uspstf/uspsdrin .htm (Accessed on April 20, 2012)

[52] USPSTF 2008. *Screening for Illicit Drug Use.* http://www.uspreventive servicestaskforce.org/uspstf/uspsdrug.htm (Accessed on April 20, 2012)

[53] Gohlke H. Is it worth offering cardiovascular disease prevention to the elderly? *Eur J Cardiovasc Prev Rehabil.* 2011 Nov 16. [Epub ahead of print]

[54] Rehm J, Mathers C, Popova S, Thavorncharoensap M, Teerawattananon Y, Patra J. Global burden of disease and injury and economic cost attributable to alcohol use and alcohol-use disorders. *Lancet.* 2009 Jun 27;373(9682):2223-33.

[55] Beaglehole R, Bonita R. Alcohol: a global health priority. *Lancet.* 2009 Jun 27;373(9682):2173-4.

[56] Allen NE, Beral V, Casabonne D, Kan SW, Reeves GK, Brown A, Green J; Million Women Study Collaborators. Moderate alcohol intake and cancer incidence in women. *J Natl Cancer Inst.* 2009 Mar 4;101(5):296-305.

[57] Gilmore I. Action needed to tackle a global drink problem. *Lancet.* 2009 Jun 27;373(9682):2174-6.

[58] Schütze M, Boeing H, Pischon T, Rehm J, Kehoe T, Gmel G, Olsen A, Tjønneland AM, Dahm CC, Overvad K, Clavel-Chapelon F, Boutron-Ruault MC, Trichopoulou A,Benetou V, Zylis D, Kaaks R, Rohrmann S, Palli D, Berrino F, Tumino R, Vineis P, Rodríguez L, Agudo A, Sánchez MJ, Dorronsoro M, Chirlaque MD, Barricarte A, Peeters PH, van Gils CH, Khaw KT, Wareham N, Allen NE, Key TJ, Boffetta P, Slimani N, Jenab M, Romaguera D, Wark PA, Riboli E, Bergmann MM. Alcohol attributable burden of incidence of cancer in eight European countries based on results from prospective cohort study. *BMJ.* 2011 Apr 7;342:d1584.

[59] Hallgren MÅ, Högberg P, Andréasson S. Alcohol consumption and harm among elderly Europeans: falling between the cracks. *Eur J Public Health.* 2010 Dec;20(6):616-7.

[60] Scafato E. Alcohol and the elderly: the time to act is now! *Eur J Public Health.* 2010 Dec;20(6):617-8.

[61] Mathews S, Oslin DW. Alcohol misuse among the elderly: an opportunity for prevention. *Am J Psychiatry.* 2009 Oct;166(10):1093-5.

[62] Bush K, Kivlahan DR, McDonell MB, Fihn SD, Bradley KA. The AUDIT alcohol consumption questions (AUDIT-C): an effective brief screening test for problem drinking. Ambulatory Care Quality Improvement Project (ACQUIP). Alcohol Use Disorders Identification Test. *Arch Intern Med.* 1998 Sep 14;158(16):1789-95.

[63] Mayfield D, McLeod G, Hall P. The CAGE questionnaire: validation of a new alcoholism screening instrument. *Am J Psychiatry.* 1974 Oct;131(10):1121-3.

[64] Lucas RM, Repacholi MH, McMichael AJ. Is the current public health message on UV exposure correct? *Bull World Health Organ.* 2006 Jun;84(6):485-91.

[65] Lucas RM, Ponsonby AL. Considering the potential benefits as well as adverse effects of sun exposure: can all the potential benefits be provided by oral vitamin D supplementation? *Prog Biophys Mol Biol.* 2006 Sep;92(1):140-9.

[66] Holick MF. Vitamin D: a d-lightful solution for health. *J Investig Med.* 2011 Aug;59(6):872-80.

[67] Fryhofer SA. *Staying Sun Safe: Confessions of a Former Tanner. Medscape Internal Medicine.* Posted: 05/03/2011. http://www.medscape.com/viewarticle/741507 (Accessed April 19, 2012)

[68] USPSTF 2003. *Counseling to Prevent Skin Cancer.* http://www. uspreventive servicestaskforce.org/uspstf/uspsskco.htm#summary (Accessed April 19, 2012)

[69] International Agency for Research on Cancer Working Group on artificial ultraviolet (UV) light and skin cancer. The association of use of sunbeds with cutaneous malignant melanoma and other skin cancers: A systematic review. Int J Cancer. 2007 Mar 1;120(5):1116-22. Review. *Erratum in: Int J Cancer.* 2007 Jun 1;120(11):2526.

[70] Weiderpass E, Veierød MB. Ultraviolet exposure and women's health. *Maturitas.* 2011 Nov;70(3):208-9.

[71] El Ghissassi F, Baan R, Straif K, Grosse Y, Secretan B, Bouvard V, Benbrahim-Tallaa L, Guha N, Freeman C, Galichet L, Cogliano V; WHO International Agency for Research on Cancer Monograph Working Group. A review of human carcinogens--part D: radiation. *Lancet Oncol.* 2009 Aug;10(8):751-2.

[72] van Schoor NM, Lips P. Worldwide vitamin D status. *Best Pract Res Clin Endocrinol Metab.* 2011 Aug;25(4):671-80.

[73] Rosen CJ. Clinical practice. Vitamin D insufficiency. *N Engl J Med.* 2011 Jan 20;364(3):248-54.

[74] Holick MF, Binkley NC, Bischoff-Ferrari HA, Gordon CM, Hanley DA, Heaney RP, Murad MH, Weaver CM; Endocrine Society. Evaluation, treatment, and prevention of vitamin D deficiency: an Endocrine Society clinical practice guideline. J Clin Endocrinol Metab. 2011 Jul;96(7):1911-30. Epub 2011 Jun 6. Erratum in: *J Clin Endocrinol Metab.* 2011 Dec;96(12):3908.

[75] IOM (Institute of Medicine). 2011. *Dietary Reference Intakes for Calcium and Vitamin D.* Washington, DC: The National Academies Press. http://books.nap.edu/ openbook.php?record_id=13050 (Accessed on April 21 2011)

[76] Elamin MB, Abu Elnour NO, Elamin KB, Fatourechi MM, Alkatib AA, Almandoz JP, Liu H, Lane MA, Mullan RJ, Hazem A, Erwin PJ, Hensrud DD, Murad MH, Montori VM. Vitamin D and cardiovascular outcomes: a systematic review and meta analysis. *J Clin Endocrinol Metab.* 2011 Jul;96(7):1931-42.

[77] Manson JE, Mayne ST, Clinton SK. Vitamin D and prevention of cancer--ready for prime time? *N Engl J Med.* 2011 Apr 14;364(15):1385-7.

[78] Sanders KM, Stuart AL, Williamson EJ, Simpson JA, Kotowicz MA, Young D, Nicholson GC. Annual high-dose oral vitamin D and falls and fractures in older women: a randomized controlled trial. JAMA. 2010 May 12;303(18):1815-22. Erratum in: *JAMA.* 2010 Jun 16;303(23):2357.

[79] Maggi S. Vaccination and healthy aging. *Expert Rev Vaccines.* 2010 Mar;9(3 Suppl):3-6.

[80] Lang PO, Govind S, Mitchell WA, Siegrist CA, Aspinall R. Vaccine effectiveness in older individuals: what has been learned from the influenza-vaccine experience. *Ageing Res Rev.* 2011 Jul;10(3):389-95.

[81] World Health Organization. Influenza vaccines: WHO position paper. *Wkly Epidemiol Rec,* 2005; 33: 279–287. Available: http://www.who.int/wer/2005/wer8033.pdf (accessed on Mar 30, 2012).

[82] Jefferson T, Di Pietrantonj C, Al-Ansary LA, Ferroni E, Thorning S, Thomas RE. Vaccines for preventing influenza in the elderly. *Cochrane Database Syst Rev.* 2010 Feb 17;(2):CD004876.

[83] Centers for Disease Control and Prevention. Influenza. In: Atkinson W, Wolfe S, Hamborsky J, eds. *Epidemiology and Prevention of Vaccine-Preventable Diseases.* Washington DC: Public Health Foundation, 20011: 151-172 (12th ed).

[84] Centers for Disease Control and Prevention (CDC). Licensure of a high-dose inactivated influenza vaccine for persons aged >or=65 years (Fluzone High-Dose) and guidance for use - United States, 2010. *MMWR Morb Mortal Wkly Rep.* 2010 Apr 30;59(16):485-6.

[85] Pitsiou GG, Kioumis IP. Pneumococcal vaccination in adults: does it really work? *Respir Med.* 2011 Dec;105(12):1776-83.

[86] World Health Organization. 23-Valent pneumococcal polysaccharide vaccine: WHO position paper. *Wkly Epidemiol Rec,* 2008; 83: 373–84. Available: www.who.int/wer/2008/wer8342.pdf (accessed on Mar 30, 2012).

[87] World Health Organization. Tetanus vaccine: WHO position paper. *Wkly Epidemiol Rec,* 2006; 20: 198–208. Available: http://www.who.int/wer/2006/wer8120.pdf (accessed on Mar 30, 2012).

[88] Centers for Disease Control and Prevention. Tetanus. In: Atkinson W, Wolfe S, Hamborsky J, eds. *Epidemiology and Prevention of Vaccine-Preventable Diseases.* Washington DC: Public Health Foundation, 2011: 291-300 (12th ed).

[89] Centers for Disease Control and Prevention. Pertussis. In: Atkinson W, Wolfe S, Hamborsky J, eds. *Epidemiology and Prevention of Vaccine-Preventable Diseases.* Washington DC: Public Health Foundation, 2011: 215-232 (12th ed).

[90] Centers for Disease Control and Prevention. Varicella. In: Atkinson W, Wolfe S, Hamborsky J, eds. *Epidemiology and Prevention of Vaccine-Preventable Diseases.* Washington DC: Public Health Foundation, 2011: 301-324 (12th ed).

[91] Shapiro M, Kvern B, Watson P, Guenther L, McElhaney J, McGeer A. Update on herpes zoster vaccination: a family practitioner's guide. *Can Fam Physician.* 2011 Oct;57(10):1127-31.

[92] Mathers CD, Boerma T, Ma Fat D. Global and regional causes of death. *Br Med Bull.* 2009;92:7-32.

[93] American Diabetes Association. Standards of medical care in diabetes--2012. *Diabetes Care.* 2012 Jan;35 Suppl 1:S11-63.

[94] Gaede P, Lund-Andersen H, Parving HH, Pedersen O. Effect of a multifactorial intervention on mortality in type 2 diabetes. *N Engl J Med.* 2008 Feb 7;358(6):580-91.

[95] Scuteri A, Lakatta EG. Bringing prevention in geriatrics: Evidences from cardiovascular medicine supporting the new challenge. *Exp Gerontol.* 2012 Mar 3.[Epub ahead of print]

[96] WHO. *Prevention of Cardiovascular Disease. Pocket Guidelines for Assessment and Management of Cardiovascular Risk.* Geneva 2007. http://www.who.int/ cardiovascular_diseases/guidelines/PocketGL.ENGLISH.AFR-D-E.rev1.pdf (Accessed on April 6 2012)

[97] WHO/ISH cardiovascular risk prediction charts. Available at http://www.who.int/ cardiovascular_diseases/publications/Chart_predictions/en/index.html (Accessed on April 6 2012)

[98] USPSTF 2008. *Screening for Type 2 Diabetes Mellitus in Adults.* http://www. uspreventiveservicestaskforce.org/uspstf/uspsdiab.htm (Accessed April 2, 2012).

[99] Shanmugasundaram M, Rough SJ, Alpert JS. Dyslipidemia in the elderly: should it be treated? *Clin Cardiol.* 2010 Jan;33(1):4-9.

[100] Taylor F, Ward K, Moore TH, Burke M, Davey Smith G, Casas JP, Ebrahim S. Statins for the primary prevention of cardiovascular disease. *Cochrane Database Syst Rev.* 2011 Jan 19;(1):CD004816.

[101] Redberg RF, Katz MH. Healthy men should not take statins. *JAMA.* 2012 Apr 11;307(14):1491-2.

[102] Blaha MJ, Nasir K, Blumenthal RS. Statin therapy for healthy men identified as "increased risk". *JAMA.* 2012 Apr 11;307(14):1489-90.

[103] National Institute for Health and Clinical Excellence 2006. *Statins for the prevention of cardiovascular events.* http://www.nice.org.uk/nicemedia/ live/11564/33151/33151.pdf (Accessed on April 6, 2012).

[104] Cooper A, Nherera L, Calvert N, O'Flynn N, Turnbull N, Robson J, Camosso-Stefinovic J, Rule C, Browne N, Ritchie G, Stokes T, Mannan R, Brindle P, Gill P, Gujral R, Hogg M, Marshall T, Minhas R, Pavitt L, Reckless J, Rutherford A, Thorogood M, Wood D(2008) *Clinical Guidelines and Evidence Review for Lipid Modification: cardiovascular risk assessment and the primary and secondary prevention of cardiovascular disease London: National Collaborating Centre for Primary Care and Royal College of General Practitioners.* http://www. nice.org.uk/CG67/FullGuideline (Accessed on April 21, 2012).

[105] Grundy SM, Cleeman JI, Merz CN, Brewer HB Jr, Clark LT, Hunninghake DB, Pasternak RC, Smith SC Jr, Stone NJ; National Heart, Lung, and Blood Institute; American College of Cardiology Foundation; American Heart Association.Implications of recent clinical trials for the National Cholesterol Education Program Adult Treatment Panel III guidelines. *Circulation.* 2004 Jul 13;110(2):227-39. Review. Erratum in: Circulation. 2004 Aug 10;110(6):763.

[106] USPSTF 2008. Screening for Lipid Disorders in Adults. http://www. uspreventiveservicestaskforce.org/uspstf/uspschol.htm (accessed on april 21, 2012)

[107] Morley JE. The cholesterol conundrum. *J Am Geriatr Soc.* 2011 Oct;59(10):1955-6.

[108] Preiss D, Sattar N. Statins and the risk of new-onset diabetes: a review of recent evidence. *Curr Opin Lipidol.* 2011 Dec;22(6):460-6.

[109] Mancia G. Antihypertensives in octogenarians. *BMJ.* 2012 Jan 4;344:d7293. doi: 10.1136/bmj.d7293.

[110] Beckett NS, Peters R, Fletcher AE, Staessen JA, Liu L, Dumitrascu D, Stoyanovsky V, Antikainen RL, Nikitin Y, Anderson C, Belhani A, Forette F, Rajkumar C, Thijs L, Banya W, Bulpitt CJ; HYVET Study Group. Treatment of hypertension in patients 80 years of age or older. *N Engl J Med.* 2008 May 1;358(18):1887-98.

[111] Beckett N, Peters R, Tuomilehto J, Swift C, Sever P, Potter J, McCormack T, Forette F, Gil-Extremera B, Dumitrascu D, Staessen JA, Thijs L, Fletcher A, Bulpitt C; HYVET Study Group. Immediate and late benefits of treating very elderly people with hypertension: results from active treatment extension to Hypertension in the Very Elderly randomised controlled trial. *BMJ.* 2011 Jan 4;344:d7541.

[112] Bangalore S, Messerli FH, Wun CC, Zuckerman AL, DeMicco D, Kostis JB, LaRosa JC; Treating to New Targets Steering Committee and Investigators. J-curve revisited: An analysis of blood pressure and cardiovascular events in the Treating to New Targets (TNT) Trial. *Eur Heart J.* 2010 Dec;31(23):2897-908.

[113] Kaplan NM. The diastolic J curve: alive and threatening. *Hypertension.* 2011 Nov;58(5):751-3.

[114] Chobanian AV, Bakris GL, Black HR, Cushman WC, Green LA, Izzo JL Jr, Jones DW, Materson BJ, Oparil S, Wright JT Jr, Roccella EJ; National Heart, Lung, and Blood Institute Joint National Committee on Prevention, Detection, Evaluation, and Treatment of High Blood Pressure; National High Blood Pressure Education Program Coordinating Committee. The Seventh Report of the Joint National Committee on Prevention, Detection, Evaluation, and Treatment of High Blood Pressure: the JNC 7 report. *JAMA.* 2003 May 21;289(19):2560-72. Epub 2003 May 14. Erratum in: JAMA. 2003 Jul 9;290(2):197.

[115] Whitworth JA; World Health Organization, International Society of Hypertension Writing Group. 2003 World Health Organization (WHO)/International Society of Hypertension (ISH) statement on management of hypertension. *J Hypertens.* 2003 Nov;21(11):1983-92.

[116] Mancia G, De Backer G, Dominiczak A, Cifkova R, Fagard R, Germano G, Grassi G, Heagerty AM, Kjeldsen SE, Laurent S, Narkiewicz K, Ruilope L, Rynkiewicz A, Schmieder RE, Struijker Boudier HA, Zanchetti A, Vahanian A, Camm J, De Caterina R, Dean V, Dickstein K, Filippatos G, Funck-Brentano C, Hellemans I, Kristensen SD, McGregor K, Sechtem U, Silber S, Tendera M, Widimsky P, Zamorano JL, Kjeldsen SE, Erdine S, Narkiewicz K, Kiowski W, Agabiti-Rosei E, Ambrosioni E, Cifkova R, Dominiczak A, Fagard R, Heagerty AM, Laurent S, Lindholm LH, Mancia G, Manolis A, Nilsson PM, Redon J, Schmieder RE, Struijker-Boudier HA, Viigimaa M, Filippatos G, Adamopoulos S, Agabiti-Rosei E, Ambrosioni E, Bertomeu V, Clement D, Erdine S, Farsang C, Gaita D, Kiowski W, Lip G, Mallion JM, Manolis AJ, Nilsson PM, O'Brien E, Ponikowski P, Redon J, Ruschitzka F, Tamargo J, van Zwieten P, Viigimaa M, Waeber B, Williams B, Zamorano JL, The task force for the management of arterial hypertension of the European Society of Hypertension, The task force for the management of arterial hypertension of the European Society of Cardiology. 2007 Guidelines for the management of arterial hypertension: The Task Force for the

Management of Arterial Hypertension of the European Society of Hypertension (ESH) and of the European Society of Cardiology (ESC). *Eur Heart J.* 2007 Jun;28(12):1462-536.

[117] Mazza A, Ramazzina E, Cuppini S, Armigliato M, Schiavon L, Rossetti C, Marzolo M, Santoro G, Ravenni R, Zuin M, Zorzan S, Rubello D, Casiglia E. Antihypertensive Treatment in the Elderly and Very Elderly: Always "the Lower, the Better?" *Int J Hypertens.* 2012;2012:590683. Epub 2011 Sep 22.

[118] National Institute for Health and Clinical Excellence 2011. *The clinical management of primary hypertension in adults.* August 2011. Available at http://www.nice.org.uk/nicemedia/live/13561/56008/56008.pdf (Accessed on April 7, 2012)

[119] Aronow WS, Fleg JL, Pepine CJ, Artinian NT, Bakris G, Brown AS, Ferdinand KC, Ann Forciea M, Frishman WH, Jaigobin C, Kostis JB, Mancia G, Oparil S, Ortiz E, Reisin E, Rich MW, Schocken DD, Weber MA, Wesley DJ, Harrington RA, Bates ER, Bhatt DL, Bridges CR, Eisenberg MJ, Ferrari VA, Fisher JD, Gardner TJ, Gentile F, Gilson MF, Hlatky MA, Jacobs AK, Kaul S, Moliterno DJ, Mukherjee D, Rosenson RS, Stein JH, Weitz HH, Wesley DJ. ACCF/AHA 2011 expert consensus document on hypertension in the elderly: a report of the American College of Cardiology Foundation Task Force on Clinical Expert Consensus Documents developed in collaboration with the American Academy of Neurology, American Geriatrics Society, American Society for Preventive Cardiology, American Society of Hypertension, American Society of Nephrology, Association of Black Cardiologists, and European Society of Hypertension. *J Am Soc Hypertens.* 2011 Jul-Aug;5(4):259-352.

[120] USPSTF 2007. Screening for High Blood Pressure in Adults. http://www.uspreventiveservicestaskforce.org/uspstf/uspshype.htm. (Accessed on April 1 2012).

[121] WHO. Health topics. *Obesity.* Available at http://www.who.int/topics/obesity/en/ (Accessed on April 7, 2012).

[122] Flegal KM, Carroll MD, Kuczmarski RJ, Johnson CL. Overweight and obesity in the United States: prevalence and trends, 1960-1994. *Int J Obes Relat Metab Disord.* 1998 Jan;22(1):39-47.

[123] Han TS, Tajar A, Lean ME. Obesity and weight management in the elderly. *Br Med Bull.* 2011;97:169-96.

[124] Chapman IM. Obesity paradox during aging. *Interdiscip Top Gerontol.* 2010;37:20-36.

[125] USPSTF 2003. *Screening for Obesity in Adults.* http://www. uspreventiveservice staskforce.org/uspstf/uspsobes.htm (Accessed April 2, 2012).

[126] Dai Y, Ge J. Clinical use of aspirin in treatment and prevention of cardiovascular disease. *Thrombosis.* 2012;2012:245037. Epub 2011 Nov 24.

[127] Seshasai SR, Wijesuriya S, Sivakumaran R, Nethercott S, Erqou S, Sattar N, Ray KK. Effect of aspirin on vascular and nonvascular outcomes: meta-analysis of randomized controlled trials. *Arch Intern Med.* 2012 Feb 13;172(3):209-16.

[128] Berger JS. Aspirin as preventive therapy in patients with asymptomatic vascular disease. *JAMA.* 2010 Mar 3;303(9):880-2.

[129] Brookes L, Ray K. *Aspirin in Primary Prevention: Interview With Kausik Ray. Medscape Cardiology.* Mar 8, 2012. Available at http://www.medscape.com/viewarticle/759883 (Accessed April 7, 2012).

[130] de Jong PT, Chakravarthy U, Rahu M, Seland J, Soubrane G, Topouzis F, Vingerling JR, Vioque J, Young I, Fletcher AE. Associations between aspirin use and aging macula disorder: the European Eye Study. *Ophthalmology.* 2012 Jan;119(1):112-8.

[131] Morimoto T, Fukui T, Lee TH, Matsui K. Application of U.S. guidelines in other countries: aspirin for the primary prevention of cardiovascular events in Japan. *Am J Med.* 2004 Oct 1;117(7):459-68.

[132] USPSTF 2009. *Aspirin for the Prevention of Cardiovascular Disease.* http://www.uspreventiveservicestaskforce.org/uspstf/uspsasmi.htm (accessed on April 1, 2012)

[133] Mant J, Edwards D. Stroke prevention in atrial fibrillation: putting the guidelines into practice. *Drugs Aging.* 2010 Nov 1;27(11):859-70.

[134] Wann LS, Curtis AB, January CT, Ellenbogen KA, Lowe JE, Estes NA 3rd, Page RL,Ezekowitz MD, Slotwiner DJ, Jackman WM, Stevenson WG, Tracy CM; 2011 Writing Group Members, Fuster V, Rydén LE, Cannom DS, Le Heuzey JY, Crijns HJ, Lowe JE, Curtis AB, Olsson SB, Ellenbogen KA, Prystowsky EN, Halperin JL, Tamargo JL, Kay GN, Wann LS; 2006 Writing Committee Members, Jacobs AK, Anderson JL, Albert N, Hochman JS, Buller CE, Kushner FG, Creager MA, Ohman EM, Ettinger SM, Stevenson WG, Guyton RA, Tarkington LG, Halperin JL, Yancy CW; ACCF/AHA Task Force Members. 2011 ACCF/AHA/HRS focused update on the management of patients with atrial fibrillation (updating the 2006 guideline): a report of the American College of Cardiology Foundation/American Heart Association Task Force on Practice Guidelines. Circulation. 2011 Jan 4;123(1):104-23. Epub 2010 Dec 20. *Erratum in: Circulation.* 2011 Aug 2;124(5):e173.

[135] European Heart Rhythm Association; European Association for Cardio-Thoracic Surgery, Camm AJ, Kirchhof P, Lip GY, Schotten U, Savelieva I, Ernst S, Van Gelder IC, Al-Attar N, Hindricks G, Prendergast B, Heidbuchel H, Alfieri O, Angelini A, Atar D, Colonna P, De Caterina R, De Sutter J, Goette A, Gorenek B, Heldal M, Hohloser SH, Kolh P, Le Heuzey JY, Ponikowski P, Rutten FH. Guidelines for the management of atrial fibrillation: the Task Force for the Management of Atrial Fibrillation of the European Society of Cardiology (ESC). Eur Heart J. 2010 Oct;31(19):2369-429. Epub 2010 Aug 29. *Erratum in: Eur Heart J.* 2011 May;32(9):1172.

[136] Cairns JA, Connolly S, McMurtry S, Stephenson M, Talajic M; CCS Atrial Fibrillation Guidelines Committee. Canadian Cardiovascular Society atrial fibrillation guidelines 2010: prevention of stroke and systemic thromboembolism in atrial fibrillation and flutter. *Can J Cardiol.* 2011 Jan Feb;27(1):74-90.

[137] Tulner LR, Van Campen JP, Kuper IM, Gijsen GJ, Koks CH, Mac Gillavry MR, van Tinteren H, Beijnen JH, Brandjes DP. Reasons for undertreatment with oral anticoagulants in frail geriatric outpatients with atrial fibrillation: a prospective, descriptive study. *Drugs Aging.* 2010 Jan 1;27(1):39-50.

[138] USPSTF 2005. *Screening for Abdominal Aortic Aneurysm.* http://www.uspreventiveservicestaskforce.org/uspstf/uspsaneu.htm (Accessed on April 1, 2012)

[139] Lim LS, Haq N, Mahmood S, Hoeksema L; ACPM Prevention Practice Committee; American College of Preventive Medicine. Atherosclerotic cardiovascular disease screening in adults: American College Of Preventive Medicine position statement on preventive practice. *Am J Prev Med.* 2011 Mar;40(3):381.e1-10.

[140] Takagi H, Goto SN, Matsui M, Manabe H, Umemoto T. A further meta-analysis of population-based screening for abdominal aortic aneurysm. *J Vasc Surg.* 2010 Oct;52(4):1103-8.

[141] Lederle FA. Screening for AAA in the USA. *Scand J Surg.* 2008;97(2):139-41.

[142] Schmidt T, Mühlberger N, Chemelli-Steingruber IE, Strasak A, Kofler B, Chemelli A, Siebert U. *Benefit, risks and cost-effectiveness of screening for abdominal aortic aneurysm. Rofo.* 2010 Jul;182(7):573-80. Epub 2010 Jun 18. Review. PubMed PMID: 20563953.

[143] WHO Media centre 2012. *Cancer, key facts.* Available at http://www.who.int/mediacentre/factsheets/fs297/en/ (Accessed on April 8, 2012).

[144] Resnick B, McLeskey SW. Cancer screening across the aging continuum. *Am J Manag Care.* 2008 May;14(5):267-76.

[145] Barrett B, McKenna P. Communicating benefits and risks of screening for prostate, colon, and breast cancer. *Fam Med.* 2011 Apr;43(4):248-53.

[146] USPSTF 2004. *Lung Cancer Screening. Recommendation Statement.* Available at http://www.uspreventiveservicestaskforce.org/3rduspstf/lungcancer/lungcanrs.htm Accessed on April 9, 2012.

[147] National Lung Screening Trial Research Team, Aberle DR, Adams AM, Berg CD, Black WC, Clapp JD, Fagerstrom RM, Gareen IF, Gatsonis C, Marcus PM, Sicks JD. Reduced lung-cancer mortality with low-dose computed tomographic screening. *N Engl J Med.* 2011 Aug 4;365(5):395-409.

[148] WHO Cancer. *Breast cancer: prevention and control.* http://www.who.int/cancer/detection/breastcancer/en/index1.html

[149] WHO Media Center. *Women's health.* http://www.who.int/mediacentre/ factsheets /fs334/en/index.html

[150] USPSTF 2009. *Screening for Breast Cancer* http://www.uspreventiveservicestaskforce.org/uspstf/uspsbrca.htm (Accessed on April 21, 2012)

[151] Türkiye'de Kanser İstatistikleri. http://www.turkkanser.org.tr/newsfiles/ 60turkiye _kanser_istatistikleri-2.pdf (Accessed on April 23, 2012)

[152] Lacey JV Jr, Kreimer AR, Buys SS, Marcus PM, Chang SC, Leitzmann MF, Hoover RN, Prorok PC, Berg CD, Hartge P; Prostate, Lung, Colorectal and Ovarian (PLCO)Cancer Screening Trial Project Team. Breast cancer epidemiology according to recognized breast cancer risk factors in the Prostate, Lung, Colorectal and Ovarian (PLCO) Cancer Screening Trial Cohort. *BMC Cancer.* 2009 Mar 17;9:84.

[153] Canadian Task Force on Preventive Health Care 2011. *Screening for Breast Cancer.* http://www.canadiantaskforce.ca/recommendations/2011_01_eng.html (Accessed on April 21, 2012)

[154] IARC (2008). World cancer report 2008. *Breast cancer.* Pages 412-417. Lyon, International Agency for Research on Cancer. http://www.iarc.fr/en/publications/pdfs-online/wcr/2008/index.php (Accessed on April 21, 2012)

[155] Danaei G, Vander Hoorn S, Lopez AD, Murray CJ, Ezzati M; Comparative Risk Assessment collaborating group (Cancers). Causes of cancer in the world: comparative risk assessment of nine behavioural and environmental risk factors. *Lancet.* 2005 Nov 19;366(9499):1784-93.

[156] McPherson K. Screening for breast cancer--balancing the debate. *BMJ.* 2010 Jun 24;340:c3106.

[157] Warner E. Clinical practice. Breast-cancer screening. *N Engl J Med.* 2011 Sep 15;365(11):1025-32.

[158] IARC (2008). World cancer report 2008. *Prostate cancer.* Pages 450-455. Lyon, International Agency for Research on Cancer. http://www.iarc.fr/en/publications/pdfs-online/wcr/2008/index.php (Accessed on April 21, 2012)

[159] USPSTF 2008 and 2011 *Screening for Prostate Cancer.* http://www.uspreventiveservicestaskforce.org/uspstf/uspsprca.htm (Accessed on April 21, 2012)

[160] Draisma G, Etzioni R, Tsodikov A, Mariotto A, Wever E, Gulati R, Feuer E, de Koning H. Lead time and overdiagnosis in prostate-specific antigen screening: importance of methods and context. *J Natl Cancer Inst.* 2009 Mar 18;101(6):374-83.

[161] Hoffman RM. Clinical practice. Screening for prostate cancer. *N Engl J Med.* 2011 Nov 24;365(21):2013-9.

[162] Wolf AM, Wender RC, Etzioni RB, Thompson IM, D'Amico AV, Volk RJ, Brooks DD, Dash C, Guessous I, Andrews K, DeSantis C, Smith RA; American Cancer Society Prostate Cancer Advisory Committee. American Cancer Society guideline for the early detection of prostate cancer: update 2010. *CA Cancer J Clin.* 2010 Mar-Apr;60(2):70-98.

[163] IARC (2008). *World cancer report 2008. Colorectal cancer.* Pages 374-379. Lyon, International Agency for Research on Cancer. http://www.iarc.fr/en/publications/pdfs-online/wcr/2008/index.php (Accessed on April 21, 2012)

[164] Qaseem A, Denberg TD, Hopkins RH Jr, Humphrey LL, Levine J, Sweet DE, Shekelle P; Clinical Guidelines Committee of the American College of Physicians. Screening for colorectal cancer: a guidance statement from the American College of Physicians. *Ann Intern Med.* 2012 Mar 6;156(5):378-86.

[165] Hewitson P, Glasziou P, Watson E, Towler B, Irwig L. Cochrane systematic review of colorectal cancer screening using the fecal occult blood test (hemoccult): an update. *Am J Gastroenterol.* 2008 Jun;103(6):1541-9.

[166] Penston J. Should we use total mortality rather than cancer specific mortality to judge cancer screening programmes? *Yes. BMJ.* 2011 Oct 13;343:d6395.

[167] USPSTF 2008. *Screening for Colorectal Cancer.* http://www. uspreventiveservices taskforce.org/uspstf08/colocancer/colors.htm (Accessed on April 12, 2011)

[168] *NHS Bowel Cancer Screening Programme.* http://www. cancerscreening.nhs.uk/ bowel/index.html (Accessed on April 12, 2012)

[169] New guidance for colorectal cancer screening. *Lancet.* 2012 Mar 17;379(9820):978.

[170] IARC (2008). World cancer report 2008. *Cervical cancer.* Pages 418-423. Lyon, International Agency for Research on Cancer. http://www.iarc.fr/en/publications/pdfs-online/wcr/2008/index.php (Accessed on April 21, 2012)

[171] USPSTF 2012. Screening for Cervical Cancer. http://www.uspreventiveservice staskforce. org/uspstf/uspscerv.htm (Accessed on April 13, 2012).

[172] Saslow D, Solomon D, Lawson HW, Killackey M, Kulasingam SL, Cain J, Garcia FA, Moriarty AT, Waxman AG, Wilbur DC, Wentzensen N, Downs LS Jr, Spitzer M, Moscicki AB, Franco EL, Stoler MH, Schiffman M, Castle PE, Myers ER. American Cancer Society, American Society for Colposcopy and Cervical Pathology, and American Society for Clinical Pathology screening guidelines for the prevention and early detection of cervical cancer. *CA Cancer J Clin.* 2012 Mar 14. doi: 10.3322/caac.21139. [Epub ahead of print]

[173] *WHO Global Burden of Disease:* 2004 Update. Geneva: World Health Organization, 2008. http://www.who.int/healthinfo/global_burden_disease/GBD_report_2004 update _full.pdf (accessed April 13, 2012).

[174] Rodda J, Walker Z, Carter J. Depression in older adults. *BMJ.* 2011 Sep 28;343:d5219. doi: 10.1136/bmj.d5219.

[175] USPSTF 2009. *Screening for Depression in Adults.* http://www. uspreventiveservices taskforce.org/uspstf/uspsaddepr.htm (Accessed April 13, 2012)

[176] Allaby M 2010. Screening for Depression: A report for the UK National Screening Committee. http://www.screening.nhs.uk/depression (Accessed April 13, 2012)

[177] Johnell O, Hertzman P. (2006). *What evidence is there for the prevention and screening of osteoporosis?* Copenhagen, WHO Regional Office for Europe (Health Evidence Network report; http://www.euro.who.int/document/e88668.pdf, Accessed April 13, 2012)

[178] Kanis JA, Oden A, Johnell O, Johansson H, De Laet C, Brown J, Burckhardt P, Cooper C, Christiansen C, Cummings S, Eisman JA, Fujiwara S, Glüer C, Goltzman D, Hans D, Krieg MA, La Croix A, McCloskey E, Mellstrom D, Melton LJ 3rd, Pols H, Reeve J, Sanders K, Schott AM, Silman A, Torgerson D, van Staa T, Watts NB, Yoshimura N. The use of clinical risk factors enhances the performance of BMD in the prediction of hip and osteoporotic fractures in men and women. *Osteoporos Int.* 2007 Aug;18(8):1033-46.

[179] National Osteoporosis Guideline Group (NOGG) 2010. NOGG Osteoporosis: Clinical guideline for prevention and treatment. *Executive Summary.* http://www. shef.ac.uk/NOGG/downloads.html (Accessed April 15, 2012)

[180] Hillier TA, Stone KL, Bauer DC, Rizzo JH, Pedula KL, Cauley JA, Ensrud KE,Hochberg MC, Cummings SR. Evaluating the value of repeat bone mineral density measurement and prediction of fractures in older women: the study of osteoporotic fractures. *Arch Intern Med.* 2007 Jan 22;167(2):155-60.

[181] Lim LS, Hoeksema LJ, Sherin K; ACPM Prevention Practice Committee. Screening for osteoporosis in the adult U.S. population: ACPM position statement on preventive practice. *Am J Prev Med.* 2009 Apr;36(4):366-75.

[182] UK NSC Policy Database. *Osteoporosis* (policy currently under review). http://www.screening.nhs.uk/osteoporosis (Accessed on April 14, 2012)

[183] *The National Osteoporosis Guideline Group** (NOGG) http://www.shef.ac.uk/NOGG/ (Accessed on April 20, 2012).

[184] National Osteoporosis Guideline Group (NOGG) 2010. ***NOGG** Guideline for the diagnosis and management of osteoporosis in postmenopausal women and men from the age of 50 years in the UK.* http://www.shef.ac.uk/NOGG/downloads.html (Accessed April 15, 2012)

[185] Panel on Prevention of Falls in Older Persons, American Geriatrics Society and British Geriatrics Society. Summary of the Updated American Geriatrics Society/British Geriatrics Society clinical practice guideline for prevention of falls in older persons. *J Am Geriatr Soc.* 2011 Jan;59(1):148-57.

[186] USPSTF 2010. *Interventions to Prevent Falls in Older Adults.* http://www. uspreventiveservicestaskforce.org/uspstf/uspsfalls.htm (Accessed on April 21, 2012)

[187] Parker MJ, Gillespie WJ, Gillespie LD. Effectiveness of hip protectors for preventing hip fractures in elderly people: systematic review. *BMJ.* 2006 Mar 11;332(7541):571-4

[188] USPSTF 2009. *Screening for Impaired Visual Acuity in Older Adults.* http://www.uspreventiveservicestaskforce.org/uspstf/uspsviseld.htm (Accessed April 2, 2012)

[189] WHO Media Centre. *Visual impairment and blindness.* http://www.who.int/mediacentre/factsheets/fs282/en/ (Accessed on April 23, 2011)

[190] Baltussen R, Sylla M, Mariotti SP. Cost-effectiveness analysis of cataract surgery: a global and regional analysis. *Bull World Health Organ.* 2004 May;82(5):338-45.

[191] Agarwal A, Kumar DA. Cost-effectiveness of cataract surgery. *Curr Opin Ophthalmol.* 2011 Jan;22(1):15-8.

[192] Taylor HR, Keeffe JE. World blindness: a 21st century perspective. *Br J Ophthalmol.* 2001 Mar;85(3):261-6.

[193] *WHO Prevention of Blindness and Visual Impairment: Priority eye diseases-Cataract.* http://www.who.int/blindness/causes/priority/en/index1.html (Accessed on April 23, 2012)

[194] *USPSTF 2011. Screening for Hearing Loss in Older Adults.* http://www.uspreventiveservicestaskforce.org/uspstf/uspshear.htm (Accessed April 2, 2012)

[195] *USPSTF 2003. Screening for Dementia.* http://www.uspreventiveservicestaskforce.org/3rduspstf/dementia/dementrr.htm#clinical (Accessed on April 15, 2012)

[196] Elsawy B, Higgins KE. The geriatric assessment. *Am Fam Physician.* 2011 Jan 1;83(1):48-56.

[197] Stuck AE, Iliffe S. Comprehensive geriatric assessment for older adults. *BMJ.* 2011 Oct 27;343:d6799.

[198] Ellis G, Whitehead MA, Robinson D, O'Neill D, Langhorne P. Comprehensive geriatric assessment for older adults admitted to hospital: meta-analysis of randomised controlled trials. *BMJ.* 2011 Oct 27;343:d6553.

[199] Wieland ML, Weis JA, Olney MW, Alemán M, Sullivan S, Millington K, O'Hara C, Nigon JA, Sia IG. Screening for tuberculosis at an adult education center: results of a community-based participatory process. *Am J Public Health.* 2011 Jul;101(7):1264-7.

[200] Hamashima C, Shibuya D, Yamazaki H, Inoue K, Fukao A, Saito H, Sobue T. The Japanese guidelines for gastric cancer screening. *Jpn J Clin Oncol.* 2008 Apr;38(4):259-67.

[201] USPSTF 2004. Screening for Thyroid Disease. http://www. uspreventiveservices taskforce.org/uspstf/uspsthyr.htm (Accessed April 16, 2011)

[202] Dharmarajan TS, Adiga GU, Norkus EP. Vitamin B12 deficiency. Recognizing subtle symptoms in older adults. *Geriatrics.* 2003 Mar;58(3):30-4, 37-8.

[203] Chui CH, Lau FY, Wong R, Soo OY, Lam CK, Lee PW, Leung HK, So CK, Tsoi WC, Tang N, Lam WK, Cheng G. Vitamin B12 deficiency--need for a new guideline. *Nutrition.* 2001 Nov-Dec;17(11-12):917-20.

[204] Watts G. Will medicine ever be able to halt the process of ageing? *BMJ* 2011;343:d4119

[205] USPSTF 2005. *Hormone Replacement Therapy for the Prevention of Chronic Conditionsin Postmenopausal Women.* http://www.uspreventiveservicestaskforce.org/uspstf/uspspmho.htm (Accessed April 2, 2012)

[206] Gestuvo M, Hung W. Common dietary supplements for cognitive health. *Aging health.* 2012 Feb;8(1):89-97.

SECTION 3: APPROACH TO COMMON SIGNS AND SYMPTOMS IN GERIATRICS

In: New Horizons in Geriatric Medicine. Volume 1
Editors: Ahmet Turan Isik, M. Refik Mas et al.
ISBN: 978-1-62808-972-1

Chapter 4

PAIN

Pakize Kirdemir
Anesthesiology, Pain Clinic
Suleyman Demirel University Medical School

ABSTRACT

The International Association for the Study of Pain (IASP) defines pain in terms of both actual or potential tissue damage and the emotional experiences associated with pain. [1]

Pain is one of the most common complaints that remains poorly treated in the elderly. As we become older, different changes occur in the body and effect how it works.

Pain that is under-recognized and undertreated can result in significant physical and social disability in the elderly long-term care population. [2] An aging adult may not respond to pain in the way that a younger person would. Their ability to recognize and report the pain often change according their illnesses, social conditions and dementia. The elderly need to detail the history of the pain, drugs and other complementaries that they have. They also need a good individual pain management plan. Most pain problems can be improved by proper assessment and careful use of analgesic drugs and nondrug strategies. [3, 4]

INTRODUCTION

There are different types of pain and the mechanism of pain based on pathophysiology. Nociceptive pain results from stimulation of pain receptors (Somatic: damage to body tissue, well localized; Visceral: from viscera, poorly localized, may have nausea). Neuropathic pain results from dysfunctions or lesions in either the central or peripheral nervous systems. Mixed pain syndromes have multiple or unknown mechanisms (e.g., headaches, vasculitic syndromes). Psychogenic pain results of somatoform disorders and conversion reactions. [5, 6, 7]

They have age related changes. There are reductions in the number and function of peripheral nociceptive neurons and also a decrease in pain receptors (50% Pacini's corpuscles, 10%-30% decrease in Meissner's/Merkle's disks). Sensory threshold for thermal and vibratory stimuli increase with age, endogenous analgesic response is diminished (endorphins). *Myelinated nerves* have decreased density, increased abnormal/degenerating fibers and slower conduction velocity. Large fibers of *unmyelinated nerves* and substance P content decrease. In the central nervous system there is a loss of neurons in dorsal horn, cortex, midbrain, brainstem and 18% loss in thalamus, endogenous inhibition altered (hyperalgesia) and catacholamines decreased (acetylcholine, GABA, serotonin).[8]

On the other hand aging also causes physiological changes such as decreased renal function, volume of distribution, liver mass and hepatic blood flow, activity of some drug-metabolizing enzymes, serum protein concentrations and pulmonary function. All age-related physiologic changes alter the pharmacokinetics and pharmacodynamics of analgesics, narrowing their therapeutic index and increasing the risk of toxicity and drug-drug interactions.

CNS changes lead to an increased risk of delirium. Pharmacokinetics' changes lead to increased plasma drug concentrations and pharmacodynamic changes lead to increased drug sensitivity in the elderly. Many of them currently take herbal/dietary supplements and are prone to drug-drug interactions related to these supplements.

Their ability to recognize pain may be blunted by illness or the use of multiple prescription drugs. Depression may also keep the older adult from reporting they are in pain. The older adult may also quit doing activities they love because it hurts too much. Decline in self-care activities (dressing, grooming, walking, etc.) may also be indicators that the older adult is experiencing pain. The older adult may refrain from reporting pain because they are afraid they will have to have surgery or will be put on a drug they become addicted to. They may not want others to see them as weak, or may feel there is something impolite or shameful in complaining about pain, or they may feel the pain is deserved punishment for past transgressions. [9, 10, 11]

Cultural barriers can also keep a person from telling someone they are in pain. They may not report pain because they feel it is a sign that death is near. Some believe that admitting they are in pain and need help make them lose respect in society while other cultures feel they should report pain right away and get immediate relief. Gender differences are usually the result of social and cultural expectations, with women expected to be emotional and show pain and men stoic, keeping pain to themselves. [12, 13, 14, 15]

Factors Affecting Perception of Pain

- Affects quality of life far beyond the local region of injury
- Feeling of loneliness is predictor of psychological distress
- Lack of intimate relationships, dependency and loss increase loneliness
- Loneliness has been shown to lower pain threshold and occurs as a risk factor for depression.
- Depression followed by lack of energy, avoidance of diversional activities, decreased engagement in treatment.
- Anxiety inhibits participating in rehabilitation efforts.

- Sleep disturbance is best predictor of pain.
- Increased health care needs.
- Isolation and reduced independence.
- Focusing one's attention on pain makes the pain worse.
- Patients who have low levels of pain generally being worse than they originally reported.
- Pain can be a learned response, rather than a purely physical problem.
- Psychosocial issues like patient's belief about their pain , their coping skills, their involvement in the "sick role", all have an impact on how much pain patients feel, and how it affects them. [16]

Prevalence of Pain in Elderly

- 1 in 5 elderly have pain 18% above 65 are taking pain medications regularly
- One-fifth of adults 65 years and older said they had experienced pain in the past month that persisted for more than 24 hours.
- Almost three-fifths of adults 65 and older with pain said it had lasted for one year or more.
- Women report severely painful joints more often than men (10 % versus 7 %).
- Greater than 50% patients dying of a variety of illnesses, including cancer, COPD, CAD.
- 31% of women & 19% of men > 75 yrs report pain in 3 or more sites. [17, 18]

How Is Pain Diagnosed?

Pain Assessment

Detailed pain history makes easier to diagnose the pain. Generally it includes onset, pattern, duration, location, intensity, and characteristics of the pain. Aggravating or palliating factors and the impact on the patient needs to be defined. Psychological state of patient also needed to be evaluated (screen for depression, anxiety, assess social networks and family involvement). Elder people may often describe pain as slow, dull and achy. No tests are available to diagnose pain. The diagnosis' of pain are based on how long and how often they have the symptoms and also need any of the following to check how much pain they have or find its causes. [19, 20]

- **Physical examination:** Looking for painful areas during a physical exam.
- **Imaging tests:** These may include x-rays, computed tomography (CT) scan, and magnetic resonance imaging (MRI).

c-Pain scales

Unidimensional Scales: A single item that usually relates to pain intensity alone. It is easy to administer and require little time or training to produce reasonably valid and reliable results but sometimes require vision, hearing and attention, pencil and paper.

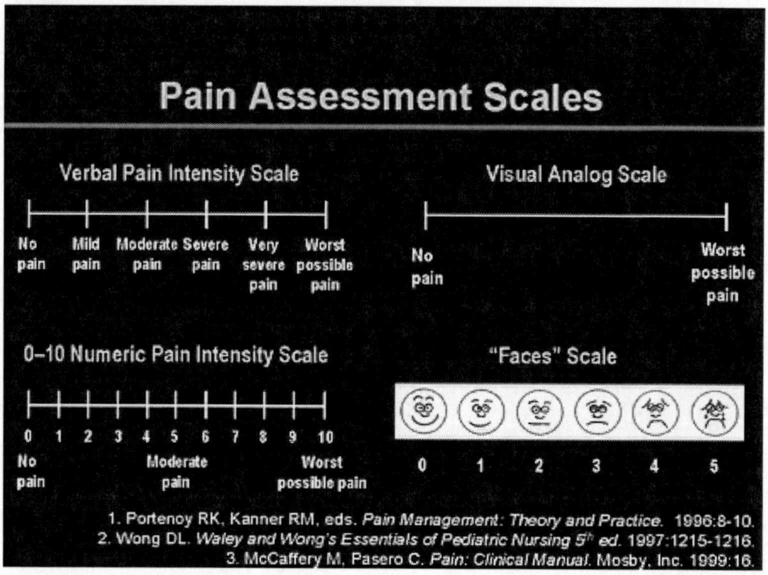

Multidimensional Scales: Evaluate pain in multiple domains (McGill Pain Questionnaire). It looks at pain in terms of intensity, affect, sensation, location, and several other domains that are not evaluable with a single question but they are long, time consuming and difficult to administer.

- **Stimulation tests:** Stimulation tests tell exactly which nerves or muscles are affected by pain.

Sometimes the elderly are not able to speak about their pain. This may be further complicated with illness or injuries like dementia, brain damage, or a stroke. This makes it very hard for caregivers and family to recognise the existence of pain. Formal pain assessments may not be sufficient for those with speech, hearing or cognitive deficits or who fear reporting pain. Close observations of behaviour may reveal expressions, movements, and activities indicative of pain. [21]

Signs that represents pain

- Normally loud and noisy patient get very quiet and withdrawn. Stop doing activities that used to do.
- Quiet and withdrawn patient get loud, act stubborn, and hit people.
- Lack of appetite. Only want to drink or eat soft foods.
- Suddenly, ceasing all the activities they used to do
- Losing bowel and bladder control.
- Acting very depressed and have a sad face.

- Blinking eyes very fast and also grimace (make strange faces).
- Being very easy going and happy or very sensitive and cry easily
- Start to walk or move differently than before. Suddenly stop walking, or start pacing all the time.
- Having knees drawn up to chest and rock like a baby
- Touch, rub, pull or pick at a body part that is hurting
- Start to pull away from peoples' touch and protect their arms or legs.
- Suddenly begin to stumble or fall, when they had no problems before.
- Sleep more or less than usual.
- Start to whimper or groan quietly.
- Becoming very confused suddenly without any problem.[22]

TREATMENT

Goals of Treatment

- Adequate pain management,
- Restoration of both physical and social function,
- Listen, Assess, Treat, Reassess often,
- Start low doses and increase slowly,

The World Health Organization (WHO) recommends a *pain ladder* for managing analgesia. It was first described for use in cancer pain, but it can be used by medical professionals as a general principle when dealing with analgesia for any type of pain. In the treatment of chronic pain, whether due to malignant or benign processes, the three-step WHO Analgesic Ladder provides guidelines for selecting the kind and stepping up the amount of analgesia. [18, 23]

Nonopioid Analgesics for Older Adults

- ***Acetaminophen*** usually used as a treatment of choice for osteoarthritis. Acetaminophen may be administered as a single medication or in combination with other analgesics (both NSAIDs and opioids). Maximum dose 4 gm/day.
- ***Nonselective NSAIDs*** inhibit prostaglandin synthesis. They are appropriate for short term use. They all have ceiling effect. They have risk of gastrointestinal bleed, renal impairment, platelet dysfunction as side effects. Selective COX-2 inhibitors reduce gastrointestinal side-effects and platelet inhibition but they have significant cardiovascular and cerebrovascular risks which have limited their utilization
- ***Tricyclic antidepressants*** (amytriptyline, desipramine) are used for neuropathic pain, depression, sleep disturbance. Not recommended for often use due to side-effects.
- ***Anticonvulsants*** are used for neuropathic pain. Carbamazepine can be used for trigeminal neuralgia, may cause pancytopenia.
- ***Muscle relaxants*** are used for muscle spasm, monitor for sedation

- ***Local anesthetics*** (lidocaine patch, topical voltaren gel, capsaicin). Capsaicin depletes substance P, may take weeks to reach full effect, adverse effects include burning and erythema. Lidocain patch approved for post herpetic neuralgia.

OPIOIDS

Show analgesic effect by stimulating mu opioid receptor. They are used for the treatment of moderate to severe pain and also used for both nociceptive and neuropathic pain. Opioid drugs have no ceiling to their analgesic effects and have been shown to relieve all types of pain. Opioids can cause drowsiness, nausea, respiratory depression. When opioids are used for prolonged periods drug tolerance, chemical dependency, diversion and addiction may occur. Tolerance develops to CNS side effects but not to constipation. Patients need prophylactic increasing fluid intake, osmotic laxatives or stimulant laxatives for constipation. Inadequately treated and un-relieved pain leading to persistent or worsening pain complaints (Pseudo-addiction). It can be prevented with frequent office visits and requests dose increase.

Elderly people, compared to younger people, may be more sensitive to the analgesic properties. Advanced age is associated with a prolonged half-life and prolonged pharmacokinetics of opioid drugs.

- ***Morphine*** has hepatic metabolism and renally excreted; it is not dialyzable. Its oral bioavailability is 30-40% and has two active metabolites. M6G is active metabolite with analgesic activity, M3G is another metabolite causes neurotoxicity. Morphine is available in varies routes such as oral (liquid and pill), topical, sublingual, parenteral, intrathecal, epidural and rectal. High doses can lead to myoclonus and hyperalgesia.
- ***Oxycodone*** is only available in oral form and more potent than morphine. Available as single agent and in combination with NSAIDs and acetaminophen.
- ***Methandone*** blocks NMDA receptors, inexpensive, no active metabolite and used for neuropathic pain. It has variable half-life and high tissue distribution.
- ***Hydrocodone*** is only available in combination with acetamenophen or NSAID
- ***Hydromorphone*** is 5 times more potent than morphine and not available in long acting preparation
- ***Propoxyphene*** has very weak analgesic effect, can cause ataxia and neurotoxicity, twofold higher risk of hip fractures.
- ***Meperidine*** is metabolized to active metabolite normeperidine. Lowers seizure threshold, risk for falls, confusion and sedation. Meperidine should be avoided for chronic use.
- ***Fentanyl Patch*** is 100 times more potent than morphine. Drug absorption altered by temperature and deposited in excess adipose tissue.
- ***Tramadol*** is a synthetic mu (opioid) agonist and inhibites serotonin and norepinephrine reuptake. 1/5th as potent as morphine. It also lowers threshold for seizure and multiple drug-drug interactions. [24, 25]

Non-Drug Treatment: *Complementary and Alternative Therapies*

- ***Education*** basic knowledge about pain (diagnosis, treatment, complications, and prognosis), other available treatment options, and information about over-the-counter medications and self-help strategies.
- ***Exercise*** tailored for individual patient needs and lifestyle; moderate-intensity exercise, 30 minutes or more 3-4 times a week and continued indefinitely.
- ***Physical modalities*** (heat, cold, and massage) cold for acute injuries in first 48 hours, to decrease bleeding or hematoma formation, edema, and chronic back pain. Heat works well for relief of muscle aches and abdominal cramping.
- ***Physical or occupational therapy*** should be conducted by a trained therapist.
- ***Chiropractic*** is effective for acute back pain. Potential spinal cord or nerve root impingement should be ruled out before any spinal manipulation.
- ***TENS unit*** can be considered for diabetic neuropathy but not for chronic low back pain
- ***Massage*** reduces pain, including release of muscle tension, improved circulation, increased joint mobility, and decreased anxiety.
- ***Acupuncture*** is performed by qualified acupuncturist. Effects may be short and require repetitive treatments
- ***Relaxation*** repetitive focus on sound, sensation, muscle tension, inattention towards intrusive thoughts. Requires individual acceptance and substantial training.
- ***Meditation*** calms the mind, allows thoughts, emotions and sensations to travel through conscious awareness without judgment.
- ***Progressive muscle relaxation*** is also tenses and relaxes certain muscle groups.
- ***Hypnosis*** reduces pain by distraction, altered pain perception, increased pain threshold.
- ***Cognitive-behavioral therapy*** pain is influenced by cognition, affect and behavior. Conducted by a trained therapist, focuses on changing individual cognitive activity to modify associated behavior, thoughts, and emotions for 10-12 weeks individual or group sessions.[26]
- ***Operant behavior therapy*** uses negative and positive consequences to modify the behaviors.
- ***Mind-body conditioning practices*** includes yoga, tai chi……
- ***Procedures***

Pulsed radiofrequency direct introduction of medication and nerve ablation may be used.

Intrathecal pump used to deliver very small quantities of medications directly to the spinal fluid. This approach allows a higher dose of the drug to be delivered directly to the site of action, with fewer systemic side effects.

Spinal cord stimulation creates electric impulses provides a paresthesia ("tingling") sensation that alters the perception of pain by the patient.

Surgery may be needed to remove the whole or a part of a tumor and also nerves or joints that may cause pain. [24, 25]

Principles of Geriatric Pain Management

- "Start low and go slow"—use low doses and titrate up slowly to achieve desired effect.
- Use analgesics with short half-lives and the fewest side effects when treating intermittent pain.
- Use around-the-clock medications for around-the clock pain.
- Monitor for adverse effects.
- Use prophylactic laxatives when administering opioids.
- Match the drug to the type of pain and pain severity.
- When possible, use a multimodal approach.
- Avoid intramuscular injections.
- Observe patients who have been on opioids preop—their postop requirement will most often be higher than the opioid naive patient.
- Evaluate effectiveness of pain management plan and modify as needed.
- Use pharmacological and non- pharmacological modalities together.

References

[1] IASP website Hix, MD. Pain Management in elderly patients, *Journal of pharmacy Practice*. 2007, 20, 49-63.

[2] Ferrell, BA. Assessing pain in the elderly. *Consult Pharm*. 2010 May, 25 Suppl A, 5-10.

[3] Ferrell, BA. Pain management. *Clin Geriatr Med*. 2000 Nov, 16(4), 853-74.

[4] Ferrell, BA. The management of pain in long-term care. *Clin J Pain*. 2004, 20(4), 240-3.

[5] Spanswick, CC; Main, CJ. *Pain management: an interdisciplinary approach*. Edinburgh: Churchill Livingstone, 2000, 93.

[6] Thienhaus, O; Cole, BE. Classification of pain. In: Weiner R. Pain management: a practical guide for clinicians. Boca Raton: CRC Press, 2002, 28.

[7] Treede, RD; Jensen, TS; Campbell, JN et al. Neuropathic pain: redefinition and a grading system for clinical and research purposes. *Neurology*. 2008, 70(18), 1630–1635.

[8] Cassel, CK; Leipzig, RM; Cohen, HJ; Larson, EB; Meier, DE. (Eds.): Geriatric medicine: An evidence based approach, 4th edition, Published by Springer-Verlay 2003.

[9] lawhorne, L; Passerini, J. Chronic Pain Management in the Long Term Care Setting: Clinical Practice Guidelines. Baltimore, Maryland: American Medical Directors Association.1999, 1–27.

[10] Stein, WM. Pain in the nursing home. *Clinics in Geriatric Medicine*. 2001, 17, 575-94.

[11] Stewart, K. et al. Assessment approaches for older people receiving social care: content and coverage. *International Journal of Geriatric Psychiatry*, 1999, 14, 147-56.

[12] Bonham, VL. Race, ethnicity, and pain treatment: striving to understand the causes and solutions to the disparities in pain treatment. *J Law Med Ethics*. 2001,29(1), 52–68.

[13] 65.Jarvis, C. Physical examination & health assessment. St. Louis, Mo: Elsevier Saunders. 2007, 180–192.

[14] Horgas, AL. et al. Pain in nursing home residents. Comparison of residents' self-report and nursing assistants' perceptions. *Journal of Gerontological Nursing*, 2001, 27, 44-53.

[15] Weiner, D et al. Chronic pain associated behaviours in the nursing home: resident versus caregiver perceptions. *Pain*, 1999, 80, 577-588.

[16] Deane, G et al., Overview of pain management in older persons. *Clin Geriatr Med*, 2008, 24, 185-201.

[17] Minner, DM et al., Evidence based assessment and treatment of persistent pain in the community dwelling elderly receiving home health services: *A pathway, Home health care management and practice*. 2005, 17, 294-301.

[18] Ferrell, B; Argoff, CE; Epplin, J; Fine, P; Gloth, FM; Herr, K; Katz, JD; Mehr, DR; Reid, C; Reisner, L. American geriatrics society(AGS) panel on the pharmacological management of persistent pain in older persons, *JAGS*, 2009, 50, 205-224.

[19] Brucenthal, P. Assessment of pain in the elderly adult. *Clinics in Geriatric Medicine*, 2008, 24(2).

[20] Bjoro, K; Herr, K. Assessment of pain in the nonverbal or cognitively impaired Older adult. *Clinics in Geriatric Medicine*, 2008, 24(2), 237-262.

[21] Feldt, KS. *Pain Manag Nurs*, 2000, 1(1), 13-21.

[22] The Australian Society for Geriatric Medicine. Pain management. February 2008.

[23] Fine, PG. Chronic pain management in older adults: special considerations, *J Pain Symptom Manage*, 2009; 38, 4-14.

[24] Jakobsson, U. et.al. Old people in pain: A comparative study. *Journal of Pain and Symptom Management*, 2003, 26, 625-636.

[25] Weiner, DK, et al., Pain in nursing home residents; management strategies. *Drugs and Aging*. 2001, 18(1), 13-19.

[26] Norelli, LJ et.al. Behavioral approaches to pain management in the elderly, *Clinics in Geriatric Medicine*, 2008, 24(2),_335–244.

In: New Horizons in Geriatric Medicine. Volume 1
Editors: Ahmet Turan Isik, M. Refik Mas et al.

ISBN: 978-1-62808-972-1

Chapter 5

ANEMIA

Cengiz Beyan and Alev Akyol Erikci
Gulhane Military Medical Academy, Department of Haematology,
Ankara, Turkey

ABSTRACT

Anemia is defined as hemoglobin levels <13 g/dl in men and <12 g/dl in women according to World Health Organization criteria. Anemia incidence is reported 11.0% in men and 10.2% in women above 65 years of age in the "National Health and Nutrition Examination Survey (NHANES) III" in United States of America. There are three major causes of anemia in the elderly: nutritional anemia, mostly iron deficiency anemia, anemia of chronic disease or anemia of chronic inflammation and unexplained anemia. NHANES III data reveals that nutritional deficiency which is the mostly iron deficiency, vitamin B_{12} and/or folate deficiency is the major cause of anemia (34% in the elderly people). Iron deficiency alone or with folate and vitamin B_{12} deficiency compromise the 20% of the anemia in the elderly. Anemia of chronic disease is common and an important cause like iron deficiency anemia. Chronic renal disease is an important cause of anemia which is commonly seen in the elderly population. Unexplained anemia is present in the 20-30% of the elderly patients according to variety of epidemiological studies. Some theories that support the high incidence of anemia in the elderly are decrease in hematopoietic stem cells, decrease in the production of hematopoietic growth factors, decrease of the sensitivity of stem cells and progenitors to growth factors, bone marrow microenvironment abnormalities, androgen deficiency, age-related decrease in renal functions and/or erythropoietin release, undiagnosed chronic renal disease or myelodysplasia or early period of anemia of chronic disease. Some of the elderly patients with unexplained anemia have myelodysplastic syndrome which is defined as ineffective hematopoiesis, cytopenias, and an increased incidence of transformation into acute myeloid leukemia. Anemia increases the risk of mortality, cardiovascular diseases, fractures, and decreases the cognitive functions and physical performance. It should be implied that these symptoms appear not only in major reduction in hemoglobin levels also in slight fluctuations from the normal values. In the management of anemia, etiology should be investigated and treated if possible in the elderly population. Management is limited to transfusion of erythrocyte suspensions and erythropoiesis stimulating agents in patients with symptomatic anemia.

Introduction

Although values vary in different laboratories, anemia is defined as hemoglobin (Hb) <14.0 g/dl in men and <12.3 g/dl in women. Alternatively, the World Health Organization (WHO) defines anemia Hb <13 g/dl in men and <12 g/dl in women [1-4]. These values are not considerable in the older population [5]. Hb and hematocrit values are significantly lower in healthy older population when compared to young ones [6].

Anemia has negative effects both on quality of life and functions in the older population. When Hb levels and all causes of death are evaluated together in women 65 years or older, the ones with Hb values 13.9 g/dl had better overall survival. In a study, including 1,156 people over 65 years old, muscular and skeletal functional results and physical performance; the ones with better results had Hb levels 1-3 g/dl more than the WHO definition of anemia [7]. Similarly, in studies evaluating the functional impairment of physical performance in 70-80 years old woman the WHO values for normal Hb were not satisfactory. People with Hb levels 13.5 g/dl had no functional impairment when compared to ones with 12 g/dl. Tests evaluating the performance status show better results in women when Hb levels increase to 13-14 g/dl from 12-13 g/dl. All these data support that even low-normal Hb values limit the physical performance in the elderly people.

Anemia Prevalence

Hb values decrease with age and anemia becomes a major health problem in the elderly. However, the prevalence of anemia varies in different studies (Table 1). Using the WHO definition of anemia (Hb <13 g/dl in men and Hb <12 g/dl in women) 11.0% of men and 10.2% of women were anemic according to the "National Health and Nutrition Examination Survey (NHANES) III" data set in people >65 years and older [8, 9]. Anemia is usually mild in the elderly; 2.8% of women and 1.6% of men have Hb values <11 g/dl. The variation of the data is a result of heterogeneous groups. Race, environmental factors and health situation have effects on the prevalence of anemia.

Table 1. Anemia prevalence in the elderly

Reference	Study Population	Anemia Criteria	Anemia Prevalence
Guralnik et al. [10]	≥65 years 5,252 subjects	Hb <13 g/dl in men and <12 g/dl in women	11.0% in men and 10.2% in women
Fleming et al. [11]	67-96 years 1,016 subjects	Hb <12.4 g/dl in men and <11.8 g/dl in women	6.1% in men and 10.5% in women
Izaks et al. [12]	≥85 years 1,016 subjects	Hb <13 g/dl in men and <12 g/dl in women	17.0% in men and 28.0% in women
Olivares et al. [13]	≥60 years 274 subjects	Hb <13 g/dl in men and <12 g/dl in women	5.4% in men and 4.4% in women
Artz et al. [14]	49-94 years 900 nursing home subjects	Hb <13 g/dl in men and <12 g/dl in women	48.0%
Cesari et al. [15]	Mean age 75 years 950 men and women	Hb <13 g/dl in men and <12 g/dl in women	10.6%
Penninx et al. [7]	≥65 years 1,156 subjects	Hb <13 g/dl in men and <12 g/dl in women	11.1% in men and 11.5% in women

Etiology and Diagnosis

There are three major causes of anemia in the elderly: nutritional anemias mostly iron deficiency, anemia of chronic disease and unexplained anemia [2, 10]. Table 2 illustrates the causes of anemia according to NHANES III data in 65 years and older subjects [8, 9, 16].

Table 2. The causes of anemia in subjects ⩾65 years according to NHANES III data [8, 9, 16]

	Prevalence (%)	Number of Cases
Nutritional Deficiency		
Folate and/or vitamin B_{12}	14%	403,608
Iron and/or folate/vitamin B_{12}	20%	561,936
Total	34%	965,544
Chronic Disease		
Chronic renal failure alone	8%	229,686
Anemia of chronic disease alone	20%	554,281
Chronic renal failure and anemia of chronic disease together	4%	120,169
Total	32%	904,136
Unexplained Anemia	34%	945,195
Total	100%	2,814,875

Iron Deficiency Anemia

NHANES III data revealed that nutritional deficiency is the 34% of anemia (iron, vitamin B_{12} and/or folate deficiency) in the elderly [9, 10]. Iron deficiency alone or folate and vitamin B_{12} deficiency make the 20% [10]. Iron deficiency anemia is characterized by microcytic and hypochromic erythrocytes classically whereas in the early stages of disease or in combination of other anemia it might be normocytic [14, 17].

Measurement of serum ferritin is the most common method for detection of iron deficiency anemia. Iron stores are depressed when ferritin value is <12 μg/l [18]. Although low ferritin levels is a marker for iron deficiency, ferritin levels might increase with age so that it is not a reliable marker when detected normal in the elderly. Therefore, higher levels of ferritin might be used for the diagnosis of iron deficiency in that special group. Optimal threshold for iron deficiency is defined as 50 μg/l in the hospitalized elderly patients [19].

In cases of inflammation or malignancies, iron indices might be affected; as a result, transferrin levels might be normal or low whereas ferritin might be normal or high [20, 21]. When inflammation is present the ratio of serum soluble transferrin receptors to log of ferritin might be helpful in the diagnosis of iron deficiency anemia [22].

Investigation of Etiology

The diagnosis of iron deficiency anemia requires investigation of the etiology in addition to iron therapy. In the developing world, as iron fortification of food items has made iron deficiency less common, definition of unknown lesions in gastrointestinal tract is important for the etiology of anemia [23]. Iron deficiency anemia might be a result of esophagitis, gastritis, ulcers, colon cancer or premalignant polyps and angiodysplasia which might result in chronic blood loss from gastrointestinal tract [24]. Gastrointestinal tract abnormalities are usually defined in some of the cases with iron deficiency anemia.

In 111 hospitalized cases 75 years or older with iron deficiency anemia were applied 92% of upper gastrointestinal endoscopy and 82% of colonoscopy. 68% had a leading lesion and 11% had synchronized lesions in these patients [25]. The 31 patients out of 43 patients (72%) with colorectal bleeding had colon cancer. Upper gastrointestinal tract examination showed lesions in 44 patients and 6 of them (14%) were malignant.

In follow-up studies, the accurate and exact time of diagnosis had a great impact on prognosis [26]. In two years follow-up studies, the prognosis of cancer cases with supplied curative treatment (28/102) (68%) were similar patients with benign lesions (80%) and undefined cause of anemia (66%). Conversely, none of the 10 patients with cancer who had palliative treatment survived.

In the presence of iron deficiency even without anemia, the bleeding site should be investigated. Upper gastrointestinal tract endoscopy and colonoscopy or both were performed in 151 elderly hospitalized patients with serum ferritin levels 50 μg/l [27]. Approximately half of the patients with anemia or non-anemia had a potential upper gastrointestinal tract lesion. Lower gastrointestinal lesion was present in 32% of cases with anemia and in 16% of cases without anemia. Upper gastrointestinal lesions were present in 6% and colon cancer in 9% of the cases without anemia.

Serum ferritin levels >50 μg/l which is defined as normal ferritin levels do not exclude the presence of a gastrointestinal tract malignancy. Colon cancer was detected in 16%, 20% and 13% of patients with serum ferritin <50 μg/l, 50-100 μg/l, and >100 μg/l, respectively in a retrospective study [28].

Folate Deficiency

A normal diet includes 500-700 mg of folate. 50-60% of dietary folate is absorbed from duodenum and jejunum. Folate deficiency is usually a result of decreased dietary intake [29, 30]. Body folate stores are enough for 4-6 months besides dietary insufficiency, drugs like methotrexate and excessive alcohol intake are other causes.

Vitamin B_{12} Deficiency

Both vitamin B_{12} and folate deficiency are commonly seen in the elderly population [20, 30]. Mostly the etiology of cobalamin deficiency is due to food-cobalamin malabsorption and pernicious anemia, rarely, deficient intake and malabsorption might be other causes in the elderly [31]. In the study of Andres et al., 200 elderly patients with cobalamin deficiency were included. 60-70% had food-cobalamin malabsorption and 15-25% had pernicious anemia in etiology [30].

Food-cobalamin malabsorption is an insufficiency in cobalamin releases of food and/or intestinal transport proteins, which is the same in hypochlorhydria. Food-cobalamin malabsorption is usually a result of atrophic gastritis. Gastric atrophy is present in 40% of population >70 years which is relevant to H. pylori infection or not [31]. Other causes of food-cobalamin malabsorption in the elderly are chronic H. pylori colonization, intestinal microbial proliferation, prolonged antacid, H_2 receptor antagonists, proton pump inhibitors, or biguanide usage, chronic alcoholism, gastric operation, and pancreatic exocrine insufficiency [32].

Anemia of Chronic Disease

Anemia of chronic disease is common and an important cause of anemia like iron deficiency [3, 21]. It is commonly seen in association with infections, rheumatologic disorders, malignancy and other chronic illnesses and is an exclusion diagnosis of these disorders. As chronic disorders are common in the elderly, it is not surprising that the diagnosis of anemia of chronic disease is common. It can coexist with iron deficiency which makes the diagnosis more difficult [24].

Anemia of chronic disease is typically mild or moderate in severity, normochromic normocytic anemia and inappropriate reticulocyte response is present [21]. Commonly the severity of anemia is correlated with the severity of the underlying disease.

The definition of anemia of chronic disease does not include the bone marrow infiltration, bleeding, hemolysis and anemia due to renal disease, in which enough ferritin levels, hypoferremia may occur. Besides low serum iron and serum iron binding capacity, normal iron stores is an important criterion for the diagnosis of anemia of chronic disease. The adequacy of iron stores is proved by high serum ferritin and stainable iron in the bone marrow. Ferritin levels ≤12 μg/l support the diagnosis of iron deficiency whereas levels ≥100 μg/l exclude the diagnosis of iron deficiency. It is claimed that serum transferrin receptors alone or its ratio to serum ferritin can be a sensitive predictor for anemia of chronic disease. Table 3 explains the predictors for differential diagnosis of iron deficiency and anemia of chronic disease [16, 21].

Table 3. The differences between anemia of chronic disease and iron deficiency

Test	Anemia of Chronic Disease	Iron Deficiency
Mean corpuscular volume	Normal or decreased	Decreased or normal
Serum iron	Decreased or normal	Decreased
Total iron binding capacity	Normal or decreased	Increased
Serum transferrin concentration	Decreased or normal	Increased
Transferrin saturation	Decreased or normal	Decreased
Serum ferritin	Normal or increased	Decreased
Serum transferrin receptor	Normal	Increased
Transferrin receptor/log ferritin	Low (<1)	High (>4)

Pathogenesis

Anemia of chronic disease has a multifactorial pathophysiology which includes decreased reuse of iron from erythrocytes, decreased of erythrocyte survival, increased apoptosis of bone marrow progenitor cells, decreased erythropoietin release and decreased response to erythropoietin [16, 21].

The impairment of iron supply and usage of iron by erythroid progenitors are the most common underlying mechanisms in anemia of chronic disease. Other important mechanisms that play role in pathophysiology are increased apoptosis of other erythroid precursors, insufficient erythropoietin production and decreased of erythrocyte survival. These mechanisms are relevant to increased proinflammatory cytokines like interleukin (IL)-1, IL-6 and tumor necrosis factor-alpha (TNFa) [21].

It is claimed that proinflammatory cytokines inhibit the erythropoiesis by increasing the apoptosis of erythroid progenitors. Erythropoietin is a critical anti-apoptotic factor in erythropoiesis. However, erythropoiesis might be ineffective and erythropoietin production might be deficient in the presence of increased proinflammatory cytokines. There is an opposite relationship between Hb and serum erythropoietin levels like Hb and reticulocyte production. Serum erythropoietin levels are significantly low in anemia of chronic disease when compared to other causes of anemia even with the same Hb levels. This situation supports the idea of anemia of chronic disease is relatively due to erythropoietin deficiency. Erythropoietin usage might be helpful in the management of anemia.

IL-6 plays a central role in the anemia of chronic disease. Like IL-1 and TNFa, IL-6 also suppresses the erythropoiesis. It causes anemia not only by increasing the plasma volume but also disturbing the usage of iron. Cytokines like interferon-gamma, IL-10 and IL-13 also suppress the erythropoietin response.

Hepcidin and Anemia of Chronic Disease

Hepcidin a recently defined amino acid peptide plays an important role in pathogenesis of anemia of chronic disease. It regulates iron absorption from intestines and secretion of iron from macrophages [21]. Hepcidin release decreases with excess iron and increases in the presence of proinflammatory cytokines. It is reported that hepcidin release increases a hundred times fold in the anemia of chronic disease.

Hepcidin inhibits intestinal iron absorption, release of iron from macrophages into the circulation, and iron transportation from the placenta. Hepcidin deficiency in hereditary hemochromatosis is related to HFE, transferrin receptor 2, hemojuvelin and mutations of hepcidin gene itself. Hepcidin is also suppressed in thalassemia and congenital dyserythropoietic anemia type I.

It is claimed that hepcidin release is stimulated by IL-6 and lipopolysaccharides are inhibited by IL-1 or TNFa [21]. Infusion of IL-6 results in a reduction of serum iron and transferrin saturation. All these observations support that hepcidin has a key regulatory role in anemia of chronic disease. Recently it is reported that recombinant human erythropoietin suppresses expression of hepcidin mRNA in mouse models. This is the result of direct effect on hepcidin gene transcription or variations in cellular iron depots secondary to increased hematopoiesis.

Serum Transferrin Receptor

Serum transferrin receptor level is a sensitive alternative for measurement of iron stores. Serum transferrin receptor is conversely related to tissue iron stores and its level increases in iron deficiency (normal values 2.6-9.9 mg/l).

Primitive erythroid cells produce enormous amounts of serum transferrin receptors when iron reactivity to cellular surfaces decreases. Receptors are expressed on the cellular membrane and it is dependant to the number of receptors on the membrane. There is no difference in serum transferrin receptor levels in men or women or postmenopausal women but it is a little bit higher in African Americans (9%). Serum transferrin receptors may increase in hemolysis; but this situation is simply differentiated from iron deficiency with reticulocyte count, reticulocyte index and serum iron stores.

Serum transferrin receptor is quite helpful in the differential diagnosis of iron deficiency anemia and anemia of chronic disease. The ratio of serum transferrin receptor levels to log of serum ferritin is the most useful marker but this test is not used routinely in clinical laboratories (Table 3). Serum transferrin receptor index was defined as the most sensitive and easy method for iron stores in a study of 129 cases (positive and negative predictive values were 1.00 and 0.98, respectively). Serum transferrin receptor index also was predicted iron deficiency alone and combination of iron deficiency and anemia of chronic disease in the study.

Differentiation of iron deficiency anemia and anemia of chronic disease in the elderly patients is difficult. Serum iron and transferrin saturation are commonly used for the diagnosis of iron deficiency; but the value of these tests is limited in the elderly population. Ferritin levels alone are not enough as these values increase with age and chronic inflammatory diseases also increase with age.

Erythropoietin Levels

Erythropoietin levels increase with age, and the most increments are observed in chronic diseases like hypertension and diabetes in the elderly. However, serum erythropoietin levels might be detected “inappropriately low” or decreased when compared to Hb levels [3, 33]. This issue depends on the comparison of the erythropoietin levels in the elderly patients with chronic anemia, young patients with anemia or just the elderly patients with iron deficiency anemia. Anemia incidence is higher in the elderly men when compared to the elderly women; however this situation does not result in difference in serum erythropoietin levels. Bone marrow reserves are also depleted in the elderly which may result in anemia. The exact reasons for decreased erythropoiesis are not clear. However, variations in cytokine levels in the elderly might explain the situation. Increased serum IL–6 level is associated with anemia which results in increased apoptosis of bone marrow and disruption of erythropoiesis.

Anemia in the elderly is typically normocytic and in most of the cases (90%) Hb levels range between 10-12 g/dl. As it is insidious with nonspecific symptoms, clinical importance of the disease might be missed.

Chronic Renal Disease and Anemia

Chronic renal disease is common in the elderly and has an important role in anemia etiology [2, 16]. In a study, Hb levels were ≤12 g/dl in 47.7% of 5,222 patients with chronic renal disease in the United States of America.

The erythropoietin hormone is mainly synthesized in peritubular interstitial cells of kidney. Normal response to decreased oxygen pressure in blood is a logarithmic increase in erythropoietin according to degree of anemia. The main cause of anemia in chronic renal failure is progressive decrease in renal erythropoietin synthesis. It has been reported that there is a direct correlation between aging, decreased renal functions, decreased erythropoietin levels and anemia [34]. Renal functions decrease with aging which is especially important [35]. Circulating erythropoietin levels are equal in both sexes. Hb and renal function gradually decrease in both men and women with aging. Mean Hb values are 15.1 g/dl in men and 13.7 g/dl in women at 65 years and in every ten years it decreases 0.75 and 0.5 g/dl, respectively. Creatinine clearance is 100 ml/min and 81.4 ml/min in men and women at 65 years, respectively and every 10 years it decreases 19.4 ml/min and 15.2 ml/min. These results support that there is a relationship between anemia incidence and renal functions; as the creatinine clearance decreases the anemia becomes worst [36, 37]. In a study of 1,005 women and men ≥65 years of age in Italy, creatinine clearance of ≤30 ml/min was associated with a significantly increased risk of anemia and significantly decreased serum erythropoietin levels [34].

Although there are contrary studies, in many of them, it is claimed that serum erythropoietin levels increase with aging [38-40]. This finding supports the idea that for the maintenance of physiological erythropoiesis more erythropoietin is needed in the elderly which might be a result of relative erythropoietin resistance. Alternatively, the increase in erythropoietin levels might be a reflection of decreased usage in the bone marrow due to bone marrow hypoplasia.

Unexplained Anemia

Unexplained anemia (idiopathic anemia of aging) is observed in 20-30 percent of the elderly anemic patients according to epidemiologic studies [10, 14, 16, 33]. The etiology could not be explained even after detailed examination of 17% of hospitalized anemic elderly patients [41].

There are many hypotheses explaining the high incidence of unexplained anemia in the elderly [10, 42, 43]. Decrease in hematopoietic stem cell reserve, growth factor production and response to growth factors of stem cells and progenitors, bone marrow microenvironment abnormalities, androgen deficiency, age-related decrease in renal functions and/or erythropoietin release, undiagnosed chronic renal failure, undefined myelodysplasia or early period of anemia of chronic disease are some of the etiologies [33-35, 44-47].

Two separate studies claim that erythropoietin levels are meaningfully lower when to compare to ones with known etiology of anemia [48]. Those studies support that major causes of anemia in unexplained ones are decreased sensitivity to hypoxia, erythropoietin production and/or bone marrow response to erythropoietin.

Anemia is hypoproliferative and has low absolute reticulocyte count and low reticulocyte index kinetically. It is known that bone marrow compensates anemia eight fold in children and five fold in adults in hemolytic anemia. However, there is no data in the elderly; in cases of unexplained anemia, there is a loss of compensatory mechanisms in erythropoiesis.

A probable mechanism is decreased response of stem cells and hematopoietic progenitors to erythropoietin as a result of increased proinflammatory cytokines like IL-6 in the elderly.

Plasma levels of IL-6 increase secondary to infection, trauma and stress and cytokine regulation becomes more irregular with aging. It is reported that serum IL-6 levels increase parallel to age in 220 healthy women between 25-104 years old; a ten times increase is detected from premenopausal woman to 100 years old women. The underlying mechanism of IL-6 increase in the elderly is not clear. It might be relevant to increased production from monocytes, T cells, endothelial cells or bone marrow cells.

Studies detailing evidence for a chronic proinflammatory state contributing to the pathogenesis of unexplained anemia in the elderly population have been a few in number as a result of an increase in IL-6 and C-reactive protein in that population [49, 50]. Three contrary studies to these findings are present. In two of them inflammatory markers (IL-6, TNFa, C-reactive protein, and hepcidin) were detected normal when compared to the non-anemic elderly controls [33, 48]. Hepcidin levels were statistically same in 18 cases with unexplained anemia when compared to patients with anemia of chronic disease it the third study [51]. Although these studies support that inflammatory mechanisms have no role in unexplained anemia, a subgroup of these patients probably have the same pathophysiology with anemia of chronic disease.

Myelodysplastic Syndromes

Myelodysplastic syndromes are clonally hematopoietic stem cell disorders defined as ineffective hematopoiesis, cytopenias and variable percentages of transformation to acute myeloid leukemia [52-54]. It is a disease of older population; the mean age of diagnosis is 65-75 years. Incidence is 20/100.000 in people ≥70 years. Some of the unexplained anemia cases have myelodysplastic syndrome.

There are small studies investigating the incidence of myelodysplastic syndrome in unexplained anemia of the elderly. In a study, 124 patients over 75 years old with macrocytosis were evaluated. Diagnosis was made with noninvasive techniques in 60% of patients whereas 49 patients had bone marrow biopsies. Six percent of 124 patients had the diagnosis of myelodysplastic syndromes. Nineteen patients (15%) had dysplasia not fulfilling the diagnostic criteria of French-American-British (FAB) classification and therefore those cases were defined as premyelodysplastic syndrome. The rest 24 patients had no morphological abnormalities [46]. In another study, 37 (15%) of 245 elderly hospitalized patients had the diagnosis of myelodysplastic syndrome according to FAB classification [47]. Thirty four had refractory anemia, 2 had "refractory anemia with ringed sideroblasts" and one had "refractory anemia with excess blasts". Seven patients had dysplastic changes in one lineage and those were defined as early myelodysplastic syndrome; 5 of the 7 patients just had dysmegakaryopoiesis [47]. During the follow up period of 1-70 months, no survival difference was reported in patients with myelodysplastic syndrome and early myelodysplastic syndrome. In another report, 178 (84%) of 732 hospitalized patients between 65-81 years due to acute complaints had anemia [41]. Bone marrow biopsies were done in 109 patients and 9 of 178 patients had myelodysplastic syndrome according to the FAB classification.

As a conclusion, 5-15% of the elderly patients with unexplained anemia have the diagnosis of myelodysplastic syndrome and a small population has minor abnormalities supporting the suspicion but not the diagnosis of myelodysplastic syndrome. The question of diagnosis must be revisited when molecular diagnostic testing for myelodysplastic syndromes improves [55].

CLINICAL EFFECTS OF ANEMIA

Anemia has plenty of bad results in the elderly; it is associated decreased functional capacity, increased cardiovascular diseases, perception defects, mortality, and falling and fracture risk [2, 3]. It has to be implied that these symptoms might be observed not only severe anemia, but in mild anemia or nearly normal Hb levels as well.

Mortality

Anemia is correlated with increased mortality in the elderly. This correlation is confirmed in a 10-year study including 1,016 elderly people ≥85 years. Mortality risk in anemia is 1.60 times more in women, 2.29 times more in men when compared to cases with normal Hb levels. Mortality risk increases with the decrease in Hb levels in both sexes [12]. The overall survival of 63 elderly patients with Hb levels <11 g/dl was meaningfully decreased when compared to ones with Hb levels >13 g/dl in 60 months follow up period (48%).

Chaves et al. investigated between Hb and all-cause mortality of 641 women with moderate or severe disability in ≥65 years old cases for 5 years. This study revealed that the threshold for Hb was 13.9 g/dl, in which levels below that showed increases in mortality rates. The results of "Established Populations for Epidemiologic Studies of the Elderly (EPESE)" study showed that definition of anemia according to WHO criteria accompanies increased mortality risk in the elderly [56]. It is claimed that there is a reverse J relationship between Hb levels and mortality in 11.2 years follow up period of 5,888 men and women ≥65 years old.

Morbidity

Cardiovascular Disease

Anemia is a strong predictor for mortality in the elderly with acute myocardial infarction (MI) [2, 3]. In a retrospective study of Wu et al., it is claimed that even mild anemia (hematocrit 36.1-39.0%) might be an important risk factor for increased 30-day mortality in over 75,000 patients' ≥65 years. Blood transfusions decrease mortality in patients with hematocrit values <33%. Silverberg et al. claimed that anemia is an independent risk factor for increased mortality in patients with compensated heart failure "Evaluation of Losartan in the Elderly (ELITE) II" study supports that anemia is an independent factor for mortality in patients with congestive heart failure [57].

Mild (Hb 11-13 g/dl) and moderate (Hb <11 g/dl) anemia resulted in diastolic dysfunction in a study including 822 patients. Anemia is a risk factor for left ventricular hypertrophy. Decrease of left ventricular mass index 2.6 g/m^2 in men and 1.8 g/m^2 in women was associated every 3% decrease in hematocrit values in 35-60% of men and 30-50% of women in Framingham follow up study of 1,376 men and 1,769 women, respectively. The risk for left ventricular hypertrophy increases 2.0 fold in men and 1.4 fold in postmenopausal women in the subjects within the lowest quartile of hematocrit levels [58].

The study of "The Atherosclerosis Risk in Communities (ARIC)" reports an increase in left ventricular diameter when Hb levels decrease in 1,968 African Americans aged between 50-75 years [59].

Falls and Fractures

Anemia has been reported as an independent and important risk factor for falls in the elderly [2, 3]. The cause for hospitalization in 6.9% of 223,085 people is involuntary falls. Independent predictors for such falls include age, sex, season, place of residence, alcohol consumption, dementia, Parkinson disease, mechanical or motor problems, and abnormalities in consciousness, convulsions/epilepsy, glaucoma and anemia.

Moreover, increased risk for falls due to anemia results in fractures. In a retrospective evaluation of 145 patients aged 60-97 years old who were hospitalized for hip fracture, anemia was significantly more common (30% vs. 13%). Anemia causes three fold risks for falls. Furthermore, each 1 g/dl rise in Hb was associated with a 23-45% reduction in the risk for falls resulting in fractures. Another recent study that evaluated 47,530 elderly subjects revealed that even mild anemia was associated with an increased risk for accidental falls and fractures. WHO-defined anemia was associated with 91% increased risk for recurrent falls and this relationship was mediated by muscle weakness, and poor physical performance in subjects with anemia.

Anemia is an important predictor for hospitalization due to femur fractures. Most recently, WHO-defined anemia results in higher number of hospital days and higher mortality in 6 and 12 months follow up period in the retrospective analysis of 395 elderly patients aged ≥65 years that treated with femoral fractures.

Cognitive Function

Cognitive failure is a common problem in the elderly [2]. Possible cognitive failure was 55.6% and 35.4% in 536 male ≥65 years who had anemia or not, respectively. This ratio was 47.5% and 40.1% in anemic or non-anemic women. The relationship between Hb levels and a cognitive test was evaluated and it was reported that low Hb levels result in decreased test performance. In another study, in 13,301 patients, it is reported that the ones with cognitive failure had more anemia risk (47%) than the ones with normal cognitive tests. "Mini-Mental State Examination" was performed in another study and the score in the elderly anemic group was lower than subjects who had normal Hb levels [60].

Hospitalization

Although the correlation between anemia and hospitalization is not certain, asymptomatic anemia (Hb <12.5 g/dl in men and <11.5 g/dl in women) during hospital admittance during hospital admittance is associated with complications in hospitalized patients due to other causes. Prospective analysis of 225 elective total hip replacement operations showed increased postoperative infections and transfusions and longer postoperative hospitalization in patients with asymptomatic anemia during hospital admittance. Moreover, the results of EPESE study support that WHO-defined anemia increases the hospitalization risk [56].

Quality of Life

There is little information about the effects of anemia on quality of life alone. However, results of multiple studies claimed that coexisting anemia with specific disease decreases the quality of life and management of anemia increases it meaningfully [2]. Erythropoietin corrects both anemia and quality of life in both cancer and renal disease patients. These analyses were performed in 2,253 renal insufficiency and 10,695 cancer patients. Meta-analyses of these patients revealed a possible correlation between treatment of anemia and quality of life.

Fatigue

The production and release of IL-6 is disturbed and the serum level of this cytokine increased in the elderly. Increased IL-6 level is an independent predictor for increased mortality in the elderly. IL-related inflammatory process is related to aging, anemia, decreasing body mass index, osteopenia, hypoalbuminemia, hypocholesterolemia, increase in inflammatory proteins like serum amyloid A and C-reactive protein, and cognitive dysfunction.

Some of the IL-6 related effects result in anemia by disturbing erythropoiesis. Results of two big studies suggest that a strong relationship is present between anemia and the disturbance of physical performance in the elderly. Presence of anemia results in reduced physical performance according to a 4 years follow up study in 1,146 people ≥71 years old. This study also suggests that even mild anemia is an important predictor for reduction in physical performance. Anemia causes reduced muscle oxygenation and muscle performance [34]. It is reported that under the same conditions, subjects with anemia have reduced their physical performance when compared non-anemic subjects.

Anemia also has negative effects on bone metabolism which results in increased fracture risk due to falls. Anemia detected together with decreased bone mineral density in 950 patients. Presence of anemia in women is related to both reductions in total and cortical bone density [34]. Moreover, low Hb levels in women are correlated with low trabecular, cortical and total bone mineral density [34]. There is a positive correlation between total and cortical bone mineral density and Hb levels in men [15]. Further studies are needed evaluating the relationship between osteoporosis or anemia or fall. Underlying inflammatory conditions might be responsible for these clinical observations in the elderly.

THERAPY AND MANAGEMENT

Underlying causes of anemia should be investigated and treated in the elderly subjects [43]. Iron, vitamin B_{12} and folate deficiencies are the most common correctable causes.

Treatment of Symptomatic Anemia

Personal approach is needed according to functional status of patients, co-existing diseases, and demands of patients in subjects with unexplained anemia. There is no threshold value for transfusions. Some patients can tolerate Hb levels <10 g/dl, whereas cases with congestive heart failure need maintenance with Hb ≥10 g/dl. Anemia is usually mild and no need for transfusions in most of the patients with unexplained anemia.

Therapy is limited to transfusion of erythrocyte suspensions and erythropoiesis stimulating agents [61].

Transfusion of Erythrocyte Suspensions

Chronic transfusions have the risk for iron deposition besides common risks of transfusion [62]. Transfusional iron overload results in severe hepatic and cardiac iron toxicity whereas status of organ toxicity is not clear in myelodysplastic syndrome [63]. Current guidelines suggests iron chelation treatment for patients 20-30 units erythrocyte suspensions transfused and need for transfusion is persisting and increased serum ferritin levels with low risk myelodysplastic syndrome. It is still yet unknown that similar recommendations are appropriate for the transfusion-dependent elderly patients with unexplained anemia.

Erythropoietin and Darbepoetin

It is defined as using erythropoiesis stimulating agents' alternative to transfusion of erythrocyte suspensions. There are three kinds of erythropoiesis stimulating agents: epoetin alpha, epoetin beta and darbepoetin. They are bound to erythropoietin receptors which is totally recombinant human erythropoietin [61]. Most of the studies about erythropoiesis stimulating agents are associated with renal disease, myelodysplastic syndrome and other malignancies.

There are plenty of studies supporting the harmful effects of overcorrection of anemia with erythropoiesis stimulating agents in patients with renal disease. Depending on these data, "Food and Drug Administration" add a black box warning to the package inserts for epoetin alpha and darbepoetin recommending that patients not to be treated to Hb level greater than 12 g/dl. Same warning is valid for the cancer patients.

The effect of erythropoietin in patients with unexplained anemia is not definite [61]. Every 2 g/dl and more increase in Hb levels results in improvement in quality of life according to randomized placebo-controlled study in African American women who had unexplained anemia or anemia of chronic disease [64]. Targeted Hb levels were 13.0-13.9 g/dl in the relevant study which is higher than recommendations of guidelines. No significant side effects were reported. Thrombotic event, pulmonary embolism was present in only one patient whose Hb level was 14.3 g/dl.

As a result, further studies are needed for evaluation of functional improvement without toxicity in the treatment of mild anemia in the elderly.

Management of Anemia of Chronic Disease

The ideal treatment is to treat the underlying chronic disease successfully. Many patients with anemia of chronic disease simply live with the effects of the anemia as part of enduring the limits placed on them by aspects of their underlying disease. Some of these diseases are not curable yet. Erythropoietin treatment is recommended in anemia of chronic disease associated with rheumatoid arthritis, AIDS, cancer and inflammatory bowel disease. There is no randomized trial for anemia of chronic disease in the elderly over 65 years of age.

Trials reporting the management of anemia of chronic disease in the elderly are limited [2, 16]. Erythropoietin treatment once a week and placebo subcutaneously were injected in 62 patients for 32 weeks in anemic subjects' ≥65 years of age (Hb ≤11.5 g/dl). At the end of 16 week, the subject passed to the other arm. The results claimed that Hb levels and quality of life were increased meaningfully in erythropoietin group. Also, erythropoietin treatment was well tolerated and no toxicity was observed including the thrombotic events.

CONCLUSION

Anemia is an important public health problem in the elderly. One fourth of the elderly men and women are anemic although there are variable results in trials. Moreover, when WHO-defined anemia (Hb <13 g/dl in men and Hb <12 g/dl in women) is considered, mild anemia and values just below the normal are major problems. Control of the hematopoiesis is deteriorated by aging. New trials support the idea that regulation of proinflammatory cytokines like IL-6 is disturbed, production of erythropoietin and erythropoietin receptors are inhibited. Some characteristics of unexplained anemia are similar to anemia of chronic disease which supports the presence of unexplained inflammatory responses in the elderly.

Complete blood count, reticulocyte count, peripheral blood smear, urea, creatinine, urine analysis, occult blood in feces, serum iron, total iron binding capacity, serum ferritin, vitamin B_{12} and folate tests should be performed in the elderly patients with anemia.

Although the etiology of anemia is not fully clear in the elderly, it has important clinical consequences. It may result in increased cardiovascular disease, deterioration of cognitive functions, more days in hospital due to hospitalization for other reasons, decrease in bone mineral density, falls and fractures besides increased mortality.

The underlying cause should be treated like the presence of iron deficiency anemia in the elderly. Asymptomatic patients with unexplained anemia need no treatment. Transfusion of erythrocyte transfusions and erythropoiesis stimulating agents might be used in symptomatic patients with unexplained anemia.

The further studies should be planned for the evaluation of underlying causes of anemia due to aging and supporting treatments which maintain the high Hb levels, so that the side effects of anemia in the long term are decreased.

REFERENCES

[1] Nandigam V, Nandigam K, Badhe BA, Dutta TK. Is adult definition of anemia applicable to a geriatric population? Study of erythrocyte parameters in Indian geriatric inpatients. *J. Am. Geriatr. Soc.* 2004; 52:1589-1590.

[2] Eisenstaedt R, Penninx BWJH, Woodman RC. Anemia in the elderly: current understanding and emerging concepts. *Blood Rev.* 2006; 20:213-226.

[3] Balducci L, Ershler WB, Krantz S. Anemia in the elderly-critical findings and impact on health. *Crit. Rev. Oncol/Hematol.* 2006; 58:156-165.

[4] World Health Organization Nutritional Anemias. Report of the World Health Scientific Group. *WHO Technical Report Series*, No. 405, Geneva-Switzerland, 1968.

[5] Beutler E, Waalen J. The definition of anemia: what is the lower limit of normal of the blood hemoglobin concentration? *Blood* 2006; 107:1747-1750.

[6] Patel KV. Epidemiology of anemia in older adults. *Semin. Hematol.* 2008; 45:210-217.

[7] Penninx BW, Pahor M, Cesari M, Corsi AM, Woodman RC, Bandinelli S, Guralnik JM, Ferrucci L. Anemia is associated with disability and decreased physical performance and muscle strength in the elderly. *J. Am. Geriatr. Soc.* 2004; 52:719-724.

[8] Guralnik JM, Ershler WB, Schrier SL, Picozzi VJ. Anemia in the elderly: a public health crisis in hematology. *Hematology Am. Soc. Hematol. Educ. Program.* 2005, 528-532.

[9] Analytic and Reporting Guidelines: The Third National Health and Nutrition Examination Survey, NHANES III (1988-94), October 1996. National Center for Health Statistics Centers for Disease Control and Prevention, Hyattsville, Maryland. Available: http://www.cdc.gov/nchs/data/nhanes/nhanes3/nh3gui.pdf. Accessed December 5, 2005.

[10] Guralnik JM, Eisenstaedt RS, Ferrucci L, Klein HG, Woodman RC. Prevalence of anemia in persons 65 years and older in the United States: evidence for a high rate of unexplained anemia. *Blood* 2004; 104:2263-2268.

[11] Fleming DJ, Jacques PF, Tucker KL, Massaro JM, D'Agostino RB Sr, Wilson PWF, Wood RJ. Iron status of the free-living, elderly Framingham Heart Study cohort: an iron-replete population with a high prevalence of elevated iron stores. *Am. J. Clin. Nutr.* 2001; 73:638-646.

[12] Izaks GJ, Westendorp RG, Knook DL. The definition of anemia in older persons. *JAMA* 1999; 281:1714-1717.

[13] Olivares M, Hertrampf E, Capurro MT, Wegner D. Prevalence of anemia in elderly subjects living at home: role of micronutrient deficiency and inflammation. *Eur. J. Clin. Nutr.* 2000; 54:834-839.

[14] Artz AS, Fergusson D, Drinka PJ, Gerald M, Bidenbender R, Lechich A, Silverstone F, McCamish MA, Dai J, Keller E, Ershler WB. Mechanisms of unexplained anemia in the nursing home. *J. Am. Geriatr. Soc.* 2004; 52:423-427.

[15] Cesari M, Pahor M, Lauretani F, Penninx BWHJ, Bartali B, Russo R, Cherubini A, Woodman R, Bandinelli S, Guralnik JM, Ferrucci L. Bone density and hemoglobin levels in older persons: results from the InCHIANTI study. *Osteoporos. Int.* 2005; 16:691-699.

[16] Woodman R, Ferrucci L, Guralnik J. Anemia in older adults. *Curr. Opin. Hematol.* 2005; 12:123-128.

[17] Punnonen K, Irjala K, Rajamäki A. Serum transferrin receptor and its ratio to serum ferritin in the diagnosis of iron deficiency. *Blood* 1997; 89:1052-1057.

[18] Carmel R. Nutritional anemias and the elderly. *Semin Hematol.* 2008; 45:225-234.

[19] Joosten E, Hiele M, Ghoos Y, Pelemans W, Boogaerts MA. Diagnosis of iron-deficiency anemia in a hospitalized geriatric population. *Am. J. Med.* 1991; 90:653-654.

[20] Ferrucci L, Balducci L. Anemia of aging: the role of chronic inflammation and cancer. *Semin Hematol.* 2008; 45:242-249.

[21] Beyan C, Beyan E. A Common Cause of Anemia in Inflammatory Disorders: Anemia of Chronic Disease. *Current Rheumatology Reviews* 2005; 1:227-230.

[22] Rimon E, Levy S, Sapir A, Gelzer G, Peled R, Ergas D, Sthoeger ZM. Diagnosis of iron deficiency anemia in the elderly by transferrin receptor-ferritin index. *Arch. Intern Med.* 2002; 162:445-449.

[23] Rockey DC, Cello JP. Evaluation of the gastrointestinal tract in patients with iron-deficiency anemia. *N. Engl. J. Med.* 1993; 329:1691-1695.

[24] Smith DL. Anemia in the elderly. *Am. Fam. Physician.* 2000; 62:1565-1572.

[25] Nahon S, Lahmek P, Aras N, Poupardin C, Lesgourgues B, Macaigne G, Delas N. Management and predictors of early mortality in elderly patients with iron deficiency anemia: a prospective study of 111 patients. *Gastroenterol. Clin. Biol.* 2007; 31:169-174.

[26] Nahon S, Lahmek P, Barclay F, Macaigne G, Poupardin C, Jounnaud V, Delas N, Lesgourgues B. Long-term follow-up and predictive factors of recurrence of anemia in a cohort of 102 very elderly patients explored for iron-deficiency anemia. *J. Clin. Gastroenterol.* 2008; 42:984-990.

[27] Joosten E, Ghesquiere B, Linthoudt H, Krekelberghs F, Dejaeger E, Boonen S, Flamaing J, Pelemans W, Hiele M, Gevers AM. Upper and lower gastrointestinal evaluation of elderly in patients who are iron deficient. *Am. J. Med.* 1999; 107:24-29.

[28] Joosten E, Meeuwissen J, Vandewinckele H, Hiele M. Iron status and colorectal cancer in symptomatic elderly patients. *Am. J. Med.* 2008; 121:1072-1077.

[29] Carmel R. Anemia and aging: an overview of clinical, diagnostic and biological issues. *Blood Rev.* 2001; 15:9-18.

[30] Andrès E, Federici L, Serraj K, Kaltenbach G. Update of nutrient-deficiency anemia in elderly patients. *Eur. J. Intern Med.* 2008; 19:488-493.

[31] Andrès E, Loukili NH, Noel E, Kaltenbach G, Ben Abdelgheni M, Perrin AE, Noblet-Dick M, Maloisel F, Schlienger JL, Blicklé JF. Vitamin B_{12} (cobalamin) deficiency in elderly patients. *CMAJ* 2004; 171:251-260.

[32] Andrès E, Affenberger S, Vinzio S, Kurtz JE, Noel E, Kaltenbach G, Maloisel F, Schlienger JL, Blicklé JF. Food-cobalamin malabsorption in elderly patients: clinical manifestations and treatment. *Am. J. Med.* 2005; 118:1154-1159.

[33] Ferrucci L, Guralnik JM, Bandinelli S, Semba RD, Lauretani F, Corsi A, Ruggiero C, Ershler WB, Longo DL. Unexplained anaemia in older persons is characterised by low erythropoietin and low levels of pro-inflammatory markers. *Brit. J. Haematol.* 2007; 136:849-855.

[34] Ble A, Fink JC, Woodman RC, Klausner MA, Windham BG, Guralnik JM, Ferrucci L. Renal function, erythropoietin and anemia of older persons : the InCHIANTI study. *Arch. Intern Med.* 2005; 165:2222-2227.

[35] Adamson JW. Renal disease and anemia in the elderly. *Semin Hematol.* 2008; 45:235-241.

[36] Cumming RG, Mitchell P, Craig JC, Knight JF. Renal impairment and anaemia in a population-based study of older people. *Intern Med. J.* 2004; 34:20-23.

[37] Hsu CY, McCulloch CE, Curhan GC. Epidemiology of anemia associated with chronic renal insufficiency among adults in the United States: results from the Third National Health and Nutrition Examination Survey. *J. Am. Soc. Nephrol.* 2002; 13:504-510.

[38] Mori M, Murai Y, Hirai M, Kawakami M, Saito T, Takanashi N, Urabe A, Takaku F. Serum erythropoietin titers in the aged. *Mech. Ageing Dev.* 1988; 46:105-109.

[39] Musso CG, Musso CA, Joseph H, De Miguel R, Rendo P, Gonzalez E, Algranati L, dos Ramos Farias E. Plasma erythropoietin levels in the oldest old. *Int. Urol. Nephrol.* 2004; 36:259-262.

[40] Ershler WB, Sheng S, McKelvey J, Artz AS, Denduluri N, Tecson J, Taub DD, Brant LJ, Ferrucci L, Longo DL. Serum erythropoietin and aging: a longitudinal analysis. *J. Am. Geriatr. Soc.* 2005; 53:1360-1365.

[41] Joosten E, Pelemans W, Hiele M, Noyen J, Verhaeghe R, Boogaerts MA. Prevalence and causes of anaemia in a geriatric hospitalized population. *Gerontology* 1992; 38:111-117.

[42] Makipour S, Kanapuru B, Ershler WB. Unexplained anemia in the elderly. *Semin Hematol.* 2008; 45:250-254.

[43] Steensma DP, Tefferi A. Anemia in the elderly: how should we define it, when does it matter, and what can be done? *Mayo Clin. Proc.* 2007; 82:958-966.

[44] Ferrucci L, Maggio M, Bandinelli S, Basaria S, Lauretani F, Ble A, Valenti G, Ershler WB, Guralnik JM, Longo DL. Low testosterone levels and the risk of anemia in older men and women. *Arch. Intern Med.* 2006; 166:1380-1388.

[45] Gazit R, Weissman IL, Rossi DJ. Hematopoietic stem cells and the aging hematopoietic system. *Semin Hematol.* 2008; 45:218-224.

[46] Mahmoud MY, Lugon M, Anderson CC. Unexplained macrocytosis in elderly patients. *Age Ageing* 1996; 25:310-312.

[47] Beloosesky Y, Cohen AM, Grosman B, Grinblat J. Prevalence and survival of myelodysplastic syndrome of the refractory anemia type in hospitalized cognitively different geriatric patients. *Gerontology* 2000; 46:323-327.

[48] Waalen J, von Löhneysen K, Lee P, Xu X, Friedman JS. Erythropoietin, GDF15, IL6, Hepcidin and Testosterone Levels in a Large Cohort of Elderly Individuals with Anaemia of Known and Unknown Cause. *Eur. J. Haematol.* 2011; 87:107-116.

[49] Ferrucci L, Semba RD, Guralnik JM, Ershler WB, Bandinelli S, Patel KV, Sun K, Woodman RC, Andrews NC, Cotter RJ, Ganz T, Nemeth E, Longo DL. Proinflammatory state, hepcidin, and anemia in older persons. *Blood* 2010; 115:3810-3816.

[50] Ganz T. Hepcidin and its role in regulating systemic iron metabolism. *Hematology Am. Soc. Hematol. Educ. Program.* 2006:29-35.

[51] Ganz T, Olbina G, Girelli D, Nemeth E, Westerman M. Immunoassay for human serum hepcidin. *Blood* 2008; 112:4292-4297.

[52] Ma X, Does M, Raza A, Mayne ST. Myelodysplastic syndromes: incidence and survival in the United States. *Cancer* 2007; 109:1536-1542.

[53] Cazzola M, Malcovati L. Prognostic classification and risk assessment in myelodysplastic syndromes. *Hematol. Oncol. Clin. North Am.* 2010; 24:459-468.

[54] Ria R, Moschetta M, Reale A, Mangialardi G, Castrovilli A, Vacca A, Dammacco F. Managing myelodysplastic symptoms in elderly patients. *Clin. Interv. Aging.* 2009; 4:413-423.

[55] Swierczek SI, Agarwal N, Nussenzveig RH, Rothstein G, Wilson A, Artz A, Prchal JT. Hematopoiesis is not clonal in healthy elderly women. *Blood* 2008; 112:3186-3193.

[56] Penninx BW, Pahor M, Woodman RC, Guralnik JM. Anemia in old age is associated with increased mortality and hospitalization. *J. Gerontol. A. Biol. Sci. Med. Sci.* 2006; 61:474-479.

[57] Sharma R, Francis DP, Pitt B, Poole-Wilson PA, Coats AJ, Anker SD. Haemoglobin predicts survival in patients with chronic heart failure: a substudy of the ELITE II trial. *Eur. Heart J.* 2004; 25:1021-1028.

[58] Amin MG, Tighiouart H, Weiner DE, Stark PC, Griffith JL, MacLeod B, Salem DN, Sarnak MJ. Hematocrit and left ventricular mass: the Framingham Heart study. *J. Am. Coll. Cardiol.* 2004; 43:1276-1282.

[59] Astor BC, Arnett DK, Brown A, Coresh J. Association of kidney function and hemoglobin with left ventricular morphology among African Americans: the Atherosclerosis Risk in Communities (ARIC) study. *Am. J. Kidney Dis.* 2004; 43:836-845.

[60] Terekeci HM, Kucukardali Y, Onem Y, Erikci AA, Kucukardali B, Sahan B, Sayan O, Celik S, Gulec M, Sanisoglu YS, Nalbant S, Top C, Oktenli C. Relationship between anaemia and cognitive functions in elderly people. *Eur. J. Intern. Med.* 2010; 21:87-90.

[61] Agarwal N, Prchal JT. Erythropoietic agents and the elderly. *Semin Hematol.* 2008; 45:267-275.

[62] Klein HG, Spahn DR, Carson JL. Red blood cell transfusion in clinical practice. *Lancet* 2007; 370:415-426.

[63] Konen E, Ghoti H, Goitein O, Winder A, Kushnir T, Eshet Y, Rachmilewitz E. No evidence for myocardial iron overload in multitransfused patients with myelodysplastic syndrome using cardiac magnetic resonance T2 technique. *Am. J. Hematol.* 2007; 82:1013-1016.

[64] Agnihotri P, Telfer M, Butt Z, Jella A, Cella D, Kozma CM, Ahuja M, Riaz S, Akamah J. Chronic anemia and fatigue in elderly patients: results of a randomized, double-blind, placebo-controlled, crossover exploratory study with epoetin alfa. *J. Am. Geriatr. Soc.* 2007; 55:1557-1565.

In: New Horizons in Geriatric Medicine. Volume 1
Editors: Ahmet Turan Isik, M. Refik Mas et al.
ISBN: 978-1-62808-972-1

Chapter 6

VERTIGO AND ITS TREATMENT IN THE ELDERLY

Ayşe Karan, Demirhan Dıraçoğlu and Cihan Aksoy
Istanbul University, School of Medicine, Department of Physical Medicine and Rehabilitation, Istanbul, Turkey

ABSTRACT

Vertigo is a term used for the complaint of disorientation in space mostly caused by an inner ear problem. It is a sense of unsteadiness or feeling of movement within the head such as giddiness or a swimming sensation. Equilibrium is affected by vision, vestibular sensation, proprioception, muscle strength and reaction time. There are many factors which may affect balance. Causes and treatment approaches of disequilibrium in elderly are discussed in this chapter.

INTRODUCTION

Vertigo is a term used for the complaint of disorientation in space mostly caused by an inner ear problem. It is a sense of unsteadiness, or feeling of movement within the head such as giddiness or a swimming sensation. Dizziness is a term used to describe non-rotator vertigo and may be due to the involvement of certain equilibrium centres and peripheral mechanisms. Patients may have difficulty in describing their dizziness and may express it as drowsiness.

In recent years, rotator and non-rotator equilibrium disorders due to vestibular and non-vestibular mechanisms are grouped under the title of vertigo [1].

DESCRIPTION, ETIOLOGY, CLASSIFICATION

Dizziness comprises a wide range of terms from the severe vertigo, mild lightheadedness, drowsiness to disorientation. Vertigo is somewhat more specific; it medically reflects movement illusions, and may be vertical, horizontal or oblique in direction.

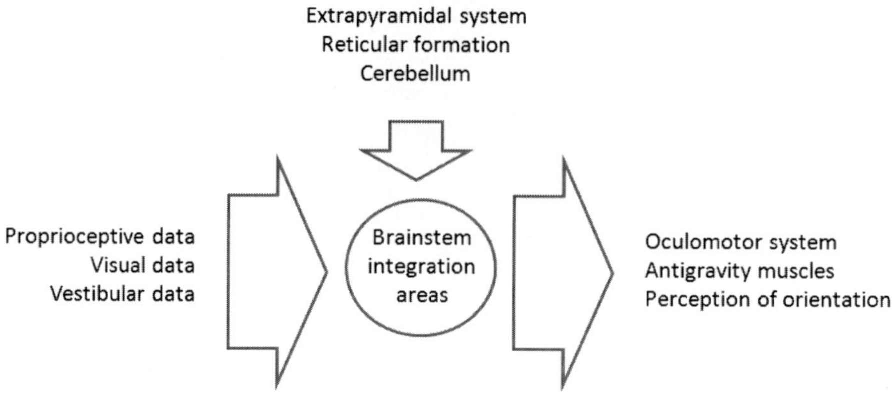

Figure 1. Components of the equilibrium.

Vertigo is mostly due to a vestibular system disorder, but dizziness may have many causes. Dizziness is quite common, its occurrence is increased especially with age, and it is the leading cause of physician visits above 65 years of age . Approximately 1/3 of the people above 70 years of age have dizziness. According to studies, the annual rates of admission to a health care unit due to vertigo and dizziness are 5/1000 and 10/1000, respectively. It is more common in women than in men [2, 3].

Equilibrium is affected by vision, vestibular sensation, proprioception, muscle strength and reaction time. The proprioceptive system provides information on spatial position of our body whereas the vestibular system sends information about the position of head to the central nervous system; and the visual system provides external information which modulates motor activity and equilibrium (Figure 1). A progressive loss of function is seen in these systems with increasing age. Among these, vision is the most important factor for equilibrium [4, 5, 6].

A. The Sensory System

1. Vision

Vision is progressively worsened after 50 years of age. Cataract (16% at >65 years), macular degeneration (9% at >65 years) and glaucoma (3% at >65 years) are the ocular disorders contributing to visual impairment. Diabetes and hypertension are frequently seen in the elderly and they cause progression of an existing retinopathy [4].

2. Vestibular Sense

The vestibular system is sensitive to the stimuli such as head position, gravity, resonance, acceleration and deceleration, and finally this information are sent to the central nervous system. During normal aging, vestibular function is weakened. Direct trauma, infection, disease of calcium carbonate accumulation in the semicircular canals, drug toxicity, migraine, cerebellar ataxia and autoimmune diseases are frequent causes of vestibular system dysfunction, especially in the elderly. These patients have dizziness, orientation problems, vertigo (illusion of rotation), and nystagmus during activities requiring head movements and the equilibrium is significantly impaired. The posture and gait are impaired in elderly patients with vestibular hypofunction. Postural instability and a faltering gait pattern with large steps in these patients increase the risk of repeated falls. Gait may be normal for a long time in subjects with a vestibular hypofunction. The gait impairment is only observed when the visual and peripheral senses are impaired. This shows that central nervous system may be adapted by using the visual and the somato sensorial inputs. Studies show that the risk of fall is not increased in these patients, since they are aware of their impaired equilibrium and they minimize risky movements [1, 4, 7, 8, 9].

3. Proprioception

In addition to the visual and vestibular information, stimuli from muscles and joints are also arrived to the central nervous system. The sensory stimuli arising from muscle, tendon and joint receptors provide feedback on joint position, movement and touching. This is called proprioception. Stimulus threshold of plantar receptors is very low. During walking, it coordinates each step and provides appropriate positioning of the feet on the floor. Loss of peripheral sensation may be due to diabetes, excess alcohol consumption, vitamin B_{12} deficiency, chemotherapy, excess administration of pyridoxine and nitric oxide. Articular facet mechanoreceptors are degraded due to cervical spondylosis, and this condition impairs postural control and predisposes patients to falls. Cervical proprioceptors are degraded in chronic neck pain and this may be a cause of equilibrium disorders. Aging may directly affect muscle spindles. These changes are more significant in distal muscles. Intact vestibular function, vision and proprioception and appropriate interaction with the central nervous system are required for a functional equilibrium. If a defect occurs in any of these systems, disequilibrium may develop. Cervical region, especially involving the first three vertebrae, is related with head movements; as the paravertebral muscles in this region are rich in receptors, this region is called the secondary labyrinth and vertigo associated with this region is called "cervical vertigo". Hands, feet and hip have special relevance in providing information from musculo-skeletal system. The plantar region is rich in superficial and deep pressoreceptors. The superficial receptors are Merkel's discs and Meissner's corpuscles, whereas the deeper ones are Golgi-Mazzoni corpuscles and Pacini-Water receptors. Ankle and hip are the most important joints during standing and walking for maintaining equilibrium. The most important muscles are the anti-gravity muscles which mainly include gastrocnemius, hamstrings, tibialis anterior, triceps surae and paravertebral muscles [1, 4, 7, 8, 9, 10].

B. Motor System

1. Muscle Strength

Muscle mass is significantly reduced between 20 to 80 years of age. This loss is especially higher in fibers which contract rapidly. Reduced re-innervation capacity with increasing age has been demonstrated in these fibers. Muscle strength is maintained until the fifth and sixth decades, then the loss is accelerated, and 50% reduction is seen at 80 years of age. Mainly, the risk of fall is significantly increased with reduced muscle strength in knee extensors, ankle dorsiflexors and hip muscles. Reduction in muscle strength of lower extremity is a significant risk factor for fall. In the osteoporotic women, equilibrium is impaired due to significant changes in body and muscle weakness; especially muscle weakness in weight bearing back extensors, hip abductor and adductor is important [4, 5].

2. Reaction Time

Reaction time is important to avoid falls and to maintain equilibrium in any case of impaired posture. Reaction time is prolonged for 25% at 20 to 60 years of age. It is significantly prolonged after this age. This is an independent cause of fall in the elderly. The reason is alteration in peripheral and central nervous systems [4].

The term "presbystasis" is used to define age-related equilibrium. This is not associated with any pathology. Dizziness may be considered within the frame of geriatric syndromes including various symptoms arising from highly different systems in the elderly. After 40 years of age, microscopic synaptic alterations are observed in vestibular nerves. During 50s of age, a significant degeneration begins in vestibular receptors. Vestibular dysfunction due to vascular problems is seen in 20% of the elderly. Falls and related injuries are increased in subjects complaining of dizziness. Vertigo and similar symptoms are indirectly effective in falls. Falls have highly negative effects on quality of life such as fractures, hospitalization, loss of independence and compromised activities. Above 65 years of age, 30% of the people will have a fall per year and 50% of these subjects will fall again. This may results in death and also limited mobility and loss of dependence. These symptoms lead to basiphobia (fear of stand and walk) in the elderly subjects [4, 5, 6, 9, 11].

Underlying causes of disequilibrium in the elderly may be classified under 3 sub-titles:

1. Age-related alterations in sensory and motor ways: Loss of ciliary structure in the labyrinth may be an example of this condition. Structure of vestibular nerves may also be impaired with aging. The proprioceptive system takes place in muscles, joints and tendons; it provides information transmission from one segment of body to another, and this system is impaired with age, and vibration and touching thresholds are reduced. In the motor system, muscle strength is reduced 20 to 40% in 70-80 years compared to younger. This is associated with reduction in the number and size of muscle fibers. Similar changes are also seen in the ocular muscles, and oculomotor functions are impaired. Central nervous system, providing integrity of these systems, may have changes with increasing age. The number of neurons is reduced and demyelinization occurs [9].
2. Benign paroxysmal positional vertigo (BPPV) has an important place among pathologies causing to dizziness at any age group. The frequency of BPPV is increased with age, since degeneration occurs in macula and autolythic organs with aging. It is the main cause of dizziness in half of the patients at 80 years of age. Méniére is another cause. Its incidence is very high after 50 years of age. Bilateral vestibular paresis may occur following an ototoxic drug administration, especially gentamycine for more than 2 weeks. Spirochetal infection of the inner ear, autoimmune diseases and changes related with age may also lead to bilateral vestibular paresis. Symptoms are oscillopsia and ataxia. Anticholinergic drug administration should be avoided for its treatment, especially in the elderly subjects. Improvement is related to the degree of vestibular loss and compensation ability of the patient [12].

   Other most frequent pathologies among the elderly subjects: Cardiovascular (cerebrovascular), peripheral vestibular and psychiatric diseases. Otological causes of central dizziness are rare; it is mostly related with changes in the brainstem and cerebellum. The most important causes of psychogenic dizziness are anxiety disorders, panic attack, agoraphobia and somatization. Anxiety disorders and panic attack frequently respond well to benzodiazepine treatment, but higher doses than used for vestibular suppression are required [9, 12].

3. Environmental and life style factors: They increase likelihood of dizziness equilibrium problems. For example, elderly patients use multiple treatments for long term and majority of these drugs have dizziness side effect. Chronic administration of benzodiazepines, antidepressants, anticonvulsive drugs, antihypertensives, anti-inflammatory drugs, hypnotics, muscle relaxants, tranquilizants and vestibular suppressants cause commonly to dizziness. Certain drugs have no effect on hearing, but may cause to ototoxicity; these are aminoglycosides, furosemide and ethacrynic acid [9, 13].

Characteristics of dizziness localizing the affected side:

1. Inner ear: loss of hearing, tinnitus, aural fullness and otalgia.
2. Nerve VIII: Impaired speech discrimination, accompanying facial weakness.
3. Cerebellopontine angle: Impaired facial sense, dysartria and incoordination.
4. Brainstem: Hemisensorial loss, hemiparesis, cranial nerve palsy, dysarthria, dysphagia, memory impairment and loss of consciousness.
5. Cerebellum: Incoordination, clumsiness and dysarthria.
6. Cerebral cortex: Loss of consciousness, olfactory and gustatory hallucination and transient hemiparesis [3].

Causes of Dizziness

1. Otological Causes

a. *Middle ear pathologies.* Peri-lymphatic fistula- may be seen following a trauma, cholesteatoma and surgery. It may be due to a glomus tympanicum tumor.
b. *Peripheral vestibular dysfunction.* Labyrinthitis and vestibular neuritis secondary to viral infections: In vestibular neuritis, there is a severe vertigo and then disequilibrium is developed. Disequilibrium may be persistent for days or weeks. If there is a loss of hearing, diagnosis is in favor of labyrinthitis. Diagnosis is made by typical history and excluding other causes such as trauma, ischemia, and basal meningitis [8].
c. *BPPV.* It is the most frequent cause of vertigo. The cause is changing place of otochonia in the utricle. Otochonial debris is in general move toward the posterior semicircular canal, and the semicircular canal may be affected in 10% of the cases. Patients have severe dizziness with the movement of head toward the affected ear or looking up. In general, it is triggered by specific head movements; examples are lying down and turning head while lying down, neck extension, leaning forward to wash hair etc. Semicircular canals are linked to inner ear and canal is activated by above-defined head movements [3, 8].

Posterior Canal BPPV: These are vertigo attacks occurring at certain positions and continuing for a few seconds. Vertigo continues in general less than 1 minute. Nausea may be seen, duration does not exceed 1 hour. Position and maneuvers provoking vertigo are used for BPPV diagnosis:

(a) Dix- Hallpike (DH) position
(b) 1 to 40 seconds delay in occurring of vertigo following moving to a provocative position.
(c) Occurrence of nystagmus also, at vertical tortional direction.
(d) Fluctuation in severity of vertigo and nystagmus for less than 60 seconds. All these are due to central adaptation.

There are two theories on the development of posterior canal BPPV: According to the *cupulolithiasis theory,* otoconia particles (calcium carbonate crystals, basophilic deposits) adhere to cupula. Cupula becomes heavier and also more sensitive to gravity by certain movements of head; disturbed particles are re-collected in patients sitting for 10 minutes. According to the *canalithiasis theory,* degenerated debris is not attached to cupula, but it freely circulates in the endolymph within semicircular canals [3, 8].

Horizontal Canal BPPV: Horizontal canal BPPV is rare; the vertigo attack is more severe and its severity increases upon lying down on the affected side; MacClure maneuver is used for diagnosis. Patient lies down and turns his/her head to right and left for 90°. When head is turned toward the affected side, a more severe horizontal nystagmus is observed. Occasionally, posterior canal BPPV is converted to horizontal canal BPPV. This may be observed by a change in direction of nystagmus [7].

d. Bilateral vestibular insufficiency.
c. Meniere syndrome. Vertigo attacks may continue for hours in Meniere, and it takes more than 1 day in very rare cases. Episodes are serious and frequently sweating, nausea and vomiting are observed. Spontaneous remission and exacerbations are typical. In general, it affects one ear, but 17% of cases are bilateral. The pathophysiology is not fully understood; endolymph pressure is increased. There is excess production of endolymph, but its absorption is insufficient. Thus, causes may include viral infection, allergy and genetic factors (3, 8).
f. Benign recurrent vertigo.
g. Vestibular migraine.

2. General Medical Causes

a. *Orthostatic hypotension.* This is a reduction of 20 mmHg or more in systolic blood pressure after 3 minutes following positional change. Prolonged bed rest, long term administration of a hypotensive drug, major tranquilisants, vasodilatators, antidepressants and beta blockers are among the frequent reasons in case of autonomic neuropathy.

b. *Vasovagal episodes.* Vision and hearing are suddenly lost;Nausea and fullness in the ear occur. The causes include standing up for a long time, noxious stimuli like pain, vertigo, emotional stress, warm and crowded places.
c. *Decreased cardiac output.* Cardiac arrhythmia, Adams Stoke attacks, carotid sinus hypersensitivity, aortic stenosis, hypertrophic obstructive cardiomyopathy.
d. *Hyperventilation.* Muscle cramps, carpopedal spasm, breathlessness, dyspnea and panic attack symptoms.
e. *Others.* Other causes may include psychological vertigo, altitude vertigo and motion sickness, hypoglycemia, chronic fatigue syndrome, acute medical disease, and anemia.

3. Neurological Causes

a. *Congenital.* Neurofibromatosis, Friedrich's ataxia, Arnold-Chiari malformation, spinocerebellar atrophy type 1-9, familial episodic ataxy type 1 and 2.
b. *Acquired.* Basillary migraine, demyelinisation, space-occupying lesions, inflammatory diseases, multisystem atrophy, vestibular epilepsy, increased intracranial pressure and drugs. Acute vertigo is present in 5 to 7% of multiple sclerosis patients. But 78% of patients have equilibrium impairment. Dizziness is present in addition to headache attacks in 27% of patients with vertigo related with migraine. Tension headache complaint is present in 8% of these patients. These patients have familial migraine history; they are sensitive to motion sickness and visual stimuli [3, 8].

Dizziness duration and possible causes were given in Table 1.

Table 1. Dizziness duration and possible causes

Duration	Possible causes
Several minutes	BPPV (less than 1 minute), vestibular epilepsy
Time varying from minutes to 2 hours	Benign recurrent vertigo, vestibular aura of migraine
2-24 hours	Meniere's disease, transischemic attack in posterior circulation and vestibular migraine
More than 24 hours	Acute peripheral vestibular dysfunction, relapse of multiple sclerosis affecting brain stem and bilateral vestibular insufficiency (3).

Other Symptoms

Unpleasant autonomic responses such as nausea, vomiting and anxiety may be observed in patients with dizziness. These side effects may be explained by associations with vestibulo-autonomic pathways. When a sensory pathway is impaired (as in the acute viral labirynthitis), significant disequilibrium is initially seen; but then, compensation is developed due to plasticity. But if two or more sensory inputs are also contributed, compensation takes more time and improvement may be incomplete. For example in the elderly, vision impairment due to cataract surgery and impaired proprioception due to diabetic neuropathy may concomitantly be present [3].

In patients complaining from other types of vertigo or dizziness, mainly postural instability is seen, postural swinging is increased, and fall and functional capacity may be reduced. Dizziness is the sensation of equilibrium dysfunction of body. But vertigo is a sign of spatial disorientation of rotator type [11].

Psychogenic signs of dizziness are anxiety, panic attack and loneliness fear. It may disturb daily life activities [11].

If both labyrinths are affected in vestibular system, bilateral vestibular weakness is seen and patients complain from oscillopsia, and walking in dark becomes difficult [8].

EVALUATION

Medical history is important. Firstly, it should be asked if vertigo attack is episodic or persistent. If this is episodic, duration of episodes is asked. Vertigo due to peripheral reasons rarely last more than a day. If vertigo shows a persistent character, and if the duration is longer than 1 day, central causes should be considered (Table 2). It should be questioned whether the attack is acute or chronic. Acute attack is for 3 days or less, while a chronic attack is a vertigo attack for more than 3 days. Frequently hearing loss, tinnitus, ear fullness and nausea are present in peripheral vestibular diseases.

Table 2. Clinical properties in discrimination of peripheral and central dizziness

Clinical properties	Peripheral	Central
Initiation	Acute	Gradual
Duration of episodes	Seconds to hours, rarely more than 24 hours	Seconds to days
Visceral symptoms such as nausea, vomiting, and sweating	+	Rare
Otic symptoms such as hearing loss, tinnitus and ear fullness	Frequent	Rare
Neurological symptoms	Rare	Frequent
Nistagmus		
Direction	Horizontal and tortional, never vertical	Horizontal, tortional, vertical and may be changed
Fatigue	+	-
Initial	Delayed	Acute
Reduction with visual fixation	+	-

Adapted from Kutz JW [13].

These are frequently seen in Meniere's disease. Visual impairment, dysarthria and headache are frequently characteristics of central type vertigo. Syncope, shortened breathing and palpitation are frequent signs of cardiovascular disease. Sweating and dyspnea are signs of anxiety disorder and panic attack [8, 13].

Physical examination of patients should be done. Whether patient uses a canadien or walker or not, may give an idea on equilibrium problems. Wearing glasses suggest that source of dizziness is ocular. Caution should be paid to nystagmus. Horizontal and tortional nystagmus are found in peripheral vestibulopathies. Vertical nystagmus suggests central vestibular impairment [8].

VOR Test

Head is turned to right and left in the horizontal plan. Patient is asked to focus his/her eyes on the nose of examining person. If patient has intact VOR, he/she remains fixed on the nose of person performing visual examination. If patient has unilateral peripheral weakness, eyes are not fixed and correcting saccade is observed [8].

Positional Test

It is performed in general at DH position. When the patient sits on an examination chair, his/her head is turned for 30-45 degree. The patient is quickly lied down by physician, the head is bended 30 degrees from the chair. Vertigo is triggered, and nystagmus is started following a latent period of 3 to 5 seconds in BPPV and takes 15 to 20 seconds. Nystagmus is toward the floor and in rotator type. The affected ear is at the inferior. Central factors also may cause nystagmus, but there is no latent period, nystagmus is not fatigued, visual fixation does not reduce nystagmus, and nystagmus is more prolonged than in BPPV [8]. If the patient is old and fragile and have some back and neck problems, this test may be modified. The patient does need to be quickly moved in this case; otolythes move by gravity, not by body movement.

The patient does not need to perform excess neck extension; symptoms may be triggered by turning the head to the right and left in bed (9). DH and other reposition maneuvers need significant neck torsion and extension and vertebral strain may be developed during these movements; vertebrobasilar insufficiency and detachment of atheroma plaque from carotid artery may occur; these patients should be well examined by medical history and physical examination [14].

Coordination, gait and posture should be evaluated for cerebellar function. Romberg test is useful for proprioception and vestibular function. The patient is asked to keep eyes closed for 10 seconds. Patients with unilateral vestibular weakness tend to fall toward the affected side. Sharpened or Tandem Romberg tests are more sensitive and similar to classical Romberg. In this case, one foot is placed in front of other [8].

Table 3. Dizziness handicap inventory

P1	Does looking up increase your problem?	Yes	No	Sometimes
E2	Because of your problem, do you feel frustrated?	Yes	No	Sometimes
F3	Because of your problem, do you restrict your travel for business or recreation?	Yes	No	Sometimes
P4	Does walking down the aisle of a supermarket increase your problem?	Yes	No	Sometimes
F5	Because of your problem, do you have difficulty getting into or out of bed?	Yes	No	Sometimes
F6	Does your problem significantly restrict your participation in social activities such as going out for dinner or to parties?	Yes	No	Sometimes
F7	Because of your problem, do you have difficulty reading?	Yes	No	Sometimes
P8	Does performing more ambitious activities like sports or dancing or household chores such as sweeping or putting dishes away increase your problem?	Yes	No	Sometimes
E9	Because of your problem, are you afraid to leave your home without having someone to accompany?	Yes	No	Sometimes
E10	Because of your problem, are you embarrassed in front of others?	Yes	No	Sometimes
P11	Do quick movements of your head increase your problem?	Yes	No	Sometimes
F12	Because of your problem, do you avoid heights?	Yes	No	Sometimes
P13	Does turning over in bed increase your problem?	Yes	No	Sometimes
F14	Because of your problem, is it difficult for you to do strenuous housework or yardwork?	Yes	No	Sometimes
E15	Because of your problem, are you afraid people may think that you are intoxicated?	Yes	No	Sometimes
F16	Because of your problem, is it difficult to walk by yourself?	Yes	No	Sometimes
P17	Does walking down a sidewalk increase your problem?	Yes	No	Sometimes
E18	Because of your problem, is it difficult for you to concentrate?	Yes	No	Sometimes
F19	Because of your problem, is it difficult for you to walk around your house in the dark?	Yes	No	Sometimes
E20	Because of your problem, are you afraid to stay home alone?	Yes	No	Sometimes
E21	Because of your problem, do you feel handicapped?	Yes	No	Sometimes
E22	Has your problem placed stress on your relationships with members of your family or friends?	Yes	No	Sometimes
E23	Because of your problem, are you depressed?	Yes	No	Sometimes
F24	Does your problem interfere with your job or household responsibilities?	Yes	No	Sometimes
P25	Does bending over increase your problem?	Yes	No	Sometimes
TOTAL	F: (38) E: (36) P: (28) TOTAL:	x4	X0	X2

Otological Evaluation

Otoscopy can reveal middle ear pathology. Rinne and Weber tests may differentiate sensorineural and conductive type hearing loss. Sensorineural and conductive type hearing losses are investigated by audiometric tests. If it is indicated, auditory evoked potential responses of brain stem are recorded to discriminate transmission in the brain stem and retrocochlear pathways, before auditory tests [3].

Vestibular Evaluation

The examination of eye movements may reveal strabismus, divergent ocular movementsand nystagmus (which may be spontaneous, evoked by vision and positional). Romberg test and gait evaluation are done to discriminate between sensorial ataxia and uncompensated vestibular lesions. Other useful tests are electro-nystagmography, video-oculography and caloric tests [3].Visual Analog Scale (VAS) is important in subjective evaluation of vertigo. Dizziness Handicap Inventory (DHI) (Table.3) may be used to evaluate negative effect of vertigo on quality of life and daily activities and Timed up and go (TUGT). DHI have 9 items for functional evaluation, 9 for emotional and 7 for physical evaluation [11, 16].

Postural control may be performed by static and active equilibrium and functional scales and computerized posturography [11].

Diagnostic Methods

Routine blood tests are not "cost effective". Selective blood tests may be performed to confirm the history Total blood count, electrolytes level, cholesterol profile and thyroid function tests may be requested [8].

Patients with typical history of peripheral vertigo (such as BPPV and vestibular neuritis), do not need imaging methods. Imaging methods may be necessary in patients with asymmetric sudden hearing loss, central vertigo with unknown causes and known neurological causes. Magnetic resonance imaging with gadolonium contrast is the most frequently used radiological method. Cerebellopontine lesions and vestibular schwannoma, meningioma are easily diagnosed. Hyperintense plates are determined in T2 sections of multiple sclerosis. If there is a problem with the bony labyrinth, computerized tomography is more sensitive [8].

Treatment

1. Pharmacological

During acute vestibular episode, antiemetics (prochlorperazine, promethazine and cyclizine) and sedatives (calcium channel antagonist cinnarizine and histamine analogue betahistine) may be used. Tardive dyskinesia may develop due to long term prochlorperazine use.

In Meniere's disease, salt restricted diet (1-2 g/day) and if necessary, thiazide diuretics are used. Regular betahistine and equilibrium exercises may be beneficial. Cases not responding to serious medical treatment may be treated by intratympanic injection of aminoglycosides.

In selected cases, vestibular neurectomy may be applied. Acute migraine attacks may be treated by tryptanes such as sumatriptane and rizatriptane. Propranolol, pizotiphene or amytriptiline may be used for prophylaxis, especially due to attack frequency. Treatment of motion sickness should be prophylactic, and hyoscine, cinnarizine or promethazine should be preferred [3].

Treatment of Meniere's disease in elderly people is very difficult due to multiple drug usage. Betahistine and cinnarizine have very well results with a few side effects. However, administration of neuroleptics and antihistamines is difficult due their side effects; they may lead to Parkinsonism and depression during long term administration. Restricted caffeine and salt diet are applied in Meniere's disease. During an acute episode, a diuretic and a benzodiazepine are administered.

Thus, symptoms are controlled in 80% of patients; surgical or non-surgical treatment is required in 20% of patients. Intratympanic steroid injection or surgical decompensation may be applied.

Ablative treatments are intratympanic gentamycine injection (chemical labirynthectomy), labirynthectomy and cutting of nerve VIII. Treatment of hearing loss and tinnitus is very difficult [8, 15].

Vestibular suppressants such as eclizine or benzodiazepines are used in vestibular neuritis. Caution should be paid when administering vestibular suppressants for more than 1 week, since they may inhibit development of vestibular compensation. If steroids are used during the acute phase, they may be beneficial. Patients with vestibular neuritis are under risk of BPPV development [8].

Diet modification and prophylaxis are fundamental in vertigo related to migraine. Tricyclic antidepressants, topiramate, calcium channel blockers and beta blockers are used for prophylaxis [8].

If vertigo attack is very severe, 25-50 mg intramuscular promethazine may be initially administered, then suppository may be applied 3 days later. This drug causes sedation and reduces nausea. Ondansetrone also is appropriate for patients with severe vertigo and nausea [13].

Risk factors should be determined and challenged to prevent chronic dizziness. These factors are depressive symptoms, anxiety, visual and auditory disturbances, equilibrium and gait disturbances, postural hypotension, administration of 5 or more drugs (for example: antihypertensive agents, antidepressants and benzodiazepines) and past history of myocardial infarction [16].

Administration of aminoglycosides should be avoided for prophylaxis against bilateral ototoxicity and alternative antibiotics should be preferred; if necessary, monitorization should include audiography or other vestibular tests [8].

2. Vestibular Rehabilitation

Recently, rehabilitation took an important place in the treatment of vertigo. Rehabilitation does not remove objective causes of vertigo, but subjective causes may be removed . Vestibular rehabilitation (VR) aims to activate adaptive and compensatory mechanisms already present in human brain. Rehabilitation should be started as early as possible. The more activated vertigo attacks, the quicker development of compensatory mechanism in the brain [1, 7, 17]. VR is a treatment modality of patients with disequilibrium of vestibular origin. Principles of VR are based on the central mechanism of neuroplasticity. This is also known as adaptation, habituation. Vestibular compensation is aimed. Purpose of vestibular exercises is to improve vestibulo-visual interaction, especially to increase static and dynamic postural stability during cephalic movement. VR is effective in improving static and dynamic equilibrium, gait, self-confidence, quality of life, dizziness, and anxiety and depression symptoms. VR provides complete resolution in 30 % of patients, and varying degree of improvement in 85% of patients [11].

Principles of Vestibular Rehabilitation

1. VR is indicated in the stable, non-compensated vestibular lesions.
2. Choice of exercise is related to both patients' symptoms and pathophysiological mechanisms; maneuvers and stability exercises should be applied according to the affected canal.
3. Exercise time is short (1-2 minutes) and exercise intensity is varied according to the symptoms.
4. Habituation exercises should be repeated (8-10 repetitions).
5. Sensorial - perceptive and motor adaptation exercises require special attention.
6. Frequency of VR should be varied [18].

In a study conducted by Jung et al., VR is applied in 103 of 240 patients with dizziness who were older than 70 years; no treatment is applied to 46 patients. Improvement in VR group was greater than in untreated group [19].

Cawthorne – Cooksey exercises include a serial of head and body movements.

Also general coordination exercises are successful in more than 90% of vestibular pathologies [3].

Table 4. Causal factors of vertigo benefiting from rehabilitation

1- BPPV
2- Cases of unilateral vestibular paresis
3- Cases of bilateral vestibular paresis
4- Significant impairment of proprioception and equilibrium in conditions such as polyneuropathy, musculo-skeletal disorders and cerebellar disorders
5- Myofacial pain syndrome (MAS) (especially sternocleidomastoid muscle)
6- Cervical osteoarthritis
7- Cervical vertebra joint blockade

Table 5. What can be done for vertigo patients in terms of rehabilitation?

1-Treatment alternatives in BBPV a- For posterior canal BPPV Brandt- Daroff habituation exercises Liberator maneuver of Semont Epley's maneuver b- For horizontal canal BPPV Long term positioning treatment of Vannucchi Lempert's maneuver
2- For acute period of unilateral vestibular paresis, electrical stimulation; coordination exercises ordered by physician and controlled by therapist; home exercise programs applied following control of symptoms
3- Gradual gait re-education program for patients with bilateral vestibular paresis
4- Proprioception and Frenkel exercises for cases with significant disequilibrium in polyneuropathy, musculo-skeletal disorders and cerebellar disorders etc.
5- Treatment in myofacial pain syndrome Training for posture and general protection Stretching, strengthening and equilibrium training between muscles following cold spray application or other physical application Trigger point injection and stretching
6- Treatment in cervical osteoarthritis cases Training for general protection principles Posture training exercise for posture and cervical region medical and physical treatment

In BPPV treatment, position provoking vertigo is repeated for many times (habituation) or an abrupt head movement is tried to reject debris from the posterior semicircular canal (7, 20). These exercises and maneuvers are provided during Brandt - Daroff habituation exercises, Semont's liberator maneuver and Epley's maneuver.

Brandt-Daroff habituation exercises: Position provoking vertigo is repeated with the patient for many times. Firstly, the patient sits and then the position provoking vertigo is applied. This position is kept until vertigo disappears or for 30 seconds, then the patient sits. Vertigo re-occurs again upon sitting. The patient sits for 30 seconds and then lies down on the other side; he/she remains at this position for 30 seconds and then sits again. Each maneuver is repeated three times daily for 10 to 20 times. If a patient is free of symptoms for two consecutive days, the maneuver is quitted. It should be performed despite nausea and vomiting. In case of nausea and vomiting, the number of maneuvers may be decreased [7, 20, 21] (Figure 2).

These exercises are important for patients with a cervical and thoracic pathology, elderly patients, patients with osteoporosis and patients with difficulties to apply below maneuvers due to any cause [22].

Semont's liberator maneuver: This is based on the theory that debris is adhered to the cupula. Initially provocative side should be revealed. In sitting position, head is turned from affected side for 45°. The patient quickly lies down toward this side. Nystagmus or vertigo is developed. This position is kept for 2 to 3 minutes. Then the patient quickly lies down toward on his/her other side, contralateral ear is underside. This position is kept for 5 minutes. Nystagmus or vertigo is re-developed. If there is no vertigo, the head is nodded several times to liberate debris. This position is kept for several minutes, and then the patient sits. The patient should stay at straight position for 48 hours and should avoid provocative positions for a week. During these 48 hours, a soft neck supporter may be recommended to these patients to keep straight position.

Epley's maneuver: It is a replacing maneuver of particle. Complaints are resolved in approximately 90% of the patients. Symptoms untreated are resolved in general within 6 months, despite recurrence. This treatment approach is based on circulation of debris within the endolymph. Firstly, Hallpike - Dix position is applied by keeping affected ear at the underside, symptoms are observed and this position is kept for 2 to 3 minutes. Then contralateral side is kept at Hallpike - Dix position. The patient keeps this position for a very short time. The patient is turned by keeping contralateral shoulder at superior. Angle of head with floor is 45°. This position is kept for 2 to 3 minutes, and then the patient sits slowly. In recurrent or persistent cases despite re-positional exercise, surgical removal of plate may be considered [8, 20, 21] (Figure 3).

The patient should be kept at sitting position for 48 hours and he/she should not be lied down on the affected side for 5 days.

In the treatment of horizontal canal BPPV, *Vannucchi's long-term positioning and Lempert's maneuver* are used. During long-term positioning, intact ear is kept at inferior for 12 hours during lying down. Lempert's maneuver is also called "Barbecue" maneuver. Maneuver is consisted of turning on total 270° by consecutive head and body movements around long axis of patients lying down. In patients subjected to these maneuvers, 5 mg Diazepam may be administered on the night before exercise day to calm patients and to help to tolerate maneuver [7, 20].

Neck and back pain may prevent these maneuvers and may increase complaints. It should be modified in patients with neck trauma and surgery in the past or it should not be applied on these subjects [7, 20].

Unilateral Vestibular Paresis

Unilateral conditions are mostly due to viral infection and bilateral conditions are usually due to aminoglycoside or chemotherapeutic drugs. In the unilateral disorder, unilateral abnormal discharge arrives to the brain and thus disequilibrium is significant. Acute unilateral vestibular paresis may be divided into 4 phases:

1. Irritation phase: Nystagmus toward affected side is present.
2. Abrupt functional loss phase: There is a typical rotator vertigo; nystagmus is toward normal side and hospitalization is common. During this period, medical treatment is recommended to initiate neurochemical compensation mechanisms. Then, vestibular electrical stimulation is applied. Exercises are initiated following the vestibular stimulation [7, 20].

3. Low frequency electrical currents are used for vestibular electrical stimulation (VES). The patient lies down on one side with his/her most comfortable position, intact side being at underside. Room should be illuminated; eyes are open and fixed to a target. Electrodes are 2 cm^2 and placed with an interval of 1 cm. One pair is placed to the area corresponding to the second cervical vertebra, contralateral to the affected side, toward spontaneous nystagmus; other pair is placed on contralateral trapezius muscle. Two stimulations per day, each at least for two hours, are applied [7, 20] (Figure 4).
4. Central compensation phase: Vertigo and nystagmus are progressively reduced. CNS compensates this inequality by two ways: [1] a labyrinth decreases to send stimulus to the other and cerebellum suppresses hyperactive vestibular nucleus. (2) An intrinsic activity slowly starts in depressed labyrinth (7, 20).
5. Remission phase: Nystagmus begins again toward affected side (7, 20).
6. Purpose of treatment is to stabilize the sight, to provide postural control and to improve general physical condition. Choice of appropriate exercises is dependent to the type of vestibular loss, symptoms and functional capacity. As psychological symptoms such as anxiety and tension are common in these patients, initially relaxation exercises are started. Massage is also performed for the same purpose. There are three exercises in these programs: Habituation, postural control and condition exercises. Exercises continue as long as vertigo continues. If programs conducted by the therapist are performed as group exercises, motivation may be improved and seeing improved patients will encourage the patient [7, 20].

Treatment Programs

Programs may be divided in two groups: Home exercise program and program driven by the therapist [7, 20].

A. Home Exercise Program

This is recommended for the patients completing acute phase, not requiring continuous observation and who have difficulty in regular visits for exercises. Purpose is to maintain well-being by therapist and to improve further. Daily 2-3 sessions and 20-30 repetitions per session are performed. A relative or a friend should be present for observation. Symptoms start to reduce within 3 to 4 weeks [1, 7]. Recommended exercises are:

Supine Position

1. When the patient lies back, he/she holds his/her knee at contralateral of lesion and compress toward his/her chest (Figure 5).
2. At above mentioned position, the patient keeps his/her arm of lesion side at complete extension on his/her head and bends identically the contralateral knee and compresses gently on his/her chest by his/her hand at that side and this position is kept for 10 seconds.
3. The patient lifts the pelvis, and at this time arms are at complete extension on head. First the arms are put down, then the pelvis returns to baseline position.

4. Patient welters. Patient elevate his/her left leg at complete extension by his/her right arm and vice versa [1, 7].

Sitting Position

1. Head movements: When sitting, the patient has feet on floor, hands on thighs, and first eyes open, then closed and he/she moves his/her head from one side to the other side firstly circularly then horizontally (Figure 6).
2. Patient holds cards at 30-35 cm in front and at eye level. Patient moves his/her eyes from one card to other by horizontal, vertical and diagonal movements.
3. Patient holds a card on which certain words are written. He/she follows up card moving horizontally, vertically and diago*n*ally with his/her eyes.
4. Patient sits and finds 3 targets in the room. One of these targets is at eye level, the second one at right shoulder level and the third one is at left shoulder level. He/she looks at the targets consecutively and gradually speeds up.
5. Focusing eye when head is turning: Patient fixes his/her eyes on a target at 25 cm away (preferably finger). Patient continues to look this fixed point while turning head from right to left and vice versa and speeds up [1, 7].

Upright Position

1. Patient stands near a table, uses his/her hands as support and transfers his/her body weight on his/her foot at lesion side by resting on tiptoe (Figure 7).
2. Now, patient stands on his/her heel at the same position by transferring body weight on lesion side foot.
3. While standing, arms are on head at complete extension position and holding an object, and then do small and large circular movements.
4. Ankle swinging: Patient stands up with the feet at shoulder distance; arms are at two side and the feet bear equal load. Then the patient bends from front to behind and then to each side to switch body weight, firstly with eyes open and then closed.
5. Ball movements: Arms at full extension holding a ball and making circular movement; eyes follow-up the ball.
6. Gait and head movements: Patient walks close to a wall at contact distance. Patient walks for three steps and look back. Then patient look back following another three steps [1, 7].

B. Program Conducted by Therapist

Above mentioned head movements, walking with ball movements and head movements are performed also here. In addition, following exercises are recommended.

Supine Position

1. Patients lifts his/her knee at extension at affected side and moves his/her knee at medial and lateral at this position without bending the knee (Figure 8) .
2. While lying back, patient places a cushion under his/her knee at affected side, a weight of 2 kg is bound to his/her ankle and asked to make his/her knee at extension [1, 7].

Sitting Position

1. At sitting position, patient fixes his/her eyes to a target in front, and then focuses on a target on ceiling and then to the target in front of him/her.
2. Therapist pushes the patient sitting on the bed in order to stimulate equilibrium (1,7) (Figure 8).

Upright Position

1. When a patient stands up, therapist pulls him/her from back and push from front.
2. Patient walks on a ramp up and down. A special cushion may be used for this maneuver and this cushion is made by a soft material to activate other compensatory mechanism by reducing stimuli coming from the footsole (Figure 9).
3. Walking on a way with obstacles: Certain obstacles such as chair, cushion is put on the way of patient.
4. Patient walks about 3 m and stops suddenly on therapist's command.
5. Patient sits on an equilibrium ball with hands swinging at both side of the ball and starts to jump slightly or the therapist slightly disturbs his/her equilibrium.
6. While standing, patient focuses his/her eyes on an object moving in front of him/her.
7. Patient throws the ball to someone and vice versa.
8. Walking with eyes closed: Patient puts his/her hand on a wall, closes his/her eyes and starts to walk laterally. This is repeated for 10 to 15 times [1, 7].

Complaints may be persistent in spite of above mentioned exercise programs. This may be defined as *decompensated vestibular insufficiency*. It would be better to continue to the program with addition of certain exercises. Then, propriocetion and equilibrium exercise may be recommended.

1. While lying back, the patient bends knees, feet are in full contact with floor and performs pelvic rotation to the right and left.
2. While standing hands and feet, the patient takes a deep breath, hunches his/her back and lowers the back while expiring [7].

Bilateral Vestibular Paresis

A gradual walking program is recommended for these patients. The purpose is preventing falls during walking, to provide gait coordination and to succeed walking in dark and on obstacle way [1, 20].

Important points to be followed during the program are:

1. If the patient has difficulty to go next step, previous step is maintained.
2. Patient should walk with an accompanying person or equipment.
3. At the beginning, walking time should be only 2 to 5 minutes and should be increased for 2 to 3 minutes per week. Total walking time should be increased to 20 to 30 minutes.
4. Walking should be done five times weekly, once daily.

5. Properties of walking floor should be as follows:

Well Illuminated Flat and Hard Floor

- Slightly illuminated flat and hard floor
- Well illuminated irregular floor (garden or beach)
- Slightly illuminated irregular floor (garden or beach) [1, 20, 23].

PROPRIOCEPTION AND FRENKEL EXERCISES

A. Proprioception Exercises: Proprioception may simply be defined as "the ability to be aware of spatial body posture at conscious and unconscious level". In other words, proprioception is a special sensory modality including joint movement sense and joint position (24). Certain exercises recommended during its impairment are shown in Figure 9 and 10.

B. Frenkel exercises: In general, they are recommended in serious disequilibrium and central vertigo.

It is started at lying back position and if patient tolerates, following steps are performed and they are finished at standing up position [25].

At Lying Back Position

1. Hip and knee are flexed, while heel being kept in touch with floor at lower extremity. Then it is repeated by the other leg.
2. Following flexion like at first exercise, hip is abducted, and then turned back to the first position.
3. Abduction and adduction are done when hip and knee are at semi-flexion.
4. When hip and knee are being flexed, patient tries to stop upon a directive at a certain moment of exercise.
5. Both lower extremities perform simultaneous flexion, abduction, adduction and then extension.
6. Both lower extremities perform semi-flexion; while this position is maintained, and abduction and adduction are done and then extension is repeated. At that moment, patient tries to stop upon a directive at a certain moment of exercise.
7. At one extremity, heel is kept 5 cm high away from the floor and hip and knee are flexed, and then the previous position is repeated.
8. While hip and knee are flexed without contacting heel to the floor, the heel is brought on contralateral knee. Then the patient tries to touch his/her heel on middle part of tibia, ankle and toes, and then to the bed on both side at level of knee and calf.
9. While knee and hip are at flexion and extension, heel is contacted on contralateral dorsal part of foot, tibia and knee, respectively.

10. During flexion, heel is randomly contacted with several points according to the therapist's directive.
11. Heel is kept 5 cm high away from the floor, leg is flexed, and then heel is contacted on contralateral knee and moved from leg to foot while extending.
12. Above exercise pattern is repeated by moving the heel up and down on contralateral knee, tibia, ankle and toes. When heel comes to level of contact with contralateral toes, contralateral knee is slightly flexed. At this stage, movement is stopped at certain points by directives.
13. While knees and malleoli are at same level, heels at both legs are kept 5 cm high away from the floor and hip and knees are flexed and extended, movement is stopped at certain points by directives.
14. Lower extremities are flexed and extended consecutively by keeping heel on the floor.
15. Above mentioned exercise program is repeated by keeping heels 5 cm high away from the floor.
16. While heels are kept 5 cm high away from the floor, both lower extremities are flexed, abducted, adducted and extended.
17. Patient tries to put heel on points indicated by therapist on bed and contralateral extremity.
18. In addition to lower extremity movement, toe is moved toward point indicated by therapist [25].

Sitting Position

1. While sitting on a chair with feet on the floor and back supported, this position is kept for 2 minutes. Then it is repeated without arm and back supports.
2. Heel is elevated and kept for a time indicated by therapist. Then foot is totally elevated and patient tries to put feet on points indicated on floor.
3. Two signs of "plus" are drawn on floor. Feet are moved on these signs to right-left and front-behind.
4. Sitting and standing are performed by keeping knees side by side [25].

Upright Position

1. Walking toward side. Equilibrium is well maintained.
2. Two parallel lines with 35 cm of interval are drawn on the floor. Patient walks straightly on the lines. A rest is taken at each 10 steps.
3. Patient walks by putting feet on footprints drawn on the floor. Footprints should be on both side of middle line and should be parallel.
4. Turning: (a) Turning right foot with heel on the floor, but without contacting toes with floor, (b) Turning left leg medially with toes contacting the floor but without touching heel on the floor, (c) Putting left foot on right foot [25].

Myofacial Pain Syndrome (MPS)

MPS shows a regional distribution, but it may also affect just only one muscle. There are trigger points in MPS. When these points are compressed, patients have severe pain which may diffuse to other regions. Patient may perceive craniocervical muscle pain as ocular, dental, auricular pain. Muscle may be palpable as a stretched band (taut band); when trigger points are compressed, patient jumps (jumping sign), and switch response is observed on muscle. Although MPS is completely improved by treatment, fibromyalgia is repeated very frequently. Most frequently considered etiological factors for MPS are cold, trauma and postural impairment [26, 27].

MPS at sternocleidomastoid muscle and dizziness: Sternocleidomastoid muscle has two divisions: sternal and clavicular. Many trigger points frequently occur on both divisions due to various causes. These may affect patient's life more negatively than pain. Stimulation of both divisions leads to diverse autonomic and proprioceptive impairments [28] (Figure 11).

At the presence of trigger points on clavicular division of sternocleidomastoid muscle, vertigo and fluctuation sensation occur. These trigger points are stimulated by abrupt head movements and complaints ranging to syncope may be developed. It may take several seconds to hours. Nausea is frequent, but vomiting is not so frequent [29].

Proprioceptive mechanisms on neckhave significant contributions to our spatial position and maintaining equilibrium. In case of MPS at sternocleidomastoid muscle, proprioceptive mechanisms of upper extremity and neck are interrupted. This muscle has a major role in head orientation. When a patient with unilateral sternocleidomastoid MPS, takes an object on his/her hang at the affected side, he/she can't correctly estimate the weight of this object, and this is improved by inactivation of trigger point on the muscle. In contrary to MPS of other muscles, pain and spasm are not typical for this muscle MPS. Main symptom triad: Frontal headache, postural dizziness and dissymmetry. Patient may not drive. This is an important unrecognized cause of traffic accident. For example, talking on the phone for a long time, lying down on a big cushion may contract sternocleidomastoid muscle and activate trigger points. Long term extension of head also leads to dizziness; for example, painting a ceiling, placing curtains, sitting at very front on theatre room. These patients have negative Romberg sign and have no nystagmus or neurological deficit [28].

MPS on digastric and superior trapezius muscle may lead also to vertigo, but this condition is also due to satellite trigger points on sternocleidomastoid muscle [28].

Treatment:

1. Prophylactic activities: Patients should not elevate their heads while waking up, this may stretch sternocleidomastoid muscle. If the condition is unilateral, patients should return to that side; if it is bilateral, patients should wake up with face turned toward bad. Cushion should not be big, no cushion should be placed on shoulder. During reading, light should be in the middle or ceiling. Patients should hold the phone by one hand and should frequently change the hand; the phone should not be placed between the head and shoulder. Excess rotation should be avoided, as this causes

excess muscle stretching and these patients should frequently perform diaphragmatic breathing to relax [26, 27, 30].
2. Applying ice like brushing and then stretching: Head is extended and rotated, face is toward opposite side. This causes to stretching of clavicular division [26, 27, 30].
3. Trigger point injection: These points may be still active in spite of injection. This is due to their property of being strong autonomic stimulation. Warm tissue should be applied following injection at home [26, 27, 30].

Cervical Osteoarthritis

Vertebral artery originates from subclavian artery on both side, and passes from interior parts of cervical vertebra transverse process. Minimal trauma of degeneration on facet joints causes compression of vertebral artery or neck hyperextension and rotation compresses vertebral artery and causes intermittent vertebrobasilar ischemia resulting in dizziness. Recently, the most accepted opinion is altered proprioception due to osteoarthritis [31].

Treatment

Goal of treatment is to reduce pain and inflammation, to maintain or to improve joint range of motion. During acute exacerbation, anti-inflammatory drugs, physical treatment and cervical collar may be used. The following simple rules should always be considered, mainly during exacerbation period:

1. Exercises such as running, jumping should be avoided.
2. Joint movement range (JMR) should be maintained by JMR exercises.
3. Muscle strength, especially neck extensor power, should be maintained,. Performing isometric exercises is important.
4. Keeping head at the same position for long term, for example driving for long-term, watching television, should be avoided.
5. Long term extension of neck should be avoided [31].

Cervical Vertebra Blockage

There is reversible especially functional movement restriction. Mobilization and manipulation may be applied in these cases [32]. An example of mobilization performed at Occiput-C1 interval block is shown in Figure 12.

Prognosis

Spontaneous remission may be seen in BPPV; but recurrence may be seen in 50% of treated patients. The course of Meniere's disease may be variable; progressive hearing loss may be observed at affected ear of many patients and bilateral symptoms may be seen in 50% of patients. Chronic disequilibrium is observed in 20% of patients with acute vestibular neuritis; but vestibular rehabilitation decreases disability; chronic dizziness may significantly affect psychological, professional and social aspects of patients and may result in long-term morbidity [3].

In Case of Following Conditions, an Otorhinolaryngologist Should be Consulted

1. Insufficient compensation within 3 months following acute dizziness attack
2. Presence of hearing loss or tinnitus
3. Presence of neurological symptoms [3].

Insufficient Compensation at Peripheral Vestibular Dysfunction, is Seen in Following Conditions

1. Undoing of exercises by patient who consider them very provocative
2. Presence of progressive vestibular pathology such as Meniere and bilateral vestibular hypofunction
3. Long-term usage of vestibular suppressants [3].

SUMMARY

Physician is frequently without solution in front of patient with dizziness. First of all medical history should be carefully obtained and discrimination between central or peripheral vertigo should be done. Peripheral dizziness is a movement sensation, this is called vertigo. Vertigo is in general episodic, and nausea, hearing loss, fullness in ear and tinnitus are frequently present. Central vertigo is continuous; it begins as gradual and less serious. Following careful medical history and physical examination, vestibular tests, imaging and laboratory evaluations are required. Magnetic resonance imaging is most important diagnostic tool to evaluate central causes such as tumor, cerebrovascular event and multiple sclerosis. Vestibular tests are required to discriminate peripheral and central causes, to make preoperative assessment, to compare unilateral post-traumatic development or to follow-up results of vestibular rehabilitation. Topical or systemic ototoxic drugs are most important causes of vestibular dysfunction. These should not be used or should be closely monitored. In patients with tympanic membrane rupture or with tympanostomy tube, polymyxine B, Neomycine or another aminoglycoside should not be used, even if in topical form. Vestibular suppressants such as scopolamine, meclisine and benzodiazepine should not be mostly used. Long-term usage may delay central compensation or improvement will not be seen. In case of chronic disequilibrium, vestibular rehabilitation is beneficial.

REFERENCES

[1] Abatzides GJ, Kitsios A. The role of rehabilitation in the treatment of balance disorders. *Journal of back and musculoskeletal rehabilitation,* 1999;12: 101-13.

[2] Sloane PD, Coeytaux RR, Beck RS, Dallara J. Dizziness: state of the science. *Ann. Intern. Med.,* 2001;134: 823-32.

[3] Pagarkar W, Davies R. Dizziness, symptoms and signs. Medicine 2004; 32(9): 18-23.

[4] Sturnieks DL, St George R, Lord SR. Balance disorders in elderly. *Clinical Neurophysiology,* 2008; 38: 467-78.

[5] Abreu DC, Trevisan DC, Costa GC, Vasconcelos FM, Gomes MM, Carneiro AA. The association between osteoporosis and static balance in elderly women. *Osteoporos Int.,* 2010; 21: 1487-91.

[6] McVey MA, Stylianou AP, Luchies CW, Lyons KE, Pahwa R, Jernigan S, Mahnken JD. *Early biomechanical markers of postural instability in Parkinson's disease. Gait&Posture,* 2009; 30: 538-42.

[7] Cesarani A, Alpini D. Vertigo and Dizziness Rehabilitation. Berlin, *Springer Co,* 1999, pp 10-168.

[8] Kutz JW. The Dizzy Patient. *Med. Clin. N. Am.,* 2010; 94: 989-1002.

[9] Barin K, Dodson EE. Dizziness in the Elderly. *Otolaryngol. Clin. N. Am.,* 2011; 44: 437-54.

[10] Yahia A, Ghroubi S, Jribi S, Malla J, Baklouti S, Ghorbel A, Elleuch MH. Chronic neck pain and vertigo: Is a true balance disorders present? *Annals of Physical and Rehabilitation Medicine,* 2009; 52: 556-67.

[11] 11-Ricci Na, Aratani MC,Dona F, Macedo C, Caovilla HH, Ganança FF. A systematic review about the effects of the vestibular rehabilitation in middle-age and older adults. *Rev. Bras. Fisioter.,* 2010; 14(5): 361-71.

[12] Hain TC, Ramaswamy T. Dizziness in the Elderly. www.galter.northwestern.edu /geriatrics/chapters/dizziness.cfm.

[13] Tusa RJ. Dizziness. *Med. Clin. N. Am.,* 2009; 93: 263-71.

[14] Angeli SI, Hawley R, Gomez O. Systematic approach to benign paroxysmal positional vertigo in the elderly. *Otolaryngol. Head Neck Surg.,* 2003; 128: 719-25.

[15] Vibert D, Caversaccio M, Hausler R. Meniere's Disease in the Elderly. *Otolaryngol. Clin. N. Am.,* 2010; 43: 1041-6.

[16] Salles N, Kressig RW, Michel JP. Managemet of chronic dizziness in elderly people. *Z. Gerontol. Geriat.,* 2003; 36: 10-5.

[17] Herdman SJ. Role of vestibular adaptation in vestibular rehabilitation. *Otolaryngology Head Neck Surgery,* 1998;119: 49-54.

[18] Boyer Fc, Macadre LP, Regrain E, Leveque M, Taiar R, Seidermann L, et al. Vestibular rehabilitation therapy. *Clinical. Neurophysiology,* 2008; 38: 479-87.

[19] Jung JY, Kim JS, Chung PS, Woo SH, Rhee CK. Effect of vestibular rehabilitation on dizziness in the elderly. American Journal of Otolarygology- *Head and Neck Medicine and Surgery,* 2009; 30: 295-9.

[20] Herdman SJ. Vestibular disorders and rehabilitation. In Lazar RB (Ed): Principles of neurologic rehabilitation. Philadelphia,The Mc Graw-Hill Co.1998, pp 267-85.

[21] Aksoy C, Karan A, Diracoglu D, Ural I, "Exercise guide of patients with vertigo", Publication of Istanbul University Istanbul Faculty of Medicine, Istanbul, 2004.

[22] Banfield GK, Wood C, Knight J. Does vestibular habituation still have a place in the treatment of benign paroxysmal positional vertigo?. *J. Laryngol. Otol.,* 2000;114: 501-5.

[23] Shepard NT, Telian SA. Vestibular Rehabilitation. Cummings CW (Ed): Otolaryngology- Head and Neck Surgery. Baltimore, Mosby Co.1993, pp 2744- 53.

[24] Diracoglu D, Aydin R, Baskent A, Celik A.Effects of kinesthesia and balance exercises in knee osteoarthritis.J. Clin. Rheumatol., 2005 Dec;11(6):303-10.

[25] Kottke FJ. Therapeutic exercise to develop neuromuscular coordination. In Wickland EH (Ed): Krusen's Handbook of Physical Medicine and Rehabilitation. Philadelphia, WB. Saunders Co.1990, pp 452-79.

[26] Berker E, Kayhan Ö. Yumuşak doku romatizması. Tuna N (Ed): Romatizmal Hastalıklar. Ankara, Hacettepe Taş Kitabevi 1994, pp 626-59.

[27] 27-Şencan S. Fibromiyalji sendromunda aerobik egzersiz ile paroksetin tedavilerinin etkinliklerinin karşılaştırılması. Uzmanlık tezi. İstanbul, İstanbul Tıp Fakültesi 1997.

[28] 28-Travell JG, Simons DG. Sternocleidomastoid Muscle. In Travell JG, Simons DG (Eds): Myofascial Pain and Dysfunction. The trigger point manuel. Baltimore, *Williams & Wilkins Co.,* 1992, pp 202-19.

[29] 29- Karan A, Diracoglu D, Erdamar B, Ellialtıoglu A, Uluğ T, Aksoy C. A Neglected reason of vertigo and a new approach to the patient with vertigo: myofascial pain syndrome. *Nobel. Med.,* 2008; 4:17-21.

[30] 30- Özaras N. Miyofasiyal ağrı sendromları ve fibromiyalji sendromu. *Ege Fiziksel Tıp ve Rehabilitasyon Dergisi,* 1998;4:55-63.

[31] 31- Braddom RL. Management of Common Cervical Pain Syndromes. In DeLisa JA, Gans BM (Eds): Rehabilitation Medicine. Philadelphia, Lippincott Co. 1993, pp 1036-47.

[32] 32- Diracoglu D, Aksoy C, "Manuel Medicine", Medical Rehabilitation, Eds: H. Oğuz, E. Dursun, N. Dursun, Nobel Tip, Istanbul, 2004. pp 383-410.

In: New Horizons in Geriatric Medicine. Volume 1
Editors: Ahmet Turan Isik, M. Refik Mas et al.
ISBN: 978-1-62808-972-1

Chapter 7

ALTERED MENTAL STATUS

Adam Mehmet Gulhan

ABSTRACT

As the population of seniors grows astoundingly, medical professionals will more frequently face to challenges in management of elderly patients with altered mental status. The general term "mental status change" has numerous synonyms. These terms are applied to a broad spectrum of conditions. Dementia, delirium, sepsis, hypoxia, hypoglycemia, depression and iatrogenic causes are common in the elderly and must be considered in differential diagnosis of altered mental status. Misdiagnosis and lack of recognition of underlying cause of altered mental status is costly to society and the family and is immeasurable in personal tragedy. Adopting an organized approach to the evaluation of mental status is therefore important for the evaluation of all older patients.

This chapter reviews the significance of altered mental status in the elderly. Specific diagnoses, including delirium, dementia, common medical conditions as a cause of altered mental status, depression and polypharmacy are discussed.

INTRODUCTION

The elderly patient with altered mental status presents a difficult diagnostic challenge. Differentiating acutely decompensated progressive dementia from other organic and reversible causes of altered mental status is challenging. [1] The *altered mental status* (AMS) label may be given to patients with seizures, speech difficulties, generalized weakness, anger management issues, hemiparesis, psychosis, etc. We need to be clear about terminology.

Normal *consciousness* requires both arousal and cognition. Arousal is mediated by the reticular activating system (RAS), housed primarily in the brainstem. Cognition is a function of properly working cortical hemispheres. Derangements of arousal can present as either depressed (lethargy, stupor, coma) or elevated (hypervigilant, agitated, - maybe seizure?). Derangements of cognition run the spectrum from "just not as sharp as usual" to confusion, amnesia, hallucination and detachment from reality.

Since you need disruption in either the RAS or both hemispheres to decrease the level of consciousness, causes due to isolated structural lesions (ischemic stroke or hemorrhage) are most often in the brainstem. It would be very rare to have multiple sudden-onset bilateral hemispheric strokes. Conversely, systemic conditions like metabolic derangements or poisonings and conditions that affect both hemispheres (CNS infections or increased intracranial pressure) are common causes of altered mental status. Keeping these conditions in mind will help to guide differential diagnosis.

Some focal neurological deficits can be mistaken for alterations in consciousness. Dysarthrias and aphasias (receptive, motor or mixed), spatial neglect syndromes, even hemianopsias and hemiparesis can be mistaken as confusion if not looked at closely. Functional (psychiatric) changes in behavior (like depression or fugue states) can be difficult to distinguish from organic causes of behavioral changes. Much of "medical clearance for psychiatry" deals with this conundrum. When in doubt, assume a medical cause until it can be clearly ruled out. [2]

EVALUATION

Mental Status Examination

The mental status examination is the tool the physician must use to access and document the current level of cognitive function accurately. The initial examination requires only that the physician talk to the patient. If a sense that something is just not quite right develops while one is taking the history, then more formal testing should be pursued. Memory is often one of the most obvious cognitive functions to be affected and can be tested with simple repetition of three times, or recall of the current and first U.S. presidents. The formal mental status evaluation consists of the assessment of appearance, level of consciousness, behavior, speech and language, mood, delusions, and frank hallucinations. The pneumonic JIM A. MOTSIG (judgment, intelligence, memory, affect, mood, orientation, thought process and content, speech, insight and grooming) may be used for a brief assessment of cognitive function. The Mini-Mental Status Examination surveys orientation, memory attention, calculation, and language functions. It is widely used and helpful in diagnosing new disease or tracking deterioration with chronic disease. Other quantitative scales, less useful in emergency setting, include the clinical dementia rating scale, the telephone interview for cognitive status, the psychogeriatric assessment scale, the cognitive assessment screening test, the confusion assessment method, and the dementia questionnaire. [3-14]

History and Physical Examination

A detailed medical history is important in elucidating the etiology of delirium. It is important to obtain information from as many sources as possible including the patient, emergency medical service providers, witnesses, family, caregivers and primary care providers. Information regarding the patient's baseline mental status and level of functioning should be ascertained. It is helpful to know if the patient has underlying dementia, if there has been an acute change and what underlying medical conditions exist. A very thorough review of medication use is important, as medications are very common precipitants of delirium in the elderly. The history should focus on causal factors related to the acute presentation such as history of trauma or fall, lack of oral intake, presence of systemic disease including metabolic and cardiopulmonary disorders, symptoms of infection, and substance use or withdrawal. [15] The careful taking of a social history and investigation of the patient's support system is also important. Is there a history of heavy alcohol use? Have there been any significant life-altering events, such as death of a spouse or recent retirement? Increasing age, lower educational level, and the presence of clinical manifestations of atherosclerotic disease have all been associated with poorer cognitive function. [16]

Vital signs should be carefully reviewed and an accurate temperature and oxygen saturation measurement obtained. A bedside glucose determination is often considered the "fifth vital sign" and is particularly important in the evaluation of the agitated patient. [15] The examination should search for evidence of medical or surgical causes for the altered mental status, including trauma, infections and focal neurological deficits. (Table 1) A comprehensive physical examination is often difficult or impossible in the confused or uncooperative patient. Clinicians should instead perform a focused assessment, concentrating upon vital signs, the state of hydration, skin condition, and potential infectious foci. The patient's general appearance may be suggestive, the dusky appearance seen with chronic pulmonary disease, the jaundiced appearance of hepatic failure, or the stigmata of renal failure. Needle tracks strongly suggest drug abuse. Cherry-red lips indicate possible carbon monoxide poisoning.

The breath may smell of alcohol, fetor hepaticus, uremic fetor or ketones. Hyperventilation offers a limited number of possible etiologies. A bitten tongue or posterior fracture-dislocation of the shoulder suggests a convulsive seizure (over 10 percent of such patients remain in nonconvulsive status epilepticus). There may also be signs of head injury. Subhyaloid or retinal hemorrhages raise the possibility of an intracranial hemorrhage, usually from a ruptured berry aneurysm. Alcohol or sedative-drug withdrawal may cause a delirium characterized by autonomic nervous system activation (tachycardia, sweating, flushing, dilated pupils) in younger persons, but these responses are blunted or absent in the geriatric population.

Anticholinergic toxicity in elders can cause delirium without peripheral signs of atropine poisoning (e.g., fever, mydriasis, tachycardia). Sepsis may present as altered mental status without obvious fever (sometimes even with hypothermia) or localizing signs (e.g., rebound tenderness from a perforated viscus).

Pitfalls in the examination must be kept in mind: temperature may be under 38.3°C (101°F) even in the presence of serious infections; auscultatory and radiographic findings of pneumonia may be subtle or absent; and abdominal catastrophes may present without peritoneal signs in frail older patients. False-positive findings occur as well (e.g., nuchal rigidity may not signify meningitis). [17] There is always the possibility of neglect or abuse of elderly, and medical staff should look for physical evidence of such. The most common problem along these lines is simple neglect, which may present with evidence of malnutrition, poor hygiene, or nonadherence with medication. [18]

Table 1. Key elements of the physical examination

Vital signs	Neurologic examination
Odors	Observation
Evidence of trauma	Cranial nerves
Toxidromes	Muscle strength
Infection	Muscle tone and bulk
Signs of abuse or neglect	Presence or absence of tremors
Malnutrition	Brief sensory evaluation
Poor hygiene	Deep tendon reflexes
Noncompliance with medications	Pathologic reflexes
Ophthalmopathy	Cerebellar signs
Bulbar palsy	Gait
Proximal muscle weakness	Station
Signs of brain herniation	Myoclonus
Meningismus	Asterixis
Mental status examination	
Appearance	
Level of consciousness	
Behavior	
Speech and language	
Mood	
Delusion	
Hallucinations	
Memory	

DIAGNOSTIC TESTS

Laboratory Tests

A number of laboratory tests may be considered in the elderly with altered mental status. Targeted testing based on acuteness of condition, historical and physical clues is appropriate in most instances. Serum electrolytes, creatinine, glucose, calcium, complete blood count, and urinalysis and urine culture are reasonable for most patients when a cause is not immediately obvious. Drug levels should be ordered where appropriate. Toxic screen of blood and urine should be obtained from patients with acute mental status change when a cause is not immediately obvious. Again, clinicians must be aware that some common drugs (e.g., risperidone) are not assessed in routine laboratory screens. Therefore, overdose of these drugs cannot be excluded by negative results from a toxic screen. Blood gas determination is often helpful. In hyperventilating patients, respiratory alkalosis is most commonly due to early sepsis, hepatic failure, early salicylate intoxication, or cardiopulmonary causes. A metabolic acidosis usually reflects uremia, diabetic ketoacidosis, lactic acidosis, late phases of sepsis or salicylate intoxication, or toxins including methanol and ethylene glycol. A chest x-ray is usually performed. Further testing, such as liver function tests, should be based upon the history and clinical examination. A report of slow cognitive decline over several months, for example, will increase the importance of evaluating thyroid function and vitamin B12 levels. [17]

Neuroimaging

All patients displaying acute, marked alteration of mental status, especially those with focal neurologic deficits, should have a CT scan as soon as possible following the initial assessment and stabilization. A retrospective study of 294 patients with acute confusion found revealed abnormal CTs in 14 percent overall [19]. However, only 4 percent of patients without focal signs had abnormal CT; the lowest yield of CT (2 percent) was in patients with premorbid dementia and no focal neurologic signs.

In a review of CT scans performed in 123 medical intensive care unit patients, new CT findings were present in 26, leading to a change in diagnosis in 11 and a new treatment plan in 6 [20]. Most studies were performed for an indication of "altered mental status" and findings included cerebral infarction in 13, intracranial hemorrhage in 2, and tumor in 3. In another review of 279 head CT scans performed in the emergency department in patients older than 70 years, 42 (15 percent) revealed an acute condition [21]. Of these, 40 were found in patients with either significantly impaired consciousness (e.g., unable to open eyes, speak, or follow simple commands) and/or new focal neurologic findings.

MRI is more sensitive than head CT for acute stroke, posterior fossa lesions, and white matter lesions. [22]. In patients with altered mental status of unknown cause and negative head CT, MRI may be useful to exclude acute or subacute stroke and multifocal inflammatory lesions (e.g., as seen in reversible posterior leukoencephalopathy. and acute disseminated encephalomyelitis).

Lumbar Puncture

A lumbar puncture is indicated to rule out subarachnoid hemorrhage after a negative CT scan or whenever meningitis or encephalitis is suspected. Older patients with bacterial meningitis are more likely to present with delirium rather than the classic triad of fever, headache, and meningismus. In a retrospective study of 81 elderly patients who were admitted to the hospital for the evaluation of fever and mental status changes, CSF cultures were negative for bacterial growth in 80 of 81 patients [23]. However, one case of bacterial meningitis and one case of aseptic meningitis were diagnosed by CSF findings. In a retrospective review of 232 lumbar punctures performed in hospitalized patients for the indication of altered mental status, 11 percent were abnormal; the yield was highest in those suspected of community-acquired meningitis [24].

Lumbar puncture is mandatory when the cause of delirium is not obvious. Clinicians should also have a low threshold for obtaining CSF in febrile patients with delirium, even when alternate explanatory conditions for delirium are present or suspected.

Neuroimaging should be obtained prior to lumbar puncture in patients with coma, focal signs, papilledema, or suspicion of increased intracranial pressure because of the very low but real risk of precipitating transtentorial herniation. If lumbar puncture is delayed and the suspicion of bacterial meningitis is high, empiric antibiotic treatment should be considered. [17]

Electroencephalography (EEG)

Electroencephalography (EEG) is useful in patients with altered consciousness in order to exclude seizures, especially nonconvulsive or subclinical seizures and to confirm the diagnosis of certain metabolic encephalopathies or infectious encephalitides that have characteristic EEG patterns. [25, 26] Nonconvulsive status epilepticus may cause continuous or fluctuating impairment of consciousness, and EEG is the only method that can make the diagnosis. One report evaluated 198 EEGs performed for the indication of altered consciousness without convulsions and found definite or probable nonconvulsive status epilepticus in 74 (37 percent) [27]. In another study, continuous EEG monitoring was performed for unexplained decrease in consciousness or detection of subclinical seizures in 570 critically ill patients [28]. Seizures were detected in 110 patients (19 percent), and the seizures were exclusively nonconvulsive in 92 percent of these individuals. Metabolic encephalopathies may show diffuse bilateral slowing of background rhythm and moderate or high wave amplitude. Triphasic waves are associated with hepatic encephalopathy but can be seen in other severe metabolic disturbances including uremic and septic encephalopathy [29, 30]. Herpes simplex encephalitis may be associated with high amplitude periodic complexes in the temporal lobe leads. EEG evaluation should be obtained for any patient with altered consciousness of unknown etiology [31].

Differential Diagnosis

Normal Physiologic Changes of Aging

Normal changes of aging include neuronal cell loss and a decrease in brain weight. All neurotransmitters show some age-related decrement. Chronic cholinergic deficiency in the CNS accompanies advancing age, increasing the patient's susceptibility to the effects of anticholinergic medications. Nervous tissue is affected by a loss of myelin and decreasing sensory nerve conduction. Autonomic dysfunction is widespread and temperature control impaired, placing the patient at increased susceptibility to environmental influences. Learned information ("crystallized intelligence") remains relatively intact, whereas problem-solving capabilities ("fluid intelligence") declines in age-related fashion. [3] An age-related memory impairment has been identified (age-associated memory impairment, or benign senescent forgetfulness), which may have a place on a continuum between normal aging and Alzheimer's senile dementia (Table 2). [18, 32]

Dementia and Delirium

Dementia is a disorder that is characterized by impairment of memory and at least one other cognitive domain (aphasia, apraxia, agnosia, executive function). These must represent a decline from previous level of function and be severe enough to interfere with daily function and independence. [33] The development of symptoms and loss of intellectual function is generally slow and gradual, versus the rapid deterioration seen in delirium. Up to 10% of the US adult population is affected by a dementing disorder by the age of 65 years, with the incidence doubling every 5 years after age 65, to reach 30% to 50% by age 85. [6, 9] The most common dementia disorder is Alzheimer's disease, followed by the dementia resulting from vascular disease. Ten percent or fewer cases are reversible. [9] The initial step in the evaluation of a patient with suspected dementia should focus upon the history. Family members or other informants who know the patient well are invaluable resources for providing an adequate history of cognitive and behavioral changes. Adequate time should be arranged for a full assessment of cognitive function, followed by a complete physical examination, including neurologic examination.

Table 2. Differential diagnosis

Delirium	Endocrinopathies
Dementia	Hyperthyroidism
Alzheimer's disease	Hypothyroidism
Vascular	Adrenal insufficiency
Dementia with Lewy bodies	Hypoparathyroidism
Infectious	Hyperparathyroidism
Sepsis	Glucocorticoid excess
Cerebral abscess	Primary neurological disorders
Meningitis	CVA/TIA
Encephalitis	Space-occupying lesion
HIV CNS infections	Subdural/epidural hematoma
Neurosyphilis	Hemorrhage
Pharmacologic/Poisoning	Subarachnoid
Medication reaction/interaction	Intracerebral
Polypharmacy	Intraventricular
Neuroleptic malignant syndrome	Epilepsy and postictal states
Lithium toxicity	Complex migraine
Salicylate poisoning	Temporal arteritis
Anticholinergic toxicity	Normal pressure hydrocephalus
Serotonin syndrome	Substance abuse
Alcohol or drug withdrawal	Alcohol
Alcohol or illicit drugs	Medications
Carbon monoxide poisoning	Withdrawal from addictive substances
Metabolic	
Hypoglycemia	Environmental
Hyperglycemia	Hypothermia
Renal failure	Hyperthermia
Hepatic failure	Cardiovascular disease
Dehydration	Myocardial ischemia
Hypercalcemia	CHF
Hypocalcemia	Arrhythmias
Hypernatremia	Hypertensive encephalopathy
Hyponatremia	Pulmonary disease
Hypermagnesemia	Hypoxia
Hypomagnesemia	Hypercarbia
Vitamin deficiency	Psychiatric disorders

The Mini-Mental State Exam is a useful screening test for dementia; a score of less than 24 points is suggestive of dementia or delirium. Neuropsychologic testing batteries are useful in identifying patients with dementia, particularly when administered to those who may be at increased risk of cognitive impairment. Screening for B12 deficiency and hypothyroidism is recommended for patients being evaluated for dementia. Screening for depression in patients with dementia is recommended because depression is a common treatable comorbidity that may also masquerade as dementia.

Genetic testing for the apolipoprotein E epsilon 4 allele is not currently recommended, nor is genetic testing for other potential causes of dementia. Structural neuroimaging with either a noncontrast head CT or MRI should be considered in the initial evaluation of all patients with dementia. [34, 35, 36]

Delirium may be defined as acute cognitive impairment with an alteration of consciousness. [7] The inability to concentrate (attention deficit) is a hallmark of delirium. The prevalence of delirium on admission can range from 10-40%. During hospitalization, it may affect an additional 25-50%. The rates of postoperative delirium are estimated at 10-52%. Even higher rates (70-87%) are seen in intensive care units. Three forms of delirium have been recognized: the hyperactive, hyperalert form; the hypoactive, hypoalert, lethargic form; and the mixed form. The hypoactive form is often unrecognized and is associated with a poorer overall prognosis. [37] Delirium as a geriatric syndrome is inherently multifactorial. Delirium may be the sole presenting symptom of life-threatening illness in the elderly, including sepsis or acute myocardial infarction. [38, 39] During an episode of delirium, the patient is generally unable to render even basic self-care, predisposing them to the development of secondary problems such as dehydration. Unfortunately, the symptoms of delirium are unrecognized as much as 70% of the time. Studies have found that at the time of admission, 15% of older patients may satisfy diagnostic criteria for delirium, and an additional 30% develop the disorder while hospitalized. [40]

Emergency physicians must rule out delirium as a cause of disturbed consciousness in all elderly patients before accepting dementia or other psychiatric conditions as the diagnosis. Development of delirium in the hospital has been associated with greater mortality rates, longer stays, increased hospital costs, greater nursing care needs, and increased discharge rates to long-term care facilities. [10, 41] Although multiple chemical problems are associated with delirium, most evidence supports failure of cholinergic transmission as the case. [40, 42]

Differentiating Delirium and Dementia

Dementia typically has an insidious onset and a progressive course. It may be difficult to determine if a change in level of functioning for a demented patient is due to the natural course of the disease or the acute superimposition of delirium or a psychiatric disturbance. Fluctuation of alertness over days, with lucid intervals, favors delirium. Rapid onset of cognitive dysfunction is highly suggestive of delirium and acute illness. Delirium frequently is misdiagnosed in a variety of situations, leading to the term *pseudodementia,* which also has been applied to misdiagnosed depressive symptoms. Hallucinations are auditory with psychoses, visual alone or visual and auditory with delirium, and generally absent in dementia. Vital signs are typically abnormal with delirium and normal with dementia. Alertness may be abnormally high or low with delirium but is usually normal with dementia.

The classic delirium patient falls asleep while speaking, whereas the demented patient may suddenly appear confused in midsentence and forget what they were saying. Dementia in itself is the single greatest risk factor for the development of delirium.(Table-3) [3, 43, 44, 45, 37]

Table 3. Differentiating dementia from delirium and depression

	Dementia	Delirium	Depression
Onset	Insidious/gradual	Abrupt	Fairly abrupt
Duration	Months-years	Days-weeks	Weeks-months
Alertness	Usually normal	Varies	Usually normal
Source of complaint	Family, caregiver	Providers, family	Patients themselves
Orientation	Disoriented later	Disoriented early	Usually normal
Attention/concentra.	Good	Poor	Poor
Effort	Good	Poor/fluctuating	Poor
"Don't know" answer	Uncommon	--	Common
Memory loss	Greater for recent	Greater for recent	Equal for both
Loss of social skills	Late	Abrupt changes	Early
Thought process/ content	Impoverished	Disorganized	May be slow
Psychomotor symptom.	Normal until late	Hyper- or hypoactive	Hypoactive

Medical Conditions

When a cause can be determined for acute altered mental status in patients of all ages, a metabolic or toxic etiology is found in 65% of cases, with focal structural lesions present in 33% of patients, and psychiatric problems accounting for the remaining 2%. [46]

Chronic subdural hematomas occur more commonly in the elderly, and those who abuse alcohol are especially at risk. Other structural causes include subarachnoid hemorrhage as well as intracerebral, cerebellar, and intraventricular hemorrhages.

Suspicion of an acute neurologic event caused by ischemic cerebrovascular disease should be heightened when there is preexisting history of hypertension or diabetes mellitus. After Alzheimer's disease, multiple infarcts are the second most common cause of dementia. Binswanger's disease, or lacunar strokes involving deep white matter typically occur in the area of the frontal lobes around the ventricles. The physician should document the presence or absence of specific signs of trauma (e.g., evidence of basilar skull fracture) and address the possibility of a recent fall or other mechanisms for head trauma.

Meningitis will present early with the variable signs of fever, headache, and stiff neck, and late with altered mental status or seizures. In addition to the usual pathogens, one must consider Listeria in the elderly patient. Encephalitis likewise presents with fever, headache, and confusion. Cerebral abscess may present secondary to trauma, from the contiguous spread of local infections, or as a distal metastasis from endocarditis, sepsis, or congenital heart disease. Immunocompromised patients, such as those with HIV disease, may harbor unusual CNS infections caused by *toxoplasmosa gondii, cryptococcus neoformans,*coccidiomycosis, or tuberculosis. These may often present as chronic meningitis. The CNS damage from HIV occurs as a result of direct cytotoxic effects or through products of HIV-infected macrophages. [47]

In the patient with a history of headache, physicians may need to consider complex migraines or temporal arteritis. Patients having space-occupying lesions also present with headache and altered mental status and may require a contrasted CT scan for detection. Brain tumors affect about 7 people per 100,000, with the highest incident occurring between the fifth and sixth decades. [46] Presentation may include headaches, focal neurologic findings, seizures, change in mental status, or acute psychiatric symptoms. Treatment of brain tumors with radiation or chemotherapeutic agents may also contribute to an altered mental status. [48]

Besides Alzheimer's and vascular disease, other progressive dementias include Parkinson's disease, Huntington's disease, progressive supranuclear palsy, amyotrophic lateral sclerosis, Kuf's disease, Creutzfeld-Jacob disease, HIV-related dementia, and postanoxic, post-traumatic, and postencephalitic dementias. Normal pressure hydrocephalus patients suffer from dementia, incontinence, and gait disorder. CT or MRI will reveal enlarged ventricles, especially in the area of the frontal horns, with alteration of the periventricular white matter. Lumbar puncture may lead to clinical improvement, and cerebrospinal fluid shunting can provide long-term reversal of symptoms. Other causes of treatable dementia include neurosyphylis, fungal infections, brain tumors, chronic alcoholism, and epilepsy.

Patients with hypertensive encephalopathy demonstrate extremely high blood pressure and altered mental status. A funduscopic examination frequently reveals papilledema. Acute myocardial infarction, congestive heart failure, and dysrhythmias are other cardiovascular causes of acutely altered mental status. Atrial fibrillation has been associated with a higher incidence of dementia, unrelated to the occurrence of cerebrovascular accidents.[49] Other common sources of infection and sepsis in the elderly are pneumonia and urinary tract infections. Fever may not be present, even with serious infections. Eighty percent of pneumonia-related deaths occur in the elderly.

A variety of metabolic and electrolyte disorders may disturb the level of consciousness, including renal or hepatic failure, dehydration, endocrinopathies, and malnutrition. Hypercalcemia is associated most commonly with malignancies or hyperparathyroidism. Mental status changes usually occur at levels over 14 mg/dL. One should consider hypocalcemia in renal failure patients, or following thyroid or parathyroid surgery. Hypercalcemia, hypocalcemia, and vitamin B12 deficiency can all cause a reversible dementia. Hypermagnesemia, seen in renal failure, or hypomagnesemia, found in malnourished patients or those on diuretics, may also alter mental status. Hyponatremia produces variable neurologic findings, depending on the rapidity of onset. The most common presentation of hypernatremia, generally accompanied by dehydration, is altered mental status. [50, 37]

Thyroid storm presents as fever, tachycardia, and delirium progressing to coma. Thyrotoxic patients are irritable, nervous, and often complain of fatigue. Reaction times are prolonged. Apathetic thyrotoxicosis in the elderly can mimic dementia or depression. Ophthalmopathy, bulbar palsies, and proximal muscle weakness can be further clues. Interestingly, hypothyroidism may manifest many of the same findings as hyperthyroidism, including fatigue, apathy, inattention, proximal muscle weakness, depression, and coma.

Myxedema madness describes the frank psychosis that may occur in up to 5% of hypothyroid patients. [13]

Major behavioral and cognitive changes occur in up to 25% of patients with hyperparathyroidism. In patients with hypoparathyroidism, 50% suffer intellectual impairment. Symptoms ranging from depression to psychosis accompany Cushing's syndrome (glucocorticoid excess) and Addison's disease (adrenal insufficiency). Both hyperglycemia (diabetic ketoacidosis, nonketotic hyperosmolar coma) and hypoglycemia cause severe alterations in mental Hypothermia and hyperthermia are common in environmental emergencies for the easily susceptible elderly person. Researching living conditions when extremes in climatic temperature are present may yield information on this.

Although society tends to believe that elderly people do not have substance problems, a surprisingly large number use both prescription drugs and illicit drugs abusively. A large number of elderly patients also misuse alcohol, perhaps owing to social isolation or difficulty in accepting life changes. These problems are generally well hidden by the patients and family and must be specifically addressed during the history. [41] Metabolic encephalopathy, infection, subdural hematoma, and withdrawal from addictive agents in the substance-abusing patient presenting with altered mental status should be considered. Autonomic signs of withdrawal may not be present in the elderly. [37, 40]

The mnemonic WHHHIMP (Wernicke's, hypoglycemia, hypertensive encephalopathy, hypoxia, intracerebral hemorrhage, meningitis, and poisoning) has been suggested to recall the life-threatening causes of altered mental status. [3]

Medication Adverse Effects and Polypharmacy

Prescribing for older patients presents unique challenges. Premarketing drug trials often exclude geriatric patients and approved doses may not be appropriate for older adults [51]. Many medications need to be used with special caution because of age-related changes in pharmacokinetics (i.e., absorption, distribution, metabolism, and excretion) and pharmacodynamics (the physiologic effects of the drug). Particular care must be taken in determining drug dosages when prescribing for older adults. An increased volume of distribution may result from the proportional increase in body fat relative to skeletal muscle with aging. Decreased drug clearance may result from the natural decline in renal function with age, even in the absence of renal disease [52]. Larger drug storage reservoirs and decreased clearance prolong drug half-lives and lead to increased plasma drug concentrations in older people.As examples, the volume of distribution for diazepam is increased, and the clearance rate for lithium is reduced, in older adults. The same dose of either medication would lead to higher plasma concentrations in an older, compared to younger, patient. Also, from the pharmacodynamic perspective, increasing age may result in an increased sensitivity to the effects of certain drugs, including benzodiazepines [53, 54] and opioids. [55]

Use of herbal or dietary supplements (e.g., ginseng, ginkgo biloba extract, and glucosamine) by older adults has been increasing, from 14 percent in older women in 1998 [56] to 26 to 27 percent in 2002 [57, 58] and 49 percent in 2006 [59]. Herbal medicines may interact with prescribed drug therapies and lead to adverse events, including altered mental status, underscoring the importance of routinely questioning patients about the use of unconventional therapies.

Polypharmacy is defined simply as the use of multiple medications by a patient which is an all too common finding in the older patient. Polypharmacy increases the possibility of "prescribing cascades" [60]. A prescribing cascade develops when an adverse drug event is misinterpreted as a new medical condition and additional drug therapy is then prescribed to treat this medical condition. The combination of side effects, decreased or altered metabolism, and drug interactions is a potential cause of anxiety, hallucinations, delirium, confusion, depression or psychosis. Many medical drugs may contribute to these symptoms. (Table 4) Benzodiazepines have been found to account for up to 29% of cases of cognitive impairment in elderly hospital inpatients. [61] Among narcotics, meperidine has been found to be the greatest offender, whereas hydromorphone is perhaps the least worrisome. [39]

The neuroleptic malignant syndrome is thought to occur with dopamine receptor blockade and can follow treatment with the high-potency neuroleptic agents such as haloperidol. The syndrome is unpredictable in its onset and course and can be lethal. Symptoms include muscular rigidity, dyskinesia, temperature elevation, and blood pressure fluctuations. Treatment includes the use of dopamine agonists such as bromocriptine, with dantrolene to control hyperthermia.

The patient suffering from lithium toxicity may present with altered mental status and coma; other symptoms include GI complaints, ataxia, and slurred speech. Dehydration, decreased renal function, and nonsteroidal anti-inflammatory (NSAID) use can precipitate acute toxicity. The emergency physician should search for evidence of chronic salicylate poisoning. Of note is that serum salicylate levels may be normal although CSF levels are high. Coma occurs frequently. The effects of anticholinergic toxicity include acute psychosis, which can be precipitated by a variety of prescription and over-the-counter (OTC) agents. Other symptoms of this toxidrome include tachycardia, dry mouth, decreased intestinal motility, urinary retention, vertigo, and increased intraocular pressure. [45]

The serotonin syndrome has been recognized increasingly over the last several years. Increased serotonin levels produce altered mental status, neuromuscular irritability, and autonomic instability. A variety of drug classes are associated with this syndrome, including the tricyclic antidepressants, monoamine oxidase (MAO) inhibitors, and most recently, the selective serotonin reuptake inhibitors. These agents are especially dangerous when combined with other drugs that affect serotonin metabolism. Although the serotonin syndrome tends to develop more quickly following drug initiation and has a milder course, there is a tremendous overlap with the symptoms of neuroleptic malignant syndrome. Muscle rigidity, tremor, hyperreflexia, and ataxia are common. Altered mental status is the most common symptom, occurring in 40% of patients. Hypertension and tachycardia are seen, although the patient may also be hypotensive. Fever is seen in 50% of cases, ranging from mild to elevations over 105°F. In severe cases, rhabdomyolysis and renal failure may result. Symptoms are generally self-limited and of brief duration, although ICU care may be required. The challenge is to recognize this disorder. [3, 62]

Various criteria have been developed by expert panels in Canada [63] and in the United States [64, 65] to assess the quality of prescribing practices and medication use in older adult individuals. The most widely used criteria for inappropriate medications are the Beers criteria. The 2012 revised *Beers criteria* are available through the American Geriatrics Society website.

In another approach, a *Drug Burden Index* has been modeled incorporating drugs with anticholinergic or sedative effects, total number of medications, and daily dosing [66, 67].

Table 4. Drugs commonly causing altered mental status

Analgesics	Dopamine Agonists
NSAID	Ropinirole
Salicylates	Amantadine
Opioids (esp. meperidine)	Bromocriptine
Anticholinergics	Levodopa
Atropine	Pergolide
Benztropine	Pramipexole
Diphenhydramine	
Scopolamine	Gastrointestinal agents
Trihexyphenidyl	Antiemetics
Corticosteroids	Antispasmodics
Antibiotics and antivirals	H-2 receptor blockers
Acyclovir	Loperamide
Aminoglycosides	Herbal preperations
Amphotericin B	Atropa belladonna extract
Antimalarials	Henbane
Cephalosporins	Mandrake
Cycloserine	Jimson weed
Fluoroquinolones	St. John's Wort
Isoniazid	Valerian
Interferon	Hypoglycemics
Linezolid	Hypnotics and sedatives
Macrolides	Barbiturates
Sulfonamids	Benzodiazepines
Rifampin	Muscle Relaxants
Penicillins	Baclofen
Nalidixic acid	Cyclobenzaprine
Metronidazole	Cardivascular and hypertension drugs
Anticonvulsants	Antiarrhythmics
Carbamazepine	Beta blockers
Levatiracetam	Clonidine
Phenytoin	Digoxin
Valproate	Diuretics
Vigabatrin	Methyldopa
Antidepressants	Other CNS-active agents
Mirtazapine	Disulfiram
SSRIs	Donepezil
Tricyclic antidepressants	Lithium
Thyroid hormones	Interleukin-2
	Phenothiazines

Psychiatric Conditions

Multiple medical problems may present masked as psychiatric conditions, mandating thorough physical and neurologic examinations in elderly patients with alteration in mental status. [3] Functional (psychiatric) changes in behavior (like depression and fugue states) can be difficult to distinguish from organic causes of behavioral changes. Depressive syndromes in the elderly can present with impairment in cognitive function, such as memory and concentration. [7] Medical conditions in the differential diagnosis of depression include Addison's disease, cirrhosis, paraneoplastic syndrome, diabetes, electrolyte disorders, renal failure, hypothyroidism and apathetic hyperthyroidism, and subdural hematomas. [41] A variety of medications effect depression, especially antihypertensives, digoxin, and cimetidine. One should be wary of lithium toxicity in bipolar patients. Major life changes (e.g., moving, retiring, death of someone close) that prompt short-term stress or grief reactions may cause a progressive and disabling depression in elderly people. A psychiatric examination may be necessary to exclude depression, anxiety, delusions, hallucinations, and psychosis. Auditory hallucinations suggest a psychiatric condition, whereas visual and other sensory hallucinations represent an organic brain disorder. In general, psychiatric disorders make their initial presentation prior to the age of 40 years. Psychiatric history must be included with all elderly patients. Components of the psychiatric examination include appearance and grooming, speech patterns (pressured or slowed), mood and affect, association of ideas (loose associations, tangential thought), and the mental status examination. [68] Thorough evaluation of a patient for delirium before diagnosing a psychiatric illness is essential. [69] Psychiatric symptoms such as depression will often coexist with chronic disease process such as dementia. [70]

Acute Management of Elderly with Altered Mental Status

Patients with a markedly altered mental status require rapid assessment of the ABCs and appropriate intervention (Table 5). [3] Acute neurologic catastrophes such as subdural hematoma, subarachnoid hemorrhage, or coma from metabolic conditions or drug ingestions may need airway management through rapid sequence intubation. Endotracheal intubation will promote oxygenation, facilitate hyperventilation and hypocapnia, reduce aspiration risk, and protect the airway. If there is a suggestion of elevated intracranial pressure, one should use lidocaine pretreatment, defasciculating doses of paralytics prior to the use of succinylcholine, and other agents (e.g., sodium pentothal) to prevent further pressure increases during intubation. Cervical spine injury precautions must be maintained if trauma is suspected. One should monitor the patient with pulse oximetry and provide supplemental oxygen as indicated.

Placing the patient on a cardiac monitor, one should then establish two large-bore IV lines and determine all vital signs, including a core temperature. Blood should be drawn and an electrocardiogram performed. A portable chest radiograph may be necessary unless the patient is determined to be stable enough to proceed to radiology after the initial assessment.

The physician should administer naloxone to a patient with a possible narcotic overdose. Initial doses up to 10 mg may be required to reverse some agents effectively (e.g., propoxyphene). Meperidine or diphenoxylate overdoses may not exhibit the classic sign of miosis. Rapid bedside glucose determination should be done but glucose should not be given routinely unless this testing is unavailable, and hyperglycemia will worsen cellular damage in acute cerebrovascular accidents. If glucose is required, D50 administration should be preceded by thiamin (100 mg IV) to avoid precipitating Wemicke's encephalopathy.

One should maintain a broad differential diagnosis, considering sepsis and meningitis in the elderly even in the absence of fever. Examine the patient for evidence of any toxidromes, treating any overdoses with GI decontamination and specific antidotes as indicated. Pertinent medication history can be obtained from family, nursing home personnel, or caretakers, prehospital personnel, or medical records in the search for causes of the patient's condition.

Table 5. Initial evaluation and disposition

Assess ABCs skin color, temperature and level of consciousness
Neck immobilization (if there is suspicious of trauma)
Chief complaint, history and physical examination
Initial diagnostic studies
Pulse oximetry
Glucose
ECG
Electrolytes
CBC
Renal (BUN/Cr)
Urinalysis
CXR
Additional tests as needed based on initial evaluation
CT of head
LP
Coagulation studies
ABG
Liver and thyroid function tests
Toxicologic screen
Drug levels
Carboxyhemoglobin
Ammonia level
Selected cultures
Selected X-rays
Further testing in selected patients
MRI
EEG
VDRL
HIV
Vitamin B12/folate
ANA
Disposition: Most patients need to be admitted

Rapid evaluation of the need for CT of the brain, lumbar puncture, cultures, and antibiotic administration is essential. If meningitis or sepsis is suspected, antibiotic administration must not be delayed for CT, X-ray, or laboratory test results. Any drug allergies should be checked for, and broad-spectrum antibiotics with CSF penetration administered. Initial fluid boluses for hypotension or dehydration should be given, with the patient monitored closely for the onset of congestive heart failure. Initiate pressor agents, such as dopamine, early if blood pressure support is indicated.

Judicious management of hypertension is necessary because elderly patients often need some degree of elevated blood pressures to ensure adequate cerebral flow, and reduction therapy may interfere with the autoregulation of blood flow to the brain. If possible, one should try to determine the patient's preinsult blood pressures. Nitroprusside and close monitoring should be used to treat hypertensive encephalopathy. Calcium channel blockage to prevent arterial spasm in the subarachnoid hemorrhage patient also should be initiated. [3]

Management of Agitated or Violent Elderly Patient

In general, nonpharmacologic strategies should be used in all agitated delirious patients. These include reorientation, encouraging the presence of family members as a stabilizing presence, and transferring the patient t o a private room or to a room closer to the nursing station for supervision. A skilled and sensitive staff can be vitally important in optimizing communication by using frequent verbal reorientation strategies, simple instruction and explanations. [73] Sensory deficits should be corrected by ensuring that assistive devices (eyeglasses, hearing aids etc.) are available, functioning and in use. All attempts should be made to minimize the use of physical restraints because they tend to worsen delirium and can aggravate or cause agitation. Improving sleep in the delirious, agitated older person is an important intervention. Coordination of the timing of medications, vital signs, and procedures may be required to achieve the uninterrupted period of sleep. [72]

Owing to the increased likelihood of side effects to all medications, changes in metabolism, and potential drug interactions in the elderly, it is prudent to avoid medication use when possible. Given that all medications used in the treatment of agitation, can also cause or worsen confusion, a general principle is to use the lowest dose possible and for the shortest period of time. The end point should be an awake and manageable patient, not a sedated patient. [71] If required, short-acting agents are preferred.

Benzodiazepines are ideal for the treatment of alcohol and sedative drug withdrawal and agitation, but they are not recommended in the primary treatment of agitation in elder persons because they may cause oversedation and exacerbation of confusion and agitation. Lorazepam has a short duration of action and is the preferred agent (0.5 mg IV, IM, or PO). Haloperidol (2.5-5.0 mg IV or IM initially) is the antipsychotic of choice when stronger tranquilization is required. Other lower-potency neuroleptics have a higher incidence of side effects (e.g., hypotension and anticholinergic effects). Haloperidol does have a higher incidence of dystonic reactions. D2-dopaminergic receptors are saturated at low dose of haloperidol. Thus, theoretically, any additional haloperidol above 5 mg over a 24 hour period is only likely to increase adverse events without providing additional clinical benefit. New, atypical neuroleptics also used in the management of agitation and delirium include risperidone, olanzapine and quetiapine; however, no sufficient comparative trials are available. Droperidol, with a higher potency, quicker onset, and reportedly fewer extrapyramidal effects, serves as an alternative to haloperidol. [39]

REFERENCES

[1] Zheng, A.: Altered Mental Status in the Elderly: Neurologic Nightmares. American College of Emergency Physicians. Scientific Assembly, Las Vegas, 2010

[2] Morrissey, T. The Approach to altered mental status. CDEM Self-Study Modules. http://www.cdemcurriculum.org/ssm/approach_to/ams.php

[3] O'Keefe, K., Sanson, T. Elderly patients with altered mental status. *Emerg Med Clin of North Am* 16: 701-715, 1998.

[4] Bauer J, Roberts MR, Reisdorff EJ: Evaluation of behavioral and cognitive changes: The mental status examination. *Emerg Med Clin North Am* 9:l-12, 1991

[5] Drachman DA, Swearer JM Screening for dementia: Cognitive Assessment Screening Test (CAST). *Am Fam Physician* 541957-1963, 1996

[6] Early Identification of Alzheimer's Disease and Related Dementia's Panel: Clinical Practice Guidelines: Early identification of Alzheimer's disease and related dementias. *Am Fam Physician* 55:1303-1314, 1997

[7] Folstein MF Differential diagnosis of dementia: The clinical process. *Psychiatr Clin North Am* 20: 45-57,1997

[8] Friedl W, Schmidt R, Stronigger WJ, et al: Mini-Mental State Examination: Influence of sociodemographic, environmental and behavioral factors and vascular risk factors. *J Clin Epidemiol* 49:73-78,1996

[9] Geldmacher DS, Whitehouse PJ: Evaluation of dementia. *N Engl J Med* 335:330-336,1996

[10] Inouye SK, van Dyck CHG, Alessi CA, et al: Clarifying confusion: The confusion assessment method: A new method for detection of delirium. *Ann Intern Med* 113: 941-948, 1994

[11] Juva K, Sulkava R, Erkinjuntti T, et al. Usefulness of the Clinical Dementia Rating scale in screening for dementia. *Psychogeriatrics* 7:17-24, 1995

[12] Kawas C, et al.: A validation study of the Dementia Questionnaire. *Arch Neurol* 51:901:906, 1994

[13] Schmitt FA, Ranseen JD, DeKosky ST: Cognitive mental status examinations. *Clin Geriatric Med* 5:545-564,1989

[14] Sturmann K: The neurologic examination. *Emerg Med Clin North Am* 15:491-506,1997

[15] Bunney EB: Altered Mental Status in the Elderly: Neurologic Nightmares. American College of Emergency Physicians. Scientific Assembly, 2008

[16] Breteler MM, Claus JJ, Grobbee DE, et al: Cardiovascular disease and distribution of cognitive function in elderly people: The Rotterdam study. *Br Med J* 1994;308:1604-1608,

[17] Francis J, Young GB: Diagnosis of delirium and confusional states. UpTo Date, 2012.

[18] Hamill RW, Pilgrim D Geriatric Neurology. In Bradley WG, Daroff RB, Fenichel GM, et al. (eds): *Neurology in Clinical Practice,* vol 2. Boston, Butterworth-Heinemann, 1996, pp 2077-2090

[19] Hufschmidt A, Shabarin V.: Diagnostic yield of cerebral imaging in patients with acute confusion. *Acta Neurol Scand* 2008; 118:245

[20] Salerno D, Marik PE, Daskalakis C, et al. The role of head computer tomographic scans on the management of MICU patients with neurological dysfunction. *J Intensive Care Med.* 2009;24(6):372

[21] Naughton BJ, Moran M, Ghaly Y, Michalakes C. Computed tomography scanning and delirium in elder patients. *Acad Emerg Med.* 1997;4(12):1107.

[22] Morandi A, Gunther ML, Vasilevskis, at al. Neuroimaging in delirious intensive care unit patients: a preliminary case series report. *Psychiatry* (Edgmont). 2010;7(9):28.

[23] Warshaw G, Tanzer F The effectiveness of lumbar puncture in the evaluation of delirium and fever in the hospitalized elderly. *Arch Fam Med.* 1993;2(3):293.

[24] Metersky ML, Williams A, Rafanan AL Retrospective analysis: are fever and altered mental status indications for lumbar puncture in a hospitalized patient who has not undergone neurosurgery? *Clin Infect Dis.* 1997;25(2):285.

[25] Jacobson SA, Leuchter AF, Walter DO, Weiner H. Serial quantitative EEG among elderly subjects with delirium. *Biol Psychiatry.* 1993;34(3):135.

[26] Hemphill JC. Disorders of consciousness in systemic diseases. In: Neurology and general medicine, Aminoff, MJ (Ed), *Churchill Livingstone*, 2001. p.1053.

[27] Privitera M, Hoffman M, Moore JL, Jester D. EEG detection of nontonic-clonic status epilepticus in patients with altered consciousness. *Epilepsy Res* 1994; 18:155

[28] Claassen J, Mayer SA, Kowalski RG, Emerson RG, Hirsch LJ Detection of electrographic seizures with continuous EEG monitoring in critically ill patients. *Neurology.* 2004;62(10):1743

[29] Fisch BJ, Klass DW The diagnostic specificity of triphasic wave patterns. *Electroencephalogr Clin Neurophysiol.* 1988;70(1):1.

[30] Young GB Metabolic and inflammatory cerebral diseases: electrophysiological aspects. *Can J Neurol Sci.* 1998;25(1):S16.

[31] Sheth RD, Drazkowski JF, Sirven JI, et al. Protracted ictal confusion in elderly patients. *Arch Neurol.* 2006;63(4):529.

[32] Schneider SM: Altered mental status in the elderly: Current assessment and management strategies for a complex clinical syndrome. *EM Reports* 1743-53, 1996

[33] American Psychiatric Association Diagnostic and Statistical Manual, 4th ed, APA Pres, Washington DC, 1994.

[34] Shadlen,MF, Larson EB, Uptodate (2012).Evaluation of cognitive impairment and dementia http://www.uptodate.com/contents/evaluation-of-cognitive-impairment-and-dementia.

[35] Knopman DS, DeKosky ST, Cummings JL, et al. Practice parameter: diagnosis of dementia (an evidence-based review). Report of the Quality Standards Subcommittee of the American Academy of Neurology. *Neurology.* 2001;56(9):1143.

[36] Petersen RC, Stevens JC, Ganguli M, et al. Practice parameter: early detection of dementia: mild cognitive impairment (an evidence-based review). Report of the Quality Standards Subcommittee of the American Academy of Neurology. *Neurology.* 2001;56(9):1133.

[37] Landefeld, CS, Palmer RM et al. Current Geriatric diagnosis and treatment. 2nd edition, McGraw Hill, New York 2004, p.53

[38] Inouye SK. The dilemma of delirium: Clinical and research controversies regarding diagnosis and evaluation of delirium in hospitalized elderly medical patients. *Am J Med* 97278-288, 1994

[39] Jacobson SA: Delirium in the elderly. *Psychiatr Clin North Am* 2091-110,1997

[40] Francis J: Delirium. In Cassel CK, Cohen HT, Larson ET, et al (eds): Geriatric Medicine, ed 3. New York, *Springer,* 1996, pp 917-922

[41] Greenstein RA, Ness DE Psychiatric emergencies in the elderly. *Emerg Med Clin North Am* 8:429-441,1990

[42] Johnson JC: Delirium in the elderly. *Emerg Med Clin North Am* 8:255-265, 1990

[43] Bross MH, Tatum NO Delirium in the elderly patient. *Am Fam Physician* 50:1325-1332, 1994

[44] Kalbfleisch N Altered mental status. In Sanders AB (ed): Emergency Care of the Elder Person. St. Louis, Beverly Cracom Publications, 1996

[45] Kennedy GJ, Lowinger R Psychogeriatric emergencies. *Geriatric Emergency Care* 9:641-653,1993

[46] Araiza J, Araiza B: Neuroimaging. *Emerg Med Clin North Am* 15:507-526, 1997

[47] Wiley CA: Pathology of neurologic diseases in AIDS. *Psychiatr Clin North Am* 17:1-15, 1994

[48] Newton HB, Shah SM Neurological syndromes and emergencies in the cancer patients: Differential diagnosis, assessment protocols, and targeted clinical interventions. *EM Reports* 18:150-158,1997

[49] Ott A, Breteler MB, de Bruyne MC, et al. Atrial fibrillation and dementia in a population- based study: The Rotterdam study. *Stroke* 28:316-321,1997

[50] Riggs JE Neurologic manifestations of fluid and electrolyte disturbances. *Neurologic Clinics* 7:509-525, 1989

[51] Cho S, Lau SW, Tandon V, et al.Geriatric drug evaluation: where are we now and where should we be in the future? *Arch Intern Med.* 2011;171(10):937.

[52] Rowe JW, Andres R, Tobin JD, et al.The effect of age on creatinine clearance in men: a cross-sectional and longitudinal study. *J Gerontol.* 1976;31(2):155.

[53] Reidenberg MM, Levy M, Warner H, Coutinho CB, et al. Relationship between diazepam dose, plasma level, age, and central nervous system depression. *Clin Pharmacol Ther.* 1978;23(4):371

[54] Herings RM, Stricker BH, de Boer A, Bakker A, Sturmans F Benzodiazepines and the risk of falling leading to femur fractures. Dosage more important than elimination half-life. *Arch Intern Med.* 1995;155(16):1801.

[55] Scott JC, Stanski DR Decreased fentanyl and alfentanil dose requirements with age. A simultaneous pharmacokinetic and pharmacodynamic evaluation. *J Pharmacol Exp Ther.* 1987;240(1):159.

[56] Kaufman DW, Kelly JP, Rosenberg L, et al. Recent patterns of medication use in the ambulatory adult population of the United States: the Slone survey. *JAMA.* 2002;287(3):337

[57] Kelly JP, Kaufman DW, Kelley K, Rosenberg L, Anderson TE, Mitchell AA Recent trends in use of herbal and other natural products. *Arch Intern Med.* 2005;165(3):281.

[58] Nahin RL, Fitzpatrick AL, Williamson JD, et al. Use of herbal medicine and other dietary supplements in community-dwelling older people: Baseline data from the ginkgo evaluation of memory study. *J Am Geriatr Soc.* 2006;54(11):1725.

[59] Qato DM, Alexander GC, Conti RM, et al.Use of prescription and over-the-counter medications and dietary supplements among older adults in the United States. *JAMA.* 2008;300(24):2867

[60] Rochon PA, Gurwitz JH Optimising drug treatment for elderly people: the prescribing cascade. *BMJ.* 1997;315(7115):1096.
[61] Foy A, OConnel D, Henry D, et al. Benzodiazepine use as a cause of cognitive impairment in elderly hospital inpatients. *J Gerontol* 1995;50:99-106
[62] LoCurto MJ: The serotonin syndrome. *Emerg Med Clin North Am* 15:665-675, 1997.
[63] McLeod PJ, Huang AR, Tamblyn RM, Gayton DC Defining inappropriate practices in prescribing for elderly people: a national consensus panel. *CMAJ.* 1997;156(3):385.
[64] Beers MH, Ouslander JG, Rollingher I, Reuben DB, Brooks J, Beck JC Explicit criteria for determining inappropriate medication use in nursing home residents. UCLA Division of Geriatric Medicine. *Arch Intern Med.* 1991;151(9):1825.
[65] Knight EL, Avorn J Quality indicators for appropriate medication use in vulnerable elders. *Ann Intern Med.* 2001;135:703.
[66] Hilmer SN, Mager DE, Simonsick EM, et al. A drug burden index to define the functional burden of medications in older people. *Arch Intern Med.* 2007;167(8):781.
[67] Hilmer SN, Mager DE, Simonsick EM,et al. Drug burden index score and functional decline in older people. *Am J Med.* 2009;122(12):1142.
[68] Landefeld, CS, Palmer RM et al. Current Geriatric diagnosis and treatment. 2nd edition, McGraw Hill, New York 2004, p.100
[69] Farrell KR, Ganzini L. Misdiagnosing delirium as depression in medically ill elderly patients. *Arch Intern Med* 155:2459-2464, 1995
[70] Lundquist RS, Bernens A, Olsen CG: Comorbid disease in geriatric patients: Dementia and depression. *Am Fam Physician* 55:2687-2694, 1997
[71] American Psychiatric Association: Practice guideline for the treatment of patients with delirium. *Am J Psychiatry* 1999; 156 (5 suppl).
[72] McDowell JA et al. A non-pharmacological sleep protocol for hospitalized older patients. *J Am Geriatr Soc* 1998; 46:700.
[73] Millisen K et al. A nurse-led interdisciplinary intervention program for delirium in elderly hip-fracture patients. *J Am Geriatr Soc* 2001,; 49:523.

In: New Horizons in Geriatric Medicine. Volume 1
Editors: Ahmet Turan Isik, M. Refik Mas et al.
ISBN: 978-1-62808-972-1

Chapter 8

DIZZINESS AND BALANCE PROBLEMS

Habib Hashemi

ABSTRACT

- Presbystasis and falling are major disasters in geriatric patients.
- The proportion of geriatric population is increasing and so are their medical expenditures.
- The causes of dizziness and falling in elderly patients are different than other age groups, and are mainly non-vestibular disorders.
- The main vestibular cause of dizziness and vertigo in elderly patients is benign paroxysmal pozisyonel vertigo.
- Dizziness accounted for one third of all visits to the primary care physician in patients over the age of 65 years.
- More than half of all elderly falls occur in the home.
- The ideal testing modality in evaluating age-related balance loss and risk factors is Computer Dynamic Posturography.
- There are many exercise protocols for vestibular balance rehabilitation therapy.

INTRODUCTION

Falls are one of the most common concerns relating to imbalance in geriatric patients. The medical costs of fall-related injuries totaled $19 billion in 2000. Moreover, falls lead to functional decline, anxiety, depression, and social withdrawal [1].

In humans and animals the vestibular systems (peripheral and central) primarily drives reflexes to maintain stable vision and posture. This important function is done by coordination between the three primary sensory systems including somatosensory, vestibular and visual systems with cerebellum, upper central brain system, spinal cord and musculoskeletal systems. These primary sensory systems provide information throughout the peripheral and central vestibular systems. Information is then compared and coordinated to the memory of central nervous system and spatial maps.

In order to maintain balance and perform activities such as walking or taking a glass of water, areas of the cortex develop a coordinated response to the different neuromusculo-skeletal systems.

As we age, there are some physiological changes in all parts of the body that gradually limit the ability to react quickly to perturbations. Weakness in the core stabilizing muscles, altered muscle activation patterns, loss of neurons in the vestibular nucleus, loss of proprioception and the inability to control normal postural sway are present. Aging also causes the inability to perform balance-sensitive physical activities like playing tennis. On the other hand social factors, such as the loss of a spouse, or changes in the living environment, can lead to further inactivity, degrading a person's ability to maintain balance.

All of these are normal physiological age related changes and social factors affecting the balance systems, occurring in every older population. But, there are also a large number of geriatric balance diseases and most of them are multifactorial. Cardiovascular, neurologic diseases, medications, joint diseases and low back pain cause degradation of the coordination between the three primary sensory systems (somatosensory, vestibular and visual systems) used in balance so that most of the balance disorders result from multiple system defects (Fig. 1).

In one study on patients older than 65 years, dizziness accounted for one third of all visits to the primary care physician and the most common complaint for those older than 75 years [2]. Since dizziness can lead to falls with serious consequences in the geriatric population, diagnosis of the underlying causes and directed therapy is mandatory [3]. Symptoms of imbalance in older populations mostly develop gradually over a number of years. This is a gradual onset of developing balance disorders in the elderly.

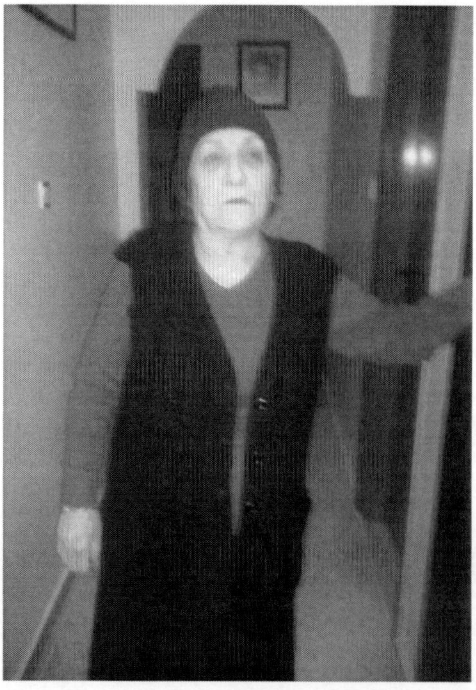

Figure 1. An 87-year old woman having coronary artery diseases, hypertension, and arthritis with typical dizziness and balance problems during walking.

Fear of falling results in a disproportionate reduction in quality of life for the elderly, and includes more visits to physicians and serious problems for the family of geriatric patients. More than half of all elderly falls occur in the home. The most common site of falls is the bedroom, mainly getting into or out of bed.

Anatomic and Neurophysiologic Basis of Vestibular and Balance System:

The vestibular system, being a very old system phylogenetically, has diffuse connections with the central nervous system. The main function of this system is to sense head movements, especially involuntary ones, and counter them with reflexive eye movements and postural adjustments that keep the visual world stable and keep us from falling.

It is important to consider the vestibular apparatus as two systems, right and left, with constant dynamic balance, one checking the other side, working as a team. They are complete systems from end organ to cortex, and do not work as two isolated end organs, each on one side.

The vestibular apparatus is enclosed within a bony labyrinth, the vestibule, in the petrous portion of the temporal bone. These vestibular end organs include three semicircular canals, each oriented in a different plane, and two maculae, one roughly in the horizontal plane (the utriculus) and one in the vertical plane (the sacculus). There are two vertical semicircular canals, the anterior (also known as the superior) and posterior canals, and one horizontal (also known as the lateral) canal. The vertical canals are oriented roughly at 45 degrees in relation to the sagittal plane, and the horizontal canal is tilted upward about 30 degrees anteriorly from the horizontal plane [4]. (Fig. 2) The three semicircular canals of the labyrinth are roughly orthogonal to each other, so that one labyrinth can sense any rotation in the three-dimensional space. Canals in the two labyrinths are arranged in complementary, coplanar pairs [5].

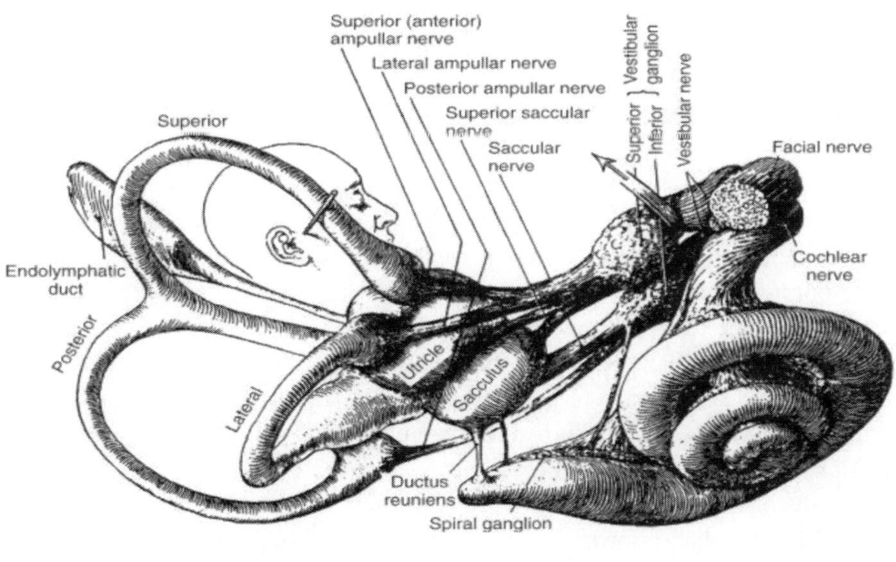

Figure 2. Vestibular end organs anatomy.

(From Brodel M. Three Unpublished Drawings of the Anatomy of the Human Ear. Philadelphia: WB Saunders; 1946.)

The five vestibular end organs, along with the cochlea, are contained within an endolymph-filled membranous labyrinth (the endolymphatic space), which is contained in the perilymph-filled bony labyrinth (the perilymphatic space) (Fig .3). The vestibule is situated between the internal auditory meatus anteromedially and the middle ear cavity laterally [4].

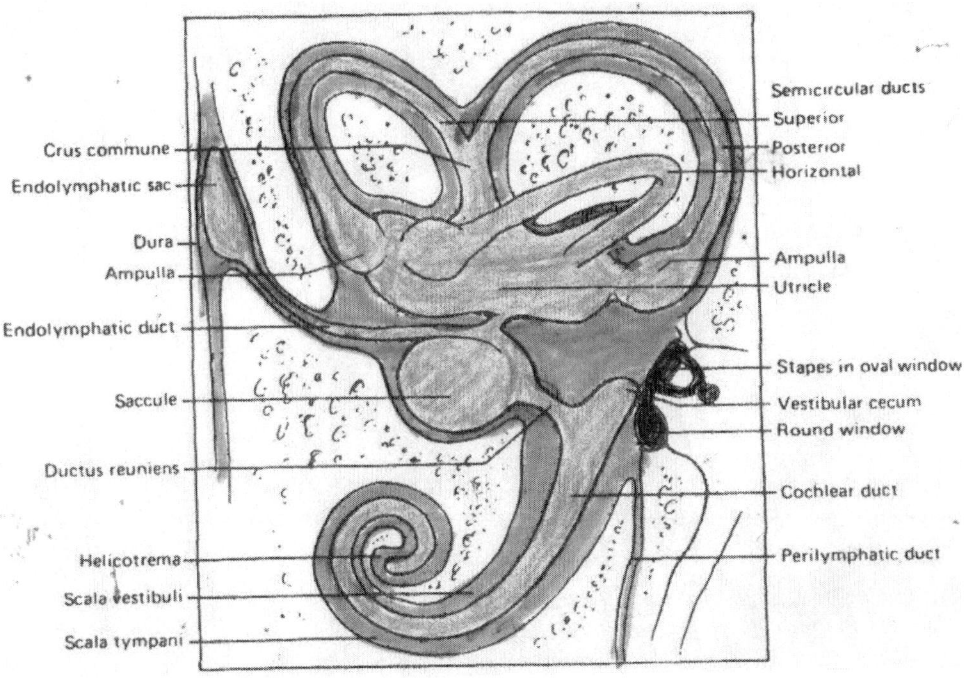

Figure 3. Membranous labyrinth (red color) situated within bony labyrinth (yellow color). Note crus commune, a duct shared by superior (anterior) and posterior ducts. Note also the endolymphatic duct originating as fusion of the utricular duct and saccular duct, and the ductus reuniens connecting vestibular apparatus with cochlear duct (uncoiled in this diagram).

(Modified from Kandel ER, Schwartz JW. Principles of Neural Science. 2nd ed. New York: Elsevier Science; 1985.)

The overall sensational work of semicircular canals: When the head accelerates in the plane of one semicircular canal, inertia causes the endolymph in the canal to lag behind the motion of the membranous canal. Relative to the canal walls, the endolymph effectively moves in the opposite direction as the head. Inside the ampulla, a swelling at the end of the canal where it meets the utricle, pressure exerted by endolymph deflects the cupula, an elastic membrane that spans a cross-section of the ampulla [6]. Vestibular hair cells are arrayed beneath the cupula on the surface of the crista ampullaris, a saddle-shaped neuroepithelium. Hair cells and stereociliary bundle activation create electrical stimulation with their synaptic afferent vestibular first order neurons [7].

The hair cells of the labyrinth of the vestibular end organ senses head rotation and linear acceleration and send that information to secondary vestibular neurons in the brainstem vestibular nuclei. There, these afferent neurons are distributed to other areas of the central nervous system to drive vestibular reflexes. Specifically, neurons encoding head movement form synapses within the ocular motor nuclei to elicit the patterns of the extraocular muscle contraction and relaxation needed for the vestibulo-ocular reflex (VOR), which stabilizes gaze (eye position in space). Other secondary vestibular neurons synapse on cervical spinal motor neurons to generate the vestibulocolic reflex (VCR), or to lower spinal motor neurons to generate the vestibulospinal reflexes (VSRs). These reflexes stabilize posture and facilitate gait. Vestibular sensory input to autonomic centers, particularly information about posture with respect to gravity, is used to adjust hemodynamic reflexes to maintain cerebral perfusion. Finally, vestibular input to the cerebellum is essential for coordination and adaptation of vestibular reflexes when changes occur such as injury to a vestibular end organ or alteration in vision (e.g., a new pair of glasses) [8, 9, 10, 11] Fig. (4, 5).

Each semicircular canal crista is stimulated by rotation in its plane in one direction and is inhibited by rotation in its plane in the opposite direction.

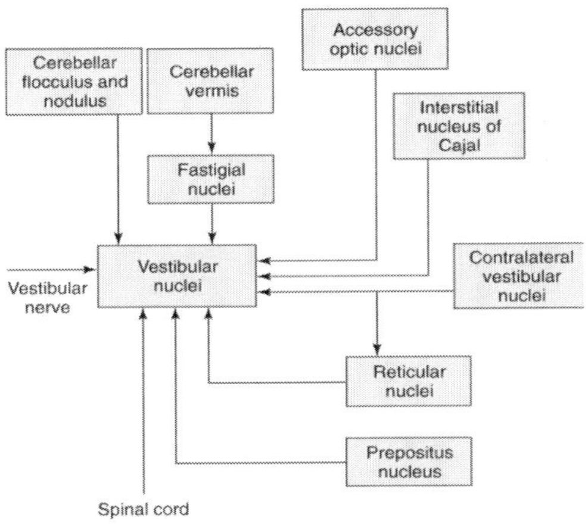

Figure 4. Afferent pathways to vestibular nuclei.

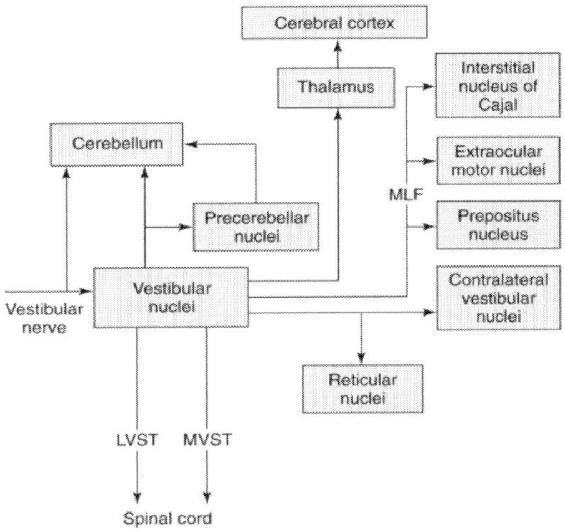

Figure 5. Efferent connections of vestibular nuclei.

Schematic courtesy of Robert McCrea (Cummings Otolaryngology-Head & Neck Surgery, 2010, MOSBY.

All vestibular receptors are tonically active. A resting, spontaneous, continual outflow of action potentials from the vestibular portion of the eighth cranial nerve has been recognized. With head motion, this spontaneous activity is modulated up or down. For example, turning the head to the right in the upright position produces an increase in activity in the nerve coming from the right horizontal semicircular canal, whereas left turns decrease activity below the resting rate from the same canal.

These paired labyrinths (one in each ear) behave in a "push-pull" fashion. The CNS compares the inputs coming from both ears. When the inputs are equal, the system is balanced, with no sense of movement. When inputs are asymmetrical, the CNS interprets this finding as a head rotation and as a result generates compensatory eye movements and postural adjustments, all of which lead to a conscious sensation relative to the perceived movement of the head [12] (Fig.6).

Of great importance, the CNS is capable of rebalancing itself—that is, compensating after an injury to the peripheral receptor. This compensation is thought to occur as a result of the organism's ability to compare other sensory, visual, and kinesthetic inputs to vestibular input.

The reflexive nature of the vestibular system is central to understanding vestibular pathophysiology.

The brainstem interprets imbalances in vestibular input due to pathologic processes in the same way that it interprets imbalances due to physiologic stimuli. Therefore, the cardinal signs of vestibular disorders are reflexive eye movements and postural changes. These reflexive signs can largely be understood as the brainstem's responses to perceived rotation around a specific axis or perceived tilting or translation of the head, even though the head is still and upright [7]. Vestibular signals also reach cortical areas to mediate the perception of movement and orientation. Nevertheless, the common head movements of everyday life usually go unnoticed, which is why the vestibular sensation is not included among the vernacular "five senses"—sight, smell, taste, touch, and hearing. Yet the loss of vestibular sensation causes distinct and often severe symptoms [13].

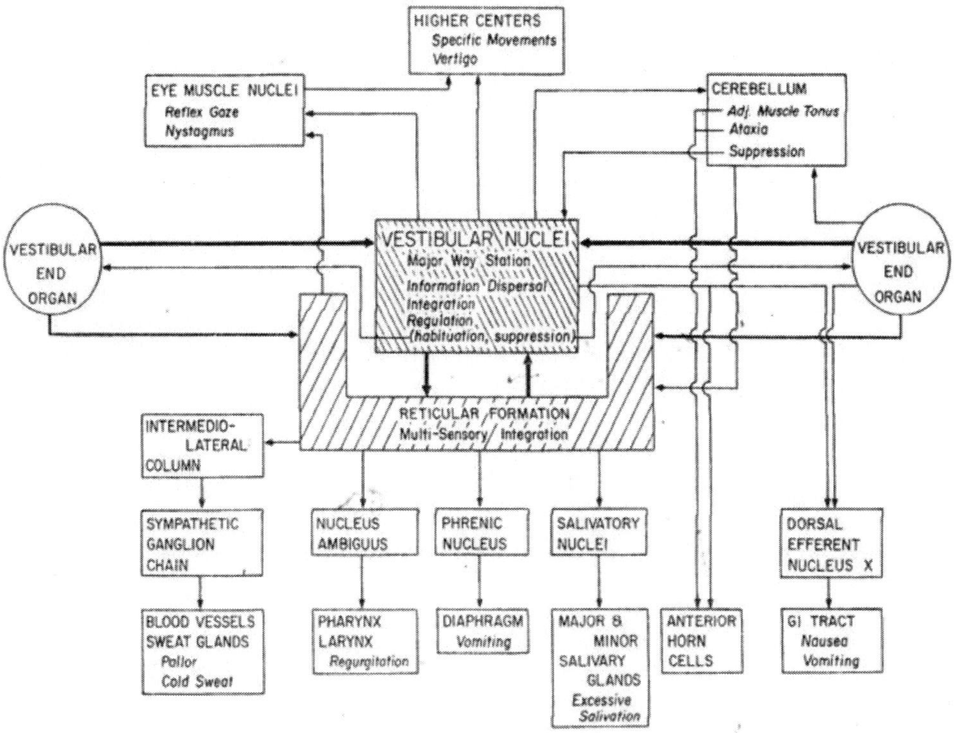

Figure 6: Schematic representation of some of the more important peripheral and central connections of vestibular nerve.

Otolaryngology/ edited by M. Paparella, 3rd ed. W.B. Saunders Company.

With the normal aging process, humans experience changes in the sensory systems, the central and peripheral nervous system, and in muscles and joints. These multisystem losses affect the functions necessary for balance [14]. Many older patients also cease to exercise; therefore, their muscle strength, proprioceptive, sensory receptors, and joint flexibility diminish. The combination of all these processes eventually culminates in a person who has difficulty with rapid movements, is slower with normal locomotion, and who develops a fear of falling and the consequences of falling and the related injuries. Reflex time decreases in the elderly, which further increases the risk of falling.

Factors Affecting Balance

Subjective orientation of the body in space is controlled by a complicated system that includes the following: The eye muscles, the proprioceptive system, the labyrinth (semicircular canals and utricle), cranial nerve VIII, the vestibular nuclei in the brain stem, the neural pathways from the vestibular nuclei to the midbrain and to the temporal bone (medial longitudinal fasciculus), the central coordinating mechanism in the cerebellum, the vestibulospinal tract (posterior columns), the afferent fibers coming from muscles and joints to the posterior columns, the end-organ of equilibrium (semicircular canals and utricles, vestibular division of cranial nerve VIII, and vestibular nuclei) [15].

Through the normal human aging process, changes occur in the sensory system, in muscles and joints, the peripheral and the central nervous system. Also, social factors such as changing in living environment, the risk of developing other diseases, gradually developing self-imposed limitation of physical activities, degradation in the visual system; all are factors for older adults causing a decrease in the vestibulo-ocular reflexes and postural control.

Most elderly patients who have balance disorders complain of dizziness or light-headedness. This leads to referrals to otolaryngologists or neurologists. In many cases, loss of balance and falling is complicated by multisensory deficits and central nervous system malfunction. To properly evaluate and manage these patients, the otolaryngologist must go beyond the usual head and neck examination and evaluate all the sensory systems that contribute to balance.

Pathophysiology

The normal process of aging affects all parts of the ear, but the greatest clinical impact is on cochlear and vestibular function [16]. Degeneration related to age has been noted in hair cells, neurons, and supporting structures of the cochlear and peripheral vestibular systems. Presbycusis, which is the loss of hearing that is associated with aging, is the most common type of auditory dysfunction. The normal changes associated with aging in the vestibular system are a reduction in the sensitivity of the semicircular canals, a decrease in the total number of peripheral vestibular neurons, and a decrease in the size of myelinated nerve fibers; these changes have been described in patients that are more than 65 years old. These changes, in the cells of the sensory epithelium, a decline in the number of first-order neurons bringing information to the vestibular nucleus, degeneration of the synaptic structures of the vestibular afferent dendrites and the cerebellum, are all age-related physiologic changes. The utricular and saccular maculae seem to be less affected. Due to the degeneration of the vestibular, proprioceptive, and visual senses, the ability to walk and drive can be reduced to the point of incapacitation; lessening spatial-orientation abilities contribute to this as well. Loss of balance is the most common manifestation of vestibular dysfunction in older adults.

Causes of Dizziness and Balance Disorders in Geriatric Patients

There are many disorders and diseases causing dizziness and vertigo in humans, such as post traumatic, otitis media, ototoxicity, panic disorders, orthostatic hypotension, mal de'barquement, motion sickness, myelopathy, and benign paroxysmal vertigo.

Falls and balance problems are more important for older populations because they are more susceptible to falls; it is a common source of morbidity and mortality for them. Falls are more common in women than men. In older patients the cause of the falling and balance disorder can be a primary disorder of the vestibular end organ or disorder of the other organ systems, especially the cardiovascular and non-vestibular neurologic systems. Sloane points out that most dizziness is non-vestibular. Vascular diseases represent the most common non-vestibular cause of balance loss and dizziness in the elderly. Small vessel ischemic disease, usually a result of small vessel atherosclerosis, is the most common cause of these.

The main responsibility of the physician is primarily to rule out life threatening causes of dizziness such as a cardiac arrhythmia or brain stem stroke, then narrowing the list of diagnoses to the most probable etiology, and then optimizing treatment:

I) Main non-vestibular causes of dizziness that may be encountered in elderly patients are:

- Life threatening: Cardiac arrhythmia, cardiac failure, shock
- Serious cause: Anemia, vertebrobasillary insufficiency, orthostatic hypotension related to use of antihypertensive therapy, prolonged bed-rest, cerebellar infarction, central lesions like brain tumors, degenerative disorders.
- Diseases affecting mobility of patients: Muscle weakness, dysequilibrium caused by alcohol and some medications like sedatives, chronic degenerative disease

Orthostatic Hypotension: Orthostatic hypotension is a particularly common cause of non-vestibular dizziness in the elderly. The venous system in healthy adults contains a ''reservoir'' of 0.3–0.8 L of blood. When additional volume is required to maintain perfusion pressure, blood from this pool is added to the circulating volume by muscle contraction. Minimal changes in arterial pressure, primarily sensed by baroreceptors in the aorta and carotid arteries, increase the sympathetic tone to maintain cerebral perfusion regardless of body position. A variety of factors can lead to significant slowing of this response in the elderly. The resultant temporary reduction in cerebral perfusion results in a number of symptoms such as light-headedness, true vertigo, blurring of vision or other visual changes, tremulousness, palpitations, cognitive dysfunction, or frank loss of consciousness. Symptoms are typically temporally related to movement to the upright position from a supine or sitting position [17].

Vertebrobasilar Insufficiency: Vertebrobasilar insufficiency is a common term used in vertebral arteries or the basilar artery or the subclavian steel syndrome, which in fact is a vestibular disorder, regardless of whether it is due to brainstem or peripheral end-organ ischemia. It can present with vertigo as the only symptom. Vertebrobasillary artery disease may be caused by atherosclerosis or cervical arthritis. Carotid artery stenosis is also fairly common in the elderly and is frequently associated with other peripheral vascular disorders. Both of these can lead to transient ischemic attacks and cerebral vascular accidents that cause slowing of the central reflexes, presyncopal sensations, and episodic feelings of loss of consciousness. Diagnosis is made on magnetic resonance angiography (MRA). As mentioned above, small vessel disease is the most common cause of non-vestibular dizziness and balance. This disorder causes increased reflex time and difficulty in processing complex tasks in the central nervous system.

Neurologic Disorders: Older patients are more likely to have some neurologic diseases like cerebellar ataxia or Alzheimer diseases vs. those that can cause dysfunction of fine motor coordination that secondarily affect balance and individuals capable of compensating for the loss of balance function.

Effects of Medication on Balance:

Many medications, including hypoglycemic agents, psychotropic agents, analgesics, narcotics, cardiovascular medications, antiepileptic medications and antihypertensive drugs have side effects, which can affect balance. Vestibular-supportive medications such as butyrophenones, benzadiazepins and antihistamines are rarely helpful in the management of balance disorders in the elderly; they can even cause a reduction in vestibular function and make symptoms worse. [18]

II) Some vestibular causes of balance disorders:

- Benign paroxysmal positional vertigo, Meniere's disease, Migraine-associated vertigo, vestibular neuritis, labyrinthine concussion.

There are some main criteria for differentiation of balance disorders:

Table 1.

Main Compliance	Main Etiology	Main Pathology	Main Site of the Lesion
Sensation of disequilibrium and vertigo especially rotational type	Peripheral vertigo	Vestibular nerve and end organ pathology	Inner ear
Mild dizziness and imbalance during walking	Central vestibular and brain disorders	Ischemic vascular and degenerative nerve diseases	Central nervous system
Imbalance exacerbated with anxiety	Psychiatric diseases	Integration with central nervous system	Psychiatric
General feeling of imbalance and dizziness	Physiologic aging and decreased motion	Normal aging related degenerative changes occurring in vestibular and proprioceptive systems	Central and peripheral vestibular, ocular and proprioceptive systems
Imbalance associated with autonomic signs and symptoms	Motion sickness	Coordination problems between cerebellum and vestibulocular, vestibulospinal systems	Endocrine, central vestibular system and inner ear
Syncope, presyncopal and related visual problems	Systemic disease and/or anemia, vascular and neurogenic disorders	Acute cerebral hypoperfusion	Cardiovascular system

Benign Paroxysmal Positional Vertigo (BPPV): It is the main type of peripheral vestibular disorder that is commonly seen in older individuals.

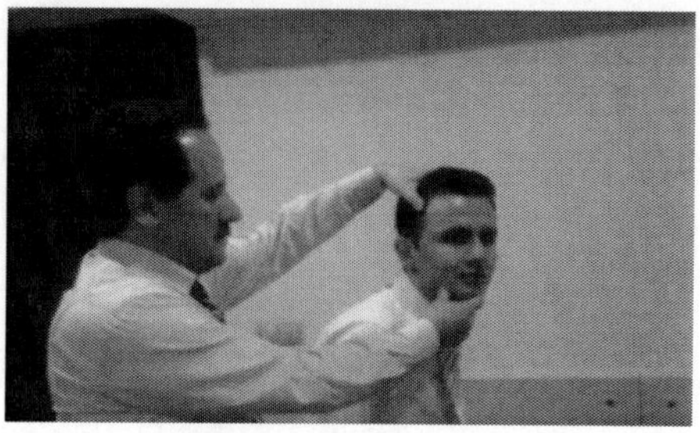

1. To test the right ear, the patient sits on a couch with the head turned to the right

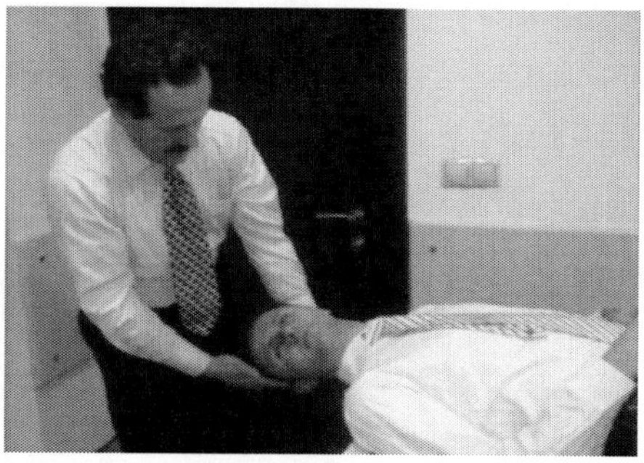

2. The clinician supports the neck, as the patient lays flat as quickly as possible, with the head slightly dangling over the edge of the couch so that the chin points slightly upwards, still turned to the right. This may produce vertigo and nystagmus. The hallmarks of nystagmus in posterior canal BPPV are delayed (by up to 20 seconds), rotational (towards the affected side), and fatigable (it gets less each time the maneuver is performed

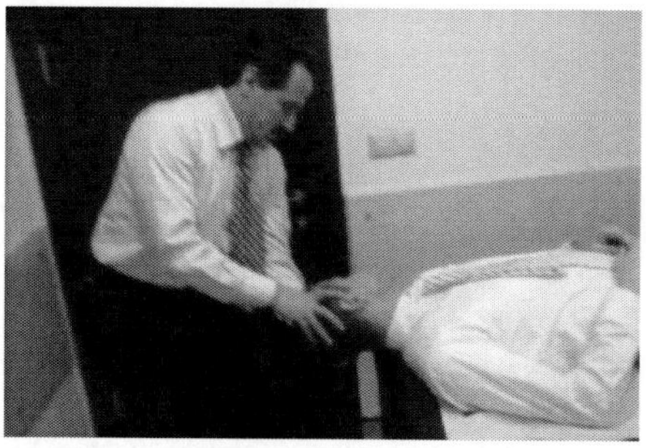

3. The vertigo and nystagmus settle after a few minutes, then the patient's head is turned to the opposite side

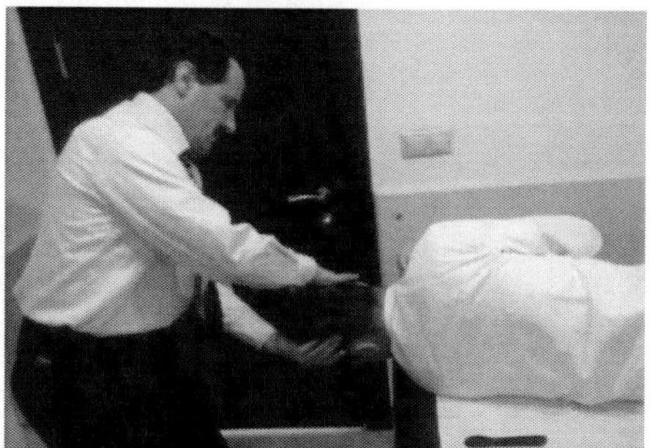

4. After a further few minutes, the patient's head is turned to look down at the floor. He has to turn on his side to do this.

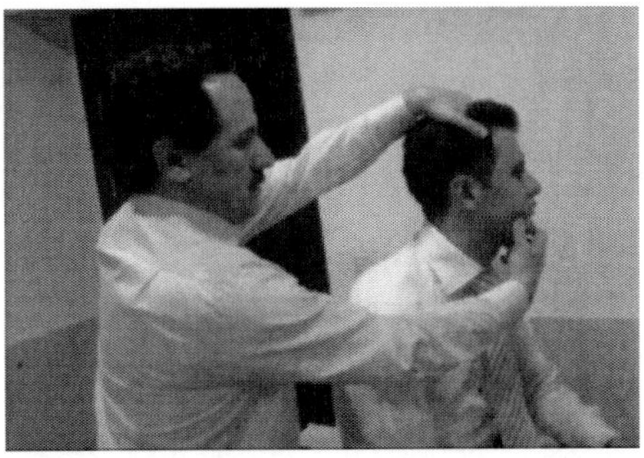

5. After a further few minutes, and with the head still turned towards the left shoulder, the patient is assisted into a sitting position.

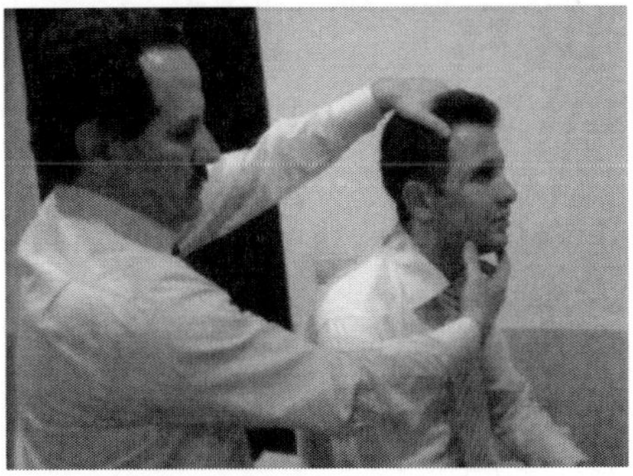

6. After a few minutes, the head turned 45 degree to the right in a straight-middle position

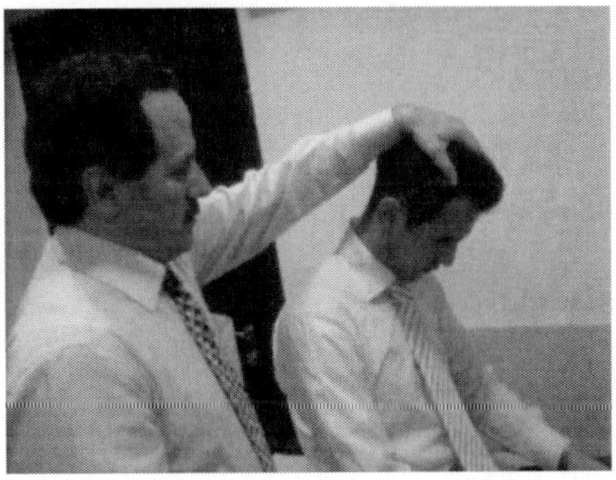

7. Once upright, the head is tilted so that the chin points slightly downward

Figure 6. The Hallpike and Epley maneuvers for BPPV. Most benign paroxysmal positional vertigo (BPPV) is caused by a problem with the posterior semicircular canal in the inner ear. It is diagnosed on the basis of history, normal neurological examination and a positive Dix–Hallpike maneuver (pictures 1 and 2) which produces transient vertigo and *characteristic* nystagmus. If positive, the clinician can go on to perform the Epley maneuver (pictures 3, 4, 5, 6 and 7), which repositions stray endolymphatic debris, which is the cause of the symptoms. In 75% of cases of BPPV, symptoms spontaneously resolve in a month or two. But for those whose symptoms persist, the Epley maneuver is extremely effective and can be performed with assistance even in frail elderly patients.

Vestibular receptors are organized to detect head motion in a specific direction or plane. Horizontal head rotation (yaw) produces a stimulus to the horizontal semicircular canals. Pitching of the head from front to back, as well as roll from side to side, is detected by the superior and posterior semicircular canals. Linear acceleration, such as gravity as well as motion along a straight trajectory, is sensed by the otolith organs located in the utricle and saccule. Canalithiasis of the posterior semicircular canal is the most frequent cause of BPPV, and it is mostly unilateral [19].

The hallmark of the disease is brief spells (lasting seconds) of often-severe vertigo, which are experienced after specific movements of the head.

The head movements that most commonly cause symptoms are the five typical features of posterior canal BPPV:

1) The canalithiasis mechanism explains the latency of nystagmus as a result of the time needed for motion of the material within the posterior canal to be initiated by gravity. Latency duration of 1-40 sec (average 3-4 sec).
2) The nystagmus duration is correlated with the length of time required for the dense material to reach the lowest part of the canal.
3) The vertical (up-beating) and torsional (top of the eyes beating toward the lowermost ear) components of the nystagmus are consistent with eye movements evoked by stimulation of the posterior canal nerve in experimental animals.
4) The reversal of nystagmus when the patient returns to the sitting upright position is due to retrograde movement of the material in the lumen of the posterior canal back toward the ampulla, with resulting ampullopetal deflection of the cupula.
5) The fatigability of the nystagmus, evoked by repeated Dix-Hallpike positional testing, is explained by dispersion of material within the canal; rolling over in bed and extreme posterior extension of the head as if looking under a sink [12].

The BPPV diagnosis can be confirmed using the Dix-Hallpike maneuver and treated using the Epley maneuver (Fig.6). These maneuvers are most helpful for diagnosis and treatment of typical BPPV, i.e., free-floating particles in the posterior semicircular canal. Performing the Dix-Hallpike maneuver can be more difficult in older individuals as a result of decreased range of motion of the neck or severe nausea during testing, musculoskeletal problems, immobility, apprehension. In such patients, a modified Dix-Hallpike maneuver may be required in which the patient's head is not extended over the edge of the examining table.

VESTIBULAR AND BALANCE FUNCTION TESTING

The evaluation of dizzy patients should proceed in a stepwise manner with the objective of discovering the site of lesion and determining the etiology of the lesion. This is accomplished by: (i) differentiating patients with visual, proprioceptive, or neuromuscular conditions from those with vestibular dysfunction; and (ii) further differentiating those with vestibular dysfunction into two groups: labyrinthine (peripheral, end organ) and retro-labyrinthine (vestibular nerve, nuclei, and central connections) [20].

It is obvious that the most important step is accurate and concise history of illness, precipitating factors such as presence of other diseases, medications, and daily life patterns of geriatric patients. In taking history, the first step is to differentiate peripheral from central vestibular disorders. A careful bedside examination, including a general otolaryngologic examination, often can be sufficient for appropriate vestibular diagnosis. The most important and well-studied inference about vestibular function testing is the eye movements (nystagmus) and its characteristic directions.

There are some different testing modalities in clinical use:

SPECIFIC TESTS: These tests show abnormalities that strongly suggest specific labyrinthine disorders.

1) The Dix-Hallpik's maneuver suggesting benign positional vertigo. The patient's head is quickly inverted in the plane of the posterior semicircular canal and then his or her eye movements are monitored.
2) The pressure test suggesting a perilymph fistula: The patient's eye movements or body sway is monitored as the external ear canal is subjected to pressure changes.

NON-SPECIFIC TESTS: They mostly indicate evidence of vestibular lesions, particularly lesions involving the labyrinth or vestibular nerve.

1) Electronystagmography consisting of the Saccade test, Tracking test, Optokinetik test, Gaze test, Positional test, Caloric test

In this group of tests the patient's eye movements are monitored as he or she undergoes a series of procedures to evaluate eye movements and to determine whether the vestibular system generates appropriate eye movements during stimulation. E.N.G. is useful in evaluating vestibular sensitivity and the eye tracking reflexes. Pursuit (Tracking) is the test in the E.N.G. battery that is most susceptible to age-related changes. Caloric testing remains the most useful laboratory investigation for determining the responsiveness of the labyrinth. It is one of the few modalities that allow one labyrinth to be studied independently of the other.

2) The rotation test, in which the patient's eye movements are monitored as he or she oscillates slowly back and forth.
3) The most commonly used system for clinical postural assessment is computerized dynamic posturography (CDP). The test subject stands on a computer-controlled movable platform with a movable visual surround. The platform and visual surround can be fixed or moved independently or concomitantly with postural sway. Anterior-to-posterior sway of the center of gravity is monitored with pressure-sensitive gauges located in each quadrant of the platform. The standard CDP test battery includes assessment of automatic postural responses to platform movements—the motor control test—and determination of effects of manipulations of visual and somatosensory information on standing balance—the sensory organization test (SOT) [21].

The two most informative subsets for elderly persons at risk of falling are the Sensory Organization Test (S.O.T.) (a type of C.D.P.) and the Limits of Stability Test (L.S.T.). In the S.O.T, the patient's sway is measured in various test conditions in which sensory information is distorted or removed. Vision and propioception may be present, absent or disturbed in various combinations. For elderly individuals, an increase in postural sway is usually seen in all tasking conditions. This is related to multisensory age-related (vestibular, visual, surface, other sensory) deficits that occur in this population.

Another important piece of information this testing provides is the use of lower-body strategies (hip, ankle and stepping foot). By awareness of loss of each of these lower-body strategies, therapists can specifically design tailored exercise programs to restore the use of the more appropriate ankle and hip strategies.

Other tests: Standing balance test, which is multifactorial sensory involving vision, vestibular propioceptive information; Romberg test, the clinical test of sensory integration in balance (CTSIB), are highly useful.

VESTIBULAR BALANCE REHABILITATION THERAPY (VBRT) IN PRESBYASTASIS AND ELDERLY PATIENTS

In the normal course of aging, humans lose sensitivity in the vestibular organs—both the rotational sensors, the semicircular canals, and the gravity receptors, the urtricle and saccule. This reduced sensitivity is due to a reduction in the number of hair cells, particularly in the superior portion of the cupula of the semicircular canals [22]. Aging also results in reduction of nerve fibers conducting vestibular information to the brain stem. Other normal changes that affect balance include slowing of central reflexes, particularly in the eye-movement control reflexes and in reflexes required to initiate body movements. Vision and hearing also decline in aging populations, and the function of proprioceptive sensory systems also declines. In addition to this, older patients tend to have less muscle mass and strength, and reduced flexibility and bone strength. Osteoporosis is particularly common in older women and further leads to more severe injuries when a fall occurs. In addition to these normal changes, there are also age-related disorders that significantly affect balance. Vascular, carotid artery, vertebral basilar, and small vessel cerebrovascular disease can significantly affect circulation to important brain structures, which are required in eye, head, and limb movements. Coronary artery disease, cardiomyopathy, and cardiac arrhythmias can also result in decreased brain perfusion, which can add to problems in balance. Many neurological disorders including stroke, degenerative diseases, head injuries, and concussion are more common in the elderly and can lead to balance disorders. Hypertension leads to accelerated arteriosclerosis, and treatment leads to postural hypotension or labile blood pressure, which results in orthostatic changes, which can also increase the risk of falling. Medications like benzodiazepines are more commonly used in the elderly populations, and many of the medications currently used can adversely affect balance [23].

Vestibular compensation is the normal physiologic response of a healthy central nervous system to vestibular pathology [24]. The central nervous system has the capacity of adjustment to asymmetries in peripheral vestibular inputs, and, to fix insults within the central vestibular pathways. This feature of the central nervous system is referred to as peripheral compensation and occurs naturally after most vestibular disorders, providing an active lifestyle for the patient. The basic physiologic components of these processes are the main elements of vestibular and balance rehabilitation programs especially for elderly patients.

Balance rehabilitation relies on innate restorative mechanisms within the brain and the body to re-establish function lost through disease, injury, medication, surgical ablation, or disuse. Balance function requires: (i) sensory information from vision, vestibular, and proprioceptive systems, (ii) integration of this information by the central nervous system, and (iii) execution of motor activities by the musculoskeletal system [23].

The use of VBRT as the primary treatment recommendation is appropriate in any condition characterized by a stable unilateral peripheral or central vestibular deficit when the patient's natural compensation process is incomplete. The final indication for the use of VBRT as a primary treatment modality is for disorders characterized by multifactorial balance difficulties, such as those seen in the elderly. Most VBRT exercises involve head movement, and head movements are essential in stimulating and retraining the vestibular system.

Most patients with chronic disequilibrium and balance disorders can significantly benefit from a balance rehabilitation program. The basis of this benefit is adaptation, compensation and restoration, and the magnitude of this benefit depends on many factors, including the characteristics of the disorder, age, and motivation. In addition to improving strength and flexibility, vestibular balance rehabilitation training attempts to re-establish functions of the vestibular system by utilizing vision and balance exercises. Some of the limitations of balance retraining include loss of vision, proprioception, and loss of vestibular sensitivity. However, balance retraining often can utilize one of these senses to overcome deficiencies in the others. The most difficult problems to manage are severe central nervous system (CNS) problems related to degenerative processes, strokes, or head injuries. It is important to assess not only the patient himself, but also family relationships, the potential for caregivers, and transportation options. Those who are likely to do well in the balance retraining exercises are those with stable vestibular dysfunction, in whom symptoms are persistent, but not progressing at a rapid rate. Poor candidates for vestibular rehabilitation are patients with rapidly progressing disease or with unstable lesions such as frequent attacks of Meniere's disease or those with demyelinating disorders and seizures. The treatment team often includes an otolaryngologist, a neurologist with a special interest in balance disorders. An audiologist, physical therapist, and occupational therapist are integral and equal members of the team [23].

The two overall goals in a VBRT program are (i) to advance the central vestibular compensation process, resulting in reduction of symptoms under static and dynamic conditions, and improvement in the function of the vestibulo-ocular reflex (VOR); and (ii) improvement in the functionality of static and dynamic balance and gait [24]. At least four distinct components of vestibular compensation are recognized: static compensation, which occurs regardless of movement, and three dynamic compensatory processes including adaptation, habituation, and sensory substitution, each of which is promoted by various exercise techniques targeted in VBFT. VBFT has been shown to be a highly effective treatment for elderly patients with presbystasis. Risk of falling must be considered in these patients and every attempt made to minimize it. In all cases, it is of paramount importance to involve other family members whenever possible. Exercises to improve reaction time, mobility, strength and gait retraining are important parts of the therapy programs. Social, environmental and living conditions of these patients are important, because most of the falls occur at home.

There are many exercise protocols in VBRT. Each protocol has been designed to fit specific balance and disequilibrium problems diagnosed by patient complaints, CDP, ENG studies.

Adaptation exercises: The principal goal of adaptation exercises is improvement in the functional performance of the VOR and accompanying gaze stability. The activities involving primarily eye-head coordinated movements called VOR (adaptation times 1, time 2) and activities involving vestibulospinal reflex.

Habituation Exercises: For most patients with positionally provoked symptoms, the primary goal is to extinguish residual pathologic responses after incomplete or disordered compensation [25]. The therapist identifies the typical movements that produce the most pronounced symptoms and provides the patient with a limited but progressive program of exercises that reproduce these movements.

Patients are counseled that symptoms are aggravated by the exercises at first but that gradual improvement will follow. If they can persevere with their program, most patients will begin to note dramatic relief of positional vertigo within 4 to 6 weeks.

Substitution Exercises: As the name implies, substitution exercises teach the patient to use alternative strategies and sensory inputs to make up for those that are deficient or absent.

Viewing of some exercise programs:

1) Adaptation time -1: Head movements in phase with target (x1 viewing): For patient with VOR deficits demonstrated in ENG testing and/or complaints of symptoms caused by head and/or eye movements:

Patient instructions: Hold a card with lettering at arm's length, with eyes focused on the letters. Move the head from side to side, increasing speed with progressions. Repeat the entire cycle 20-30 times. Can also be done vertically and diagonally. Progress from sitting to standing (feet shoulder width apart) to standing (feet together) to standing partially pointed (one foot half way ahead of the other) to standing pointed (one foot completely in front of the other). Progress from standing on firm surface to compliant surface. Post the card on the wall, with a plain background, progressing to a card with a busy patterned background.

2) Adaptation time -2: Head movement out of phase with target (x2 viewing): For patients with VOR deficits demonstrated in ENG testing and /or complaints of symptoms caused by head and/or eye movements:

Patient instructions: Hold a card with lettering at arm's length, with eyes focused on the letters. Move the head to the right, the card to the left, keeping the eyes focused on the letters. Then move the head to the left, the card to the right, keeping the eyes focused on the letters. Begin slowly and increase speed as you progress, but keep the letters in focus. Repeat the entire cycle 20-30 times. Can also be done in vertical direction. Progress from sitting to standing to sharpened stance.

3) Adaptation for vestibulospinal reflex(standing balance exercise): For patients with balance complaints and/or difficulty standing without disequilibrium; also for patients with deficits seen in CDP testing:

Patient instructions: Stand with feet together, maintaining the balance by reaching out and touching the wall in front of you. Take the hands off the wall for longer periods of time. Begin by taking one hand at a time off the wall, alternating hands. Sharpen the stance.

4) Exercise to increase pursuit gain: For patients who have pursuit abnormalities or subjective complaints in pursuit (tracking) ENG test:

Patient İnstructions: Hold a card with lettering at arm's length. Move the card left and right across the visual field, tracking with eye movement, keeping the head still. Repeat the full cycle 20-30 times. Do this in the vertical and diagonal directions as well, increasing speed, but being certain to keep the letters in focus. Progress from sitting to sharpened stance.

5) Exercise to improve saccade latency, velocity, and accuracy: For patients who have abnormalities or subjective complaints in saccade ENG test:

Patient instructions: Hold a card with lettering in each hand at arm's length, about 15 inches apart. Keeping the head still, move the eyes back and forth from card to card, 1 second per card. Repeat 20-30 times for the complete cycle. Can also be done in the vertical and diagonal planes. Progress from sitting to standing to sharpened stance.

6) Wall walking - side stepping: For patient with abnormal or ataxic gait; also for patients who cannot walk without symptoms of imbalance and disequilibrium, and for patients unable to walk without assistance, and/or with a history of falls when walking:

Patient instructions: Stand with your back against a flat wall for support. Standing still, with your feet together, slide your left leg to the side about 6-8 inches. Then slide your right leg to the left so that both feet are touching. Repeat the process by sliding your right leg to the side about 6-8 inches. Then slide your left leg to the right so that both feet are touching. Repeat process by moving your feet further apart each time, by moving more rapidly, and by moving away from the wall.

7) Walking chair to chair (sitting to standing): For patients with abnormal or ataxic gait; also for patients who cannot walk without symptoms of imbalance and disequilibrium, and for patients unable to walk without assistance, and/or with a history of falls when walking:

Patient instructions: With two chairs approximately 10 feet apart, walk from one to the other. When you reach the first chair, sit without using your hands, rising without using hands after 5 seconds. Go to the second chair touch it, and with support, practice standing on one leg for 5 seconds. Repeat the entire cycle 10 times. Add head movements as you progress and increase walking speeds and decrease the width of the gait [14].

EFFECTIVENESS OF VESTIBULAR BALANCE REHABILITATION THERAPY IN GERIATRIC PATIENTS

In recent years for geriatric patients suffering from vestibular diseases, VBRT has been one of the main treatment modalities. There are vestibular rehabilitation special interest groups that provide a health promotion for optimal function in elderly patients with balance and vestibular disorders. These patients are referred for VBRT in order to relieve their symptoms of dizziness, gaze stability, treatment of vertigo, to improve their functional status and increase their quality of life.

References

[1] Karen H. Calhoun and David E. Eibling: Geriatric Otolaryngology. Clinical approach to the geriatric patients New York: Taylor& Francis, 2006; 1: 1-4.

[2] Sloane PD, Balzer D, George LK. Dizziness in a community elderly population. JAGS 1989; 37.101–108.

[3] United Nations: An aging world population. In: World economic and social survey 2007: development in an aging world.

[4] Anna lyskowski: Cummings Otolaryngology-Head & Neck Surgery, Textbook, 5th ed. Vol.2 Mosby USA. 130: 1850-1854.

[5] Della Santina CC, Potyagaylo V, Migliaccio AA, et al: Orientation of human semicircular canals measured by three-dimensional multiplanar CT reconstruction. JARO 2005; 6.191-206.

[6] Hillman DE, McLaren JW: Displacement configuration of the semicircular canal cupula. J Neurosci 1979; 4: 1989.

[7] John P. Carey& Charles C. Della Santina: Cummings Otolaryngology- Head & Neck Surgery, Textbook, 5th ed. Vol.3 Mosby USA. 163: 2276- 2281.

[8] Baloh RW, Honrubia V: Clinical Neurophysiology of the Vestibular System. New York, Oxford University Press, 2001.

[9] Halmagyi GM, Baloh RW: Disorders of the Vestibular System. New York, Oxford University Press, 1996.

[10] Leigh RJ, Zee DS: The Neurology of Eye Movements. New York, Oxford University Press, 1999.

[11] Wilson VJ, Melvill Jones G: Mammalian Vestibular Physiology. New York, Plenum Press, 1979.

[12] Benjamin T. Carne, David A. Schessel, Julian Nedzelski, and Lıyod B. Minor: Cummings Otolaryngology- Head & Neck Surgery, Text book, 5th ed. Vol.3 Mosby USA. 165:2328-2345.

[13] Living without a balancing mechanism. N Engl J Med 1952; 246:458.

[14] Marian Girardi, Horst R. Konrad: Cummings Otolaryngology- Head & Neck Surgery, Text book, 4th ed.Vol. 4-1 Mosby USA. 141: 3199-3208.

[15] David D. Deweese: Paparella Text book of Otolaryngology, Third ed. Vol. 2 W.B. Saunders Philadelphia USA. 48: 1683- 1689.

[16] Matthew L. Kashima: Cummings Otolaryngology- Head & Neck Surgery, Text book, 4th ed. Vol.1 Mosby USA. 17: 351-357.

[17] David E. Eibling: Geriatric Otolaryngology, Taylor & Francis USA. 12: 147-153.

[18] Johns M and others: Goals and mechanisms for training otolaryngologists in the area of geriatric medicine, Otolaryngol Head Neck Surg 100:4, 1989.

[19] Longridge NS, Barber HO: Bilateral paroxysmal positioning nystagmus. J Otolaryngol 1978; 7.395.
[20] j.B. Nadol, H.F. Schuknecht: Surgery of the Ear and Temporal bone, evaluation of the vestibular system; Raven press, New York, 1993:57-70.
[21] Timothy E. Huller, David S. Zee, Lıyod B. Minor: Cummings Otolaryngology - Head & Neck Surgery, Textbook, 5th ed. Vol.3 Mosby USA. 164: 2305-2320.
[22] Nakayama M, Helfert RH, Konrad HR, Caspary DM. Scanning electron microscopic evaluation of age-related changes in the rat vestibular epithelium. Otolaryngology Head Neck Surg. 1994; 111:799–806.
[23] Horst R. Konrad, Meiho Nakayama: Geriatric Otolaryngology, Taylor& Francis USA. 14: 165-170.
[24] Neil T. Shepard, Steven A. Telian, Audery B. Erman: Cummings Otolaryngology-Head & Neck Surgery, Textbook, 5th ed. Vol.3 Mosby USA. 168: 2372-2380.
[25] Telian SA, Shepard NT, Smith-Wheelock M, et al: Bilateral vestibular paresis: diagnosis and treatment. *Otolaryngology Head Neck Surg* 1991; 104,67.

In: New Horizons in Geriatric Medicine. Volume 1
Editors: Ahmet Turan Isik, M. Refik Mas et al.
ISBN: 978-1-62808-972-1

Chapter 9

TREMORS

Gulay Kenangil
Department of Neurology, Erenkoy Psychiatry Hospital, Istanbul, Turkey

ABSTRACT

A tremor is a rhytmic, oscillatory movement produced by alternating or synchronous contractions of antagonist muscles. It is the most common form of involuntary movements and is common in the elderly population. The cause of the tremor in old age ranges from a benign physiological tremor to a more serious tremor of neurodegenerative disorders like Parkinson's disease (PD). We can classify tremors according to their phenomenology (rest or action tremors), distribution (hand, head, jaw,tongue, leg,trunk), frequency (slow, medium or fast) or etiology (physiologic, semptomatic, degenerative). The prevelance of tremors in people aged 50-85 was found to be 15 % where the most common type of tremor was physiological tremor or Essential Tremor (ET) and tremor related to parkinsonism was only 2.75%. The prevelance of the postural tremor increases with age. Beta blockers and antiepileptic drugs can be used for ET or physiological tremor, while dopaminergic drugs are used for the tremor of patients in PD. It is important to be aware of the side effects of these drugs in the elderly. Semptomatic tremors, like the serebellar tremor, can also be seen in the elderly and are mostly the result of a stroke or a tumor. Neuropathic and ortostatic tremors are less frequent tremors which may also be seen in old age.

INTRODUCTION

A tremor is a rhytmic, oscillatory movement produced by alternating or synchronous contractions of antagonist muscles. It is the most common form of involuntary movements, but only a few people ask for medical help. Tremors are common in the elderly. The cause of the tremor in old age ranges from a benign physiological tremor to a more serious tremor of neurodegenerative disorders like Parkinson's disease.

We can classify tremors according to their phenomenology, distribution, frequency or etiology [1-8].

Tremors can be divided into two major categories phenomenologically: rest tremors and action tremors. A rest tremor is present when the affected body part is fully supported against gravity and not actively contracting; It is diminished or absent during voluntary muscle contractions and during movement of that extremity. Instead, an action tremor occurs with the voluntary contraction of muscles, and it can be subdivided into the postural, kınetic, task-specific or position-specific isometric tremor. The postural tremor is evident during maintenance of an antigravity posture, such as holding the arms in an outstretched horizontal position in front of the body [9]

Tremors can also be divided according to their anatomic distribution; for example head, tongue, voice and trunk. Orolingual tremors include physiological, essential, task-and-position-specific, dystonic, orthostatic, parkinsonian, palatal, drug-induced, hereditary and psychogenic tremors [10-11]

REST TREMORS

Rest tremors are typically present in Parkinson's disease. Several studies suggested that the natural course of PD is in part related to the presence or absence of a tremor. About 32% of patients never had rest tremor during the course of their disease [12]. The tremor dominant PD has a more favorable prognosis than PD manifested by postural instability and gait difficulty [9]. Rest tremors involving the fingers, hands, lips, jaw and tongue in the same individual with a common frequency may suggest that they are of central origin [13]. Rest tremors also had other causes. Other parkinsonian disorders like multiple system atrophy (MSA), progressive supranuclear palsy (PSP), corticobasal ganglionic degeneration (CGD), Parkinsonism-dementia-ALS complex, diffuse Lewy body disease (DLBD) can be manifested by rest tremor. In addition, patients with heredodegenerative disorders such as Huntington disease, Wilson disease, Neuroacanthocytosis, Neurodegeneration with brain ıron accumulation (NBIA 1), Gerstmann-Straussler-Scheinker disease, ceroid lipofucsinosis may also have rest tremors. Patients with secondary parkinsonism (drug induced, vascular, trauma, tumor, paraneoplastic, infectious, metabolic, normal pressure hydrocephalus), severe ET, midbrain rubral tremor, tardive tremor, myorhythmia and spasmus nutans may have rest tremors, too [9]. The PD tremor has a frequency of 4-8 Hz, while the rubral tremor (2-5 Hz) and myorhythmia (1-3 Hz) is more slower.

We can use dopaminergic drugs for the treatment of tremors in PD. Although anticholinergic drugs are one of the most effective drugs for the treatment of tremors, clinicans should be aware of its side effects like confusion and be cautious when using them in the elderly. Clozapin also can be used effectively, but it has potentially serious side effects like agranulositosis. In some cases, botulunim toxin injections in the involved muscles have shown to be effective in reducing the amplitude of the tremor [14-16]. The ventral lateral intermediate nucleus of thalamus (VIM) is recently a widely used target for the treatment of distal tremor in PD and also for ET [17-18].

Postural Tremors

Physiologic tremor is a benign postural tremor that occurs in everyone but is usually not visible to the naked eye. It can increase and become visible in the presence of a sympathetic nervous system stimulation from drugs (e.g., beta-adrengeric agonists, amphetamine-like drugs, caffeine) and certain disease states (e.g., hyperthyroidism, hypoglycemia). Anxiety can also produce this type of tremor. This tremor is reversible when the stimulus is removed.

A physiologic tremor and the enhanced physiologic tremor are the most common forms of postural tremors and they rarely need to be treated. In contrast to ET the frequency of physiologic tremors can be slowed by mass loading [19].

In a study of people aged 50-89, the prevelance of tremors was found to be 15 %, where the frequency of the exagrated physiological tremor or ET was found to be 12.5%, while tremors related to parkinsonism were 2.75% [20].

The prevelance of postural tremors increase with age. In a population based study, including patients older than 65 years, postural tremors were found in 16% of those between 65-74 years, 20.7% in 75-84 years, and 25.6% in those older than 85 years [21]. Moreover, parkinsonian rest tremors were examined in 5-6 % of all the ages of the study group where only half of them had PD [21].

Essential Tremor

The age of onset for essential tremors (ET) shows bimodal distribution which peaks in the second and sixth decades [22]. Patients with older onset ET sometimes are called senile tremors and they have a more rapid progression and a more degenerative pathology than the younger onset ones [23].

Meta-analysis of epidemiologic studies has found the prevelance of ET in people older than 65 is 4.6 % and may be as high as 21.7 % in people older than 95, and the prevelance is higher in men [24]. Symptoms may begin at any age but the incidence increases markedly with advancing age, and the most prevalent cases are at age 60 and older.

ET usually begins in one upper extremity and soon affects the other. It rarely extends from the upper extremity to the ipsilateral leg. A mild degree of asymmetry is not unusual. In about 30% of cases, a tremor involves the cranial musculature; the head is involved most frequently, followed by voice, jaw, and face. Tremors may be intermittent initially, emerging only during periods of emotional activation. Over time, the tremor becomes persistent and it resolves during sleep. A family history of essential tremors is noted in 50-60% of cases.

ET is the result of an abnormally functioning central oscillator, which is located in the Guillain Mollaret triangle near the brain stem and involves the inferior olivary nucleus. The cerebellar-brainstem-thalamic-cortical circuits are probably involved. The pathophysiology of essential tremors is heterogeneous [25-26].

Alcohol can reduce the amplitude of ET in two thirds of patients. Propranolol is the most effective drug for the treatment of ET and enhanced physiologic tremors, but other beta-blockers may also be used to treat postural tremors [27-29]. The major side effects of these drugs are fatigue, sedation, depression and sexual impotence. These drugs are contraindicated in the presence of asthma, second-degree atrioventricular blocks, and insulin dependent diabetes, so they should be used cautiously in older age. Primidon and benzodiazepin drugs can also be used for the treatment of ET.

Kinetic Tremors: Cerebellar Tremor

This kind of tremor is associated with lesions of the cerebellum and its outflow pathways. It can be considered a symptomatic tremor. There also may be a postural component, seen as a head tremor, which appears a "bobbing" to-and-fro movement of the head called titubation. The key to distinguishing a cerebellar tremor from an essential tremor is usually the presence of other cerebellar signs, such as ataxia and dysmetria. Patients with cerebellar tremors may have abnormalities on neuroimaging, such as stroke, tumor, or demyelination [9, 30]. Traumas can also cause postural or kinetic tremors [31-34].

Neuropathic Tremors

Neuropathic tremors are seen in various types of peripheric neuropathy [35-36]. Patients with dysgammaglobulinemic polyneuropathies and both hereditary motor and sensory neuropathy have different types of tremor [37-38].

Orthostatic Tremor

The frequency of orthostatic tremors (OT) is fast (14-16 Hz), mainly involves the legs and trunk, and appears when the patient stands still. It is often associated with calf cramps and a feeling of unsteadiness. It disappears when the patient sits or is in a supine position. The pathophysiology of OT is not well understood. The presence of postural tremors is identical to ET, and the family history of ET in majority of OT patients support its relation with ET [39]. A form of an orthostatic tremor with a slower frequency than classical OT can be seen in various disorders like parkinsonism, ET, head trauma andpontine lesions [40-41]. An OT may improve with clonozepam and gabapentin [42].

References

[1] Hallett, M. Classification and treatment of tremor. *JAMA* 1991; 266: 115 – 117.

[2] Lou JS, Jankovic J. Tremors. In: Appel S.H. (Ed.), *Current Neurology,* vol.11. Mosby Year Book, Chicago, 1991, pp.199 – 232.

[3] Bain P. A combined clinical and neurophysiologic approach to the study of patients with tremor. *J Neurol Neurosurg Psychiatry* 1993: 69; 839 – 844.

[4] Deuschl G, Bain P, Brin M. Ad Hoc Scientific Committee: Consensus statement of the Movement Disorder Society on Tremor. *Mov Disord* 1998; 13 (suppl.3): 2 – 23.

[5] Jankovic J. Essential tremor: Clinical characteristics. *Neurology* 2000; 54 (suppl.4): 22 – 26.

[6] Deuschl G, Raethjen J, Lindemann M, Krack P. The pathophysiology of tremor. *Muscle and Nerve* 2001; 24: 716 – 735.

[7] Jankovic J, Lang AE. *Movement disorders: Diagnosis and assessment.* In: Bradley WG, Daroff RB, Fenichel GM, Jankovic J (eds.): Neurology in Clinical Practice, fifth ed. Butterworth-Heinemann (Elsevier), Philadelphia,2008, pp. 293 – 325.

[8] Deuschl G, Elble R. Essential tremor– neurodegenerative or nondegenerative disease towards a working definition of ET. *Mov Disord* 2009; 24: 2033 – 2041.

[9] Fahn S, Jankovic J, Hallett M. Tremors. In Fahn S, Jankovic J, Hallett M (eds): *Principles and practice of movement disorders*, 2011, second ed. Saunders Elsevier, China, pp. 388- 414.

[10] Erer S, Jankovic J. Hereditary chin tremor in Parkinson's disease. *Clin Neurol Neurosurg* 2007; 109: 784-785.

[11] Silverdale MA, Schneider SA, Bhatia KP, Lang AE. The spectrum of orolingual tremor – a proposed classification system. *Mov Disord* 2008; 23: 159-167.

[12] Hughes AJ, Daniel SE, Blankson S, Lees AJ. A clinicopathologic study of 100 cases of Parkinson's disease. *Arch Neurol* 1993; 50: 140-148.

[13] Hunker CJ, Abbs JH. Uniform frequency of parkinsonian resting tremor in the lips, jaw, tongue, and index finger. *Mov Disord* 1990; 5: 71-77.

[14] Jankovic J, Schwartz K. Botulinumtoxin treatment of tremors. *Neurology* 1991; 41: 1185 – 1188.

[15] Jankovic J, Schwartz K, Clemence W, et al. A randomized, double-blind, placebo-controlled study to evaluate botulinum toxin type A in essential hand tremor. *Mov Disord* 1996; 11: 250 -256.

[16] Hou JG, Jankovic J. Botulinum toxin in the treatment of tremors. In: Brin MF, Hallett M, Jankovic J (eds.): *Scientific and Therapeutic Aspects of Botulinum Toxin,* 2002. Lippincott Williams & Wilkins,Philadelphia, pp. 323 -336.

[17] Benabid AL, Pollak P, Gervason C, et al. Long-term suppression of tremor by chronic stimulation of the ventral intermediate thalamic nucleus. *Lancet* 1991; 1: 403 – 406.

[18] Jankovic J, Cardoso F, Grossman RG, Hamilton WJ. Outcome after stereotactic thalamotomy for parkinsonian, essential and other types of tremor. *Neurosurgery* 1995; 45: 1743-1746.

[19] Elble RJ, Koller WC. The measurement and quantification of tremor. In: Elble RJ, Koller WC (eds.): *Tremor,*1990. Johns Hopkins University Press, Baltimore, pp. 10 – 36, 54 – 89.

[20] Wenning GK, Kiechl S, Seppi K, et al. Prevalence of movement disorders in men and women aged 50-89 years (Bruneck Study cohort): a population-based study. *Lancet Neurol* 2005; 4: 815-820.

[21] Bennett DA, Beckett LA, Murray AM, Shannon, KM, Goetz CG, Pilgrim DM, Evans DA. Prevalance of parkinsonian signs and associated mortality in a community population of older people. *N Eng J Med* 1996; 334:71-76.

[22] Lou JS, Jankovic J. Essential tremor: Clinical correlates in 350 patients. *Neurology* 1991; 41: 234-238.

[23] Louis ED, Faust PL, Vonsattel JP, Louis ED, Faust PL, Vonsattel JPG, Honig LS, et al. Older onset essential tremor: More rapid progression and more degenerative pathology. *Mov Disord* 2009; 24: 1606-1612.

[24] Louis ED, Ferreira JJ. How common is the most common adult movement disorder? Update on the worldwide prevalence of essential tremor. *Mov Disord* 2010; 25: 534 - 541.

[25] Louis ED, Vonsattel JP. The emerging neuropathology of essential tremor. *Mov Disord*. 2008; 23: 174-82.

[26] Shill HA, Adler CH, Sabbagh MN, Connor DJ, Caviness JN, Hentz JG, Beach TG. Pathologic findings in prospectively ascertained essential tremor subjects. *Neurology* 2008; 70: 1452-1455.

[27] Caccia MR, Osio M, Galimberti V, Cataldi G, Mangoni A. Propranolol, clonidine, urapidil and trazodone infusion in essential tremor: A double-blind crossover trial. *Acta Neurol Scand* 1989; 79: 379-383.

[28] Calzetti S, Sasso E, Baratti M, Fava R. Clinical and computer-based assessment of long-term efficacy ofpropranolol in essential tremor. *Acta Neurol Scand* 1990; 81: 392-396.

[29] Koller WC, Busenbark K, Miner K. The relationship of essential tremor to other movement disorders: Report on 678 patients. *Ann Neurol* 1994; 35:717-723.

[30] Deuschl G, Volkman J, Raethjen J. Tremors: Differential diagnosis, pathophysiology and theraphy. In Jankovich J, Tolosa E (Eds), *Parkinson's disease and movement disorders,* 2007, fifth ed. Lippincott Williams &Wilkins, Philadelphia,pp: 308-309.

[31] Biary N, Cleeves L, Findley L, Koller W. Post-traumatic tremor. *Neurology* 1989; 39: 103-106.

[32] Goetz CG, Pappert EJ. Trauma and movement disorders. *Neurol Clin* 1992; 10: 907-919.

[33] Jankovic J. Posttraumatic movement disorders: Peripheral and central mechanisms. *Neurology* 1994; 44: 2008-2014.

[34] Krauss JK, Wakhloo AK, Nobbe F, Tränkle R, Mundinger F, Seeger W. Lesion of dentatothalamic pathways in severe post-traumatic tremor. *Neurol Res* 1995; 17:409-416.

[35] Said G, Bathien N, Cesaro P. Peripheral neuropathies and tremor. *Neurology* 1982; 32: 480-485.

[36] Shahani BT. Tremor associated with peripheral neuropathy. In: Findley LJ, Capildeo R. (Eds.), *Movement Disorders: Tremor,* 1984. Oxford University Press, New York,pp. 389-398.

[37] Bain PG, Britton TC, Jenkins IH, Thompson PD, Rothwell JC, Thomas PK, et al. Tremor associated with benign IgM paraproteinaemic neuropathy. *Brain* 1996; 119: 789-799.

[38] Cardoso FC, Jankovic J. Hereditary motor-sensory neuropathy and movement disorders. *Muscle and Nerve* 1993; 16: 904-910.

[39] Fitzgerald PM, Jankovic J. Orthostatic tremor: An association with essential tremor. *Mov Disord* 1991; 6: 60-64.

[40] Gabellini AS, Martinelli P, Gulli MR, Ambrosetto G, Ciucci G, Lugaresi E. Orthostatic tremor: Essential and symptomatic cases. *Acta Neurol Scand* 1990; 81: 113-137.

[41] Benito-León J, Rodriguez J, Orti-Pareja M,_Ayuso-Peralta L, Jiménez-Jiménez FJ, Molina JA. Symptomatic orthostatic tremor in pontine lesions. *Neurology* 1997; 49:1439-1441.

[42] -Rodrigues JP, Edwards DJ, Walters SE,_Byrnes ML, Thickbroom GW, Stell R and Mastaglia FL. Blinded placebo crossover study of gabapentin in primary orthostatic tremor. *Mov Disord* 2006; 21: 900-905.

SECTION 4: COMMON DISEASES IN GERIATRICS

In: New Horizons in Geriatric Medicine. Volume 1
Editors: Ahmet Turan Isik, M. Refik Mas et al.
ISBN: 978-1-62808-972-1

Chapter 10

HYPERTENSION

A. Seref Demırel
Istanbul University, Istanbul School of Medicine,
Department of Internal Medicine, Istanbul, Turkey

ABSTRACT

The prevention and management of systemic arterial hypertension (HT) remains a major public health challenge worldwide due to its high prevalance and importance as a cardiovascular disease (CVD) risk factor.

DEFINITION AND CLASSIFICATION

HT is defined as a systolic blood pressure (SBP) above 140 and diastolic blood pressure (DBP) above 90 mmHg according to 2 popular guidelines (Table 1, 2) [1, 2]. The classification based on these arbitrary cutoff values was for simplifying diagnostic and treatment approaches in daily practice. When a patient's SBP and DBP fell into different categories the higher category should be used. While DBP remained <90 mmHg, isolated systolic hypertension (ISH) could be graded in the same way like systolic-diastolic HT. The threshold for HT and need for drug treatment should be considered as flexible based on the level and profile of total cardiovascular risk [1]. The seventh report of the Joint National Committee on Prevention, Detection, Evaluation, and Treatment of High Blood Pressure (JNC 7) introduced a new term, namely prehypertension because of the new data on lifetime risk of HT and the increase in the CVD risk associated with levels of blood pressure (BP) previously considered to be normal. The intention was to identify people in whom early intervention with lifestyle changes could reduce BP, decrease the rate of progression of BP to hypertensive levels with age, or prevent HT entirely. The second major change from JNC 6 was the combining of stage 2 and stage 3 HT into a single stage 2 category due to the similarity of the management of the former two groups [2].

Table 1. Definitions and classifications of blood pressure levels (mm Hg)

Category	SBP		DBP
Optimal	< 120	and	<80
Normal	120-129	and/or	80-84
High normal	130-139	and/or	85-89
Grade 1 hypertension (mild)	140-159	and/or	90-99
Grade 2 hypertension (moderate)	160-179	and/or	100-109
Grade 3 hypertension (severe)	> 180	and/or	> 110
Isolated systolic hypertension	> 140	and	< 90

SBP: Systolic blood pressure, DBP: diastolic blood pressure

Table 2. Classification of blood pressure (BP) for adults 18 years and older

BP Classification	SBP (mm Hg)	DBP (mm Hg)
Normal	< 120	< 80
Prehypertension	120-139	80-89
Stage 1 hypertension	140-159	90-99
Stage 2 hypertension	> 160	> 100

SBP: Systolic blood pressure, DBP: diastolic blood pressure.

JNC 7 emphasized that in people older than age 50, SBP of >140 mmHg is a more important CVD risk factor than DBP. Beginning at 115/75 mmHg, CVD risk doubles for each increment of 20/10 mmHg. Normotensive people at 55 years of age will have a more than 90% lifetime risk of developing HT. The first choice of therapy in uncomplicated HT is thiazide diutetics, drugs other than thiazide diuretic may be used in high-risk conditions, i.e., in compelling indications. For patients whose BP is >20 mmHg above the SBP goal or >10 mmHg above the DBP goal, initiation of therapy using two agents should bc considered [2]. 2007 European Society of Hypertension-European Society of Cardiology (ESH-ESC) guidelines for the management of arterial hypertension differed in some aspects from JNC 7. ESH-ESC Committee decided to treat total cardiovascular risk which is the absolute change of having a cardiovascular event usually over 10 years. In Europe, in stead of Framingham data, Systemic Coronary Risk Evaluation (SCORE) charts were used which estimate the risk of dying from cardiovascular (not just coronary) disease over 10 years and allow calibration of the charts for individual countries [3, 4]. The terms ''low, moderate, high and very high risk'' are used to indicate an approximate risk. The term ''added'' is used to emphasize that in all categories relative risk is greater than average risk. In younger people relative risk, i.e., the existing risk compared to their peers was used as a guide to the need and the intensity of therapeutic interventions while in older people absolute risk was accepted. Subclinical organ damage as an intermediate stage in the continuum of vascular disease and as a determinant of overall CVD risk was first time cited in a guideline and will be used not only for screening, but also for follow-up of treatment. Low diastolic pressures (< 70 mmHg) was accepted as an added risk and indicates due to large artery stiffness subclinical organ damage [1].

EPIDEMIOLOGY AND PATHOPHYSIOLOGY

The relationship between high BP and risk of CVD and renal disease events is continuous, positive, and independent of other risk factors [5, 6, 7]. The Framingham study has shown that beginning at 110-115/75-80 mm Hg, CVD risk starts, and increases particularly above 140/90 mm Hg dramatically. SBP is superior to DBP in predicting the risk of all clinical forms of coronary heart disease (CHD) [5]. In the Multiple Risk Factor Intervention Trial (MRFIT), SBP levels of 150 to 159 mm Hg conferred a greater relative risk for CHD events than DBP levels of 95 to 100 mm Hg; for coronary deaths increasing SBP showed 3.7-fold, DBP showed 2.8-fold relative risk, and for stroke 8.2-fold, and 4.2-fold, respectively [6]. In the MRFIT study also, the relationship between the rise in BP and end stage renal disease is continuous and positive [7]. In a meta-analysis in people 40-69 years of age CVD and stroke relative risk doubles for each increment of 20 mmHg of SBP. Between 80-89 years of age this risk declines by half, but the absolute risk is of course higher in this age range [8]. BP consists of two components, i.e., mean arterial pressure (MAP) and pulse pressure (PP). MAP is more steady and depends on ventricular ejection and peripheral vascular resistance. PP (SBP-DBP) is more pulsatile, and has two components. The direct component depends on ventricular ejection and large artery stiffness while the indirect component is the result of wave reflections. Age-related increase in large artery stiffness and in amplitudes of wave reflections caused an increase in SBP and PP (Table 3) [9].

SBP, the overall prevalance of HT and the proportion of hypertensives with ISH increases with age [9, 10]. In contrast, DBP increases in paralell with SBP until about age 55, after which it declines (Table 3). By age 60, about two-thirds of those with HT have ISH; by age 75, almost all hypertensive individuals have systolic HT and about three-fourths have ISH. SBP provides more appropiate classification and risk stratification than DBP in the elderly. In the Framingham Heart Study, SBP alone correctly classified the BP stage in 94% of adults over the age of 60, while DBP alone correctly classified 66% [10].

Even in normotensive people between 55 and 65 years of age, there remains a lifetime risk of developing HT that exceeds 90 percent [11]. At the same time, there is three- to fourfold increase in CVD risk in older compared to younger individuals. Therefore, a clinical advisory statement in May 2000 was issued with the intention that SBP should be the primary target for the diagnosis and management of older people with HT [12].

Table 3. Age-related blood pressure changes and hemodynamic pattern

Age	SBP	DBP	PP	Hemodynamic pattern
30-49	↑	↑	↑ →	small artery resistance > large artery stiffness
50-59	↑	→	↑↑	small artery resistance = large artery stiffness
> 60	↑	↓	↑↑↑	small artery resistance < large artery stiffness

Table 4. Differentiating characteristics of atherosclerosis and arteriosclerosis

Characteristics	Atherosclerosis	Arteriosclerosis
Distribution	Focal	Diffuse
Localization	Intima	Media, adventitia
Geometry	Occlusive	Dilatation
Pathology	Plaque	↓ Elastin, ↑ Collagen
Physiology	Inflamation	Large artery stiffness
Hemodynamic	Ischemia	↑ Left ventricular workload

PP is only marginally stronger than SBP for risk stratification in individuals over age 60, but under age 60, PP is not useful as a CVD risk predictor [8]. PP generally decreases as a result of SBP lowering, but no prospective clinical trial has used PP as the primary clinical endpoint [13, 14]. Currently, BP control rates (systolic < 140 mmHg and diastolic < 90 mmHg) are only about 20 percent in older hypertensive individuals, largely due to poor control of SBP [15].

Both, atherosclerosis and arteriosclerosis can be found in the same old individual. Age-related vascular and neurohumoral changes leads to structural and mechanical alterations in the vessel intima and media (Table 4). Consequently, arterial compliance diminishes and the so called ''windkessel function''of the large arteries decreases. PP and pulse wave velocity increase with an earlier reflection of pressure waves from the periphery to a disproportionate increase in SBP. Cardiac output, stroke volume, intravascular volume, renal blood flow and plasma renin activity decrease, while left ventricular mass, circulating catecholamines, particularly noradrenaline, and total peripheral vascular resistance increase [16]. Baroreceptor sensitivity to BP changes also decreases causing a higher BP variability [17]. Sluggish baroreceptor function and reduced cardiovascular sensitivity to catecholamines make the elderly more sensitive to natural or drug-induced falls in BP.

Diagnostic Evaluation

When compared with JNC 7, ESH-ESC 2007 guideline will be chosen by Pickering mentioned in his paper titled JNC 7.5 for using its contents in any future guideline [18].

The diagnostic procedures consist of establishing BP levels, identifying secondary causes of HT, and evaluating the total CVD risk by searching for other risk factors, target organ damage, and concomitant diseases or accompanying clinical conditions [1].

A. Blood Pressure Measurements

BP is characterized by large spontaneous variations both during the day and between days, months and seasons [19]. Office BP should be used as reference. Normal values are different for office, home, and ambulatory BP (Table 5) [1].

An accurate and representative BP reading is a prerequisite, regardless of which technique is used. An accurate device should be subjected to independent evaluation according to one of the recognized protocols. BP is influenced by the circumstances of measurement itself, emotion, exercise, meals, tobacco, alcohol, temperature, respiration, bladder distension, pain, race, and age etc. [20].

Table 5. Blood pressure thresholds (mm Hg) for definition of hypertension with different types of measurement

	Systolic blood pressure	Diastolic blood pressure
Office or clinic	140	90
24-hour	125-130	80
Day	130-135	85
Night	120	70
Home	130-135	85

During conventional (office) BP measurement special attention must be paid for children, pregnant women, patients with arrhythmias, obese people with ‘‘cuff hypertension’’, and elderly, who often have ISH or autonomic failure with postural hypotension. The possible observer error are terminal digit preference, systematic error, observer prejudice or bias. The mercury sphygmomanometer is a reliable device, whereas the aneroid manometer is not generally as accurate. Automated devices should eliminate errors of interpretation, abolish observer bias and terminal digit preference [20].

Ambulatory BP has been found to be a significant predictor of cardiovascular morbidity, independent of office BP and other risk factors in elderly subjects and those with ISH [21, 22]. In most people, BP falls at night between two extremes, the extreme dippers and the non dippers. The nocturnal dip is less marked with increasing age [23, 24, 25] and disappears in centenarians [24]. Accepted indications for ambulatory BP monitoring (ABPM) are suspected white-coat effect and white-coat HT, suspected nocturnal and masked HT, to establish dipper status, resistant HT, and HT of pregnancy. As a guide to antihypertensive drug treatment, type 1 diabetes, evaluation of symptoms suggesting orthostatic hypotension (OH), autonomic failure, and elderly patient are potential indications [20].

In the Ohasama study, home BP had greater predictive power for mortality and stroke than screening BP [26]. Self BP measurement using oscillometric electronic devices is becoming more popular and are replacing the auscultatory technique due to requiring less training, conditions like arthritis and deafness, and store, transmit or printing capacities. Devices that measure BP at the finger are not recommended because peripheral vasoconstriction, alteration in BP in more distal site of recording, and a particularly relevant effect of limb position on BP lead to important inaccuracies. Although sharing same limitations including distal site and limb position wrist devices are more accurate than finger measuring devices, but inaccurate BP readings can occur during not helding the wrist at the heart level, and due to flexion and hyperextension of the wrist. Furthermore, as there are two arteries contributing to the oscillometric signal it is difficult to produce an accurate algorithm to estimate SBP and DBP. Upper arm (brachial artery) devices have been shown to be the most reliable in clinical practice and research and therefore their use is recommended for home BP monitoring (HBPM). Automated measurement is not possible in patients with arrhythmias and in some for no obvious reason [20, 27]. In special populations, such as obese or elderly individuals, monitoring using the upper arm is more difficult to perform, therefore wrist measuring devices should be used [28].

Several features of HT in elderly people make ABPM necessary. First, white-coat HT is more common in elderly hypertensive patients than younger hypertensive patients [29]. Second, elderly individuals are characterized by a more pronounced BP variability compared with younger individuals [19], which by itself may be associated with an elevated CVD risk [30], especially when such high variability is related to an excessive BP surge in morning hours [31]. Third, in elderly individuals, autoregulation of the circulation of target organs during excessive BP reduction is impaired and excessive antihypertensive medication targeting office BP can cause symtomatic hypotension, which may worsen treatment compliance. Although ABPM appears the most suitable technique to diagnose the above problems, HBPM may also be useful [32] (Table 6). In elderly people HBPM data are very limited, therefore the threshold for diagnosis of HT and the target level of antihypertensive medication should be the same as in other adults, that is 135/85 mmHg [27]. Physical and intellectual limitations make HBPM in elderly people difficult. Additionally, BP must be measured both in the sitting and standing positions, whenever OH is suspected [27].

Table 6. Comparison of main features of ABPM and HBPM

Feature	ABPM	HBPM
Daytime BP	++	++
Nighttime BP and dipping	++	–
Morning BP	++	+
24-h BP variability	++	±
Long-term BP variability	±	++
WCH and MH diagnosis	++	++
Placebo effect	–	–
Reproducibility	++	++
Prognostic value	++	++
Patient involvement	–	++
Patient training	±	++
Physician involvement	++	+
Patients' acceptance	±	++
HT control improvement	+	++
Cost	High	Low
Availability	Low	High
Monitoring treatment effects	Extensive information on diurnal BP profile, cannot be repeated frequently	Appropriate for long-term monitoring, limited information on BP profile

ABPM: Ambulatory blood pressure monitoring, HBPM: Home blood pressure monitoring, BP: Blood pressure, WCH: White-coat hypertension, MH: Masked hypertension, HT: Hypertension.

BP measurements are typically recorded in the sitting position. Normally, standing is accompanied by a small increase in DBP and a small decrease in SBP when compared to lying. OH is present when there is a supine-to-standing BP decrease >20 mm Hg systolic or > 10 mm Hg diastolic. This practice, while convenient for the physicians, limits the ability to diagnose OH. OH occurred in about 7% of men over 70 years of age in the Honolulu Heart Study, was highly age-dependent, and carried with it a 64% increase in age-adjusted mortality compared with a control population [33]. There is a strong correlation between the severity of OH and premature death as well as increased incidents of falls and fractures [33, 34, 35]. The causes of OH include severe volume depletion, baroreflex dysfunction, autonomic insufficiency, and certain venodilator antihypertensive drugs, especially α-blockers and α+β-blockers. Diuretics and nitrates may further aggravate OH. Exaggerated BP drops may occur in the elderly also after meals [36], and after exercise [37].

Therefore BP should be measured 1 and 5 minutes after assumption of the standing position in elderly subjects, diabetic patients, and in other conditions in which postural hypotension may be frequent or suspected since there is a high frequency, i.e., as much as 30% of a 20 mmHg or greater fall in BP in patients with a SBP over 160 mm Hg [1]. In these circumstances standing BP should be used to guide treatment decisions. Side effects like dizziness and light-headedness should alert the physicians of possible over-treatment. If present, drug therapy should be adjusted accordingly and appropiate warnings should be given to patients. Pseudohypertension, suggested to be more common among elderly, is defined as a condition in which the cuff pressure is inappropriately high compared to the intraarterial pressure because of thickened, stiff, or calcified brachial artery which can not be compressed by the BP cuff. Lack of target organ involvement despite high auscultatory BP values or symptoms of hypotension in a patient with apparent resistant HT may indicate pseudohypertension [38]. Osler's maneuver proposed as a screening method proved to have little predictive value [39]. A relatively small percentage of elderly patients have a reversible form of HT, most commonly due to renovascular disease, which is seen most often in smokers [40].

B. Central Blood Pressure

PP is a derived measure which combines the imperfection of the original measures. No practical cutoff values separating PP normality from abnormality at different ages have been produced, but some values such as 50 or 55 mmHg have been suggested [41]. Central PP taking into account the ''amplification phenomena'' between the peripheral arteries and the aorta, is more precise and may improve on these limitations (Figure 1).

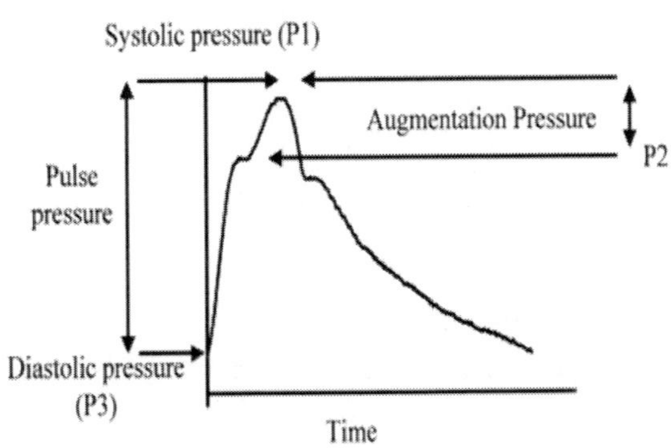

Figure 1. Carotid pressure waveform is recorded by applanation tonometry. The height of the late systolic peak (P1) above the inflection (P2) defines the augmentation pressure, and the ratio of augmentation pressure to pulse pressure (PP) defines the augmentation index in percent [41].

Aortic SBP and PP, i.e., the pressure exerted at the level of the heart, brain, and the kidney, may be different from the conventionally measured brachial pressure because of the variable superimposition of incoming and reflected waves along the arterial tree [42]. Peripheral and central systolic and PP may be differently affected by antihypertensive drugs [43]. Because of its invasive nature central BP was confined only to research until a non-invasive method which estimates aortic BP by calculating the augmentation index from the pulse wave contour recorded from a peripheral artery [44, 45]. In two studies use of this method has confirmed that BP reduction was not the same at central and brachial artery level [46, 47], and central PP was significantly related to CVD events [46].

C. Family and Clinical History

A comprehensive family and clinical history should be taken with particular attention to HT, diabetes, dyslipidaemia, premature CHD, stroke, peripheral artery or renal disease which should include as follows [1]:

- Duration and previous levels of high BP
- Previous antihypertensive therapy, its efficacy and adverse effects
- Symptoms suggestive of secondary causes of HT (muscle weakness and tetany for aldosteronism etc.) and intake of drugs or substances that can raise BP (cyclosporine etc.)
- Lifestyle factors (smoking and dietary habits, snoring etc.)
- Symptoms of organ damage: past history or current symptoms (brain and eyes, heart, kidney, peripheral arteries)
- Personal, family and environmental factors

D. Physical Examination

Physical examination should search for evidence of additional risk factors, for signs suggesting secondary HT, and for evidence of organ damage as follows [1]:

- Signs suggesting secondary HT and organ damage (palpation of enlarged kidneys for polycyctic kidney disease etc.)
- Signs of organ damage (brain, retina (fundoscopic abnormalities), heart, peripheral arteries, carotid arteries (systolic murmurs etc.))
- Heart rate
- Evidence of visceral obesity

  Increased waist circumference (standing position): 102 cm for men, 88 cm for women

  Increased body mass index: body weight (kg)/ height (m^2):

  Overweight $\geq$ 25 kg/m^2, Obesity $\geq$ 30 kg/m^2

E. Laboratory Investigations

Laboratory investigations are directed at providing evidence for additional risk factors, searching for secondary HT and looking for the absence or presence of organ damage. Investigations should progress from the most simple to the more complicated. The younger the patient, the higher the BP and the faster the development of HT, the more detailed the diagnostic work-up should be. On the basis of a number of criteria (prognostic importance, prevalence in the population, availability and cost etc.) detection of organ damage consists of relatively simple and cheap procedures for routine search and of more complex procedures or instrumentations. However, the minimum laboratory investigations needed remain a matter of debate. Laboratory investigations are divided into 3 categories [1]:

a) Routine Tests

- Fasting plasma glucose
- Serum total cholesterol
- Serum LDL-cholesterol
- Serum HDL-cholesterol
- Fasting serum triglycerides
- Serum potassium
- Serum uric acid
- Serum creatinine (an imprecise measure of renal function)
- Estimated creatinine clearance (Cockroft-Gault formula) or glomerular filtration rate (eGFR) (MDRD formula)
- Haemoglobin and haematocrit
- Urinanalysis (complemented by microalbuminuria via dipstick and microscopic examination)
- Electrocardiogram (ECG)

b) Recommended Tests

- Echocardiogram
- Carotid ultrasound
- Quantitative proteinuria (if dipstick test positive)
- Ankle-brachial BP index
- Fundoscopy
- Glucose tolerance test (if fasting plasma glucose > 5.6 mmol/L (100 mg/dl)
- HBPM and ABPM
- Pulse wave velocity measurement (where available)

c) Extended Evaluation (Domain of the Specialist)

- Further search for cerebral, cardiac, renal and vascular damage is mandatory in complicated HT
- Search for secondary HT when suggested by history, physical examination or routine tests: measurement of renin, aldosterone, corticosteroids, catecholamines in plasma and/or urine; arteriographies; renal and adrenal ultrasound; computer tomography (CT); magnetic resonance imaging (MRI)

In the rather uniform European context, where CVDs are the primary cause of morbidity and mortality, the tests above should be done. Although high sensitivity C reactive protein (hsCRP) has been reported to predict the incidence of CVD events in several clinical settings [48], its added value in determining total CVD risk is uncertain [49], except in patients with metabolic syndrome in whom hsCRP values have been reported to be associated with a further marked increase in risk [50]. The value of other inflammatory markers (fibrinogen, cytokines, homeocysteine and brain natriuretic peptide levels etc.) for CVD risk stratification is the object of active research, but at present their measurement for clinical guidance in HT cannot be recommended [51].

F. Genetic Analysis

Essential HT is a highly heterogeneous disorder, which points to a multi-factorial aetiology and polygenic abnormalities [52, 53]. A number of mutations in genes encoding for major BP controlling systems has been recognized in humans, but their exact role in the pathogenesis of essential HT is still unclear. Several rare monogenic forms of HT have been described such as glucocorticoid-remediable aldosteronism, Liddle's syndrome and others where single gene mutation fully explains the pathogenesis of HT and dictates the best treatment modality [54].

G. Subclinical Organ Damage

Signs of organ involvement should be sought carefully because subclinical organ damage (SOD), at the intermediate stage in the continuum of vascular disease is a strong predictor of total cardiovascular risk. Without ultrasound investigations for left ventricular hypertrophy (LVH) and vasular thickening or plaques, up to 50% of hypertensive subjects may be mistakenly classified at low or moderate added risk, whereas the presence of cardiac and vascular damage classifies it within a higher risk group [55]. Treatment-induced reductions in proteinuria and LVH leading to reduced incidence of CVD events make SOD investigation not only to quantify total cardiovascular risk initially but also to monitor treatment-induced protection [56, 57, 58, 59]. Appropriate techniques are as follows:

- **Heart:** ***ECG:*** LVH detected by the Sokolow-Lyons index ($SV_1+RV_{5\text{-}6} > 38$ mm) or by the Cornell voltage QRS duration product > 2440 mm*ms as cardiac damage diagnostic-monitoring marker appears to be valuable, at least in patients over 55 years of age [56]; *echocardiography* can be considered as recommended test, particularly when not detected by ECG and in the elderly in whom LVH is frequent. Although the relation between left ventricular mass index and CVD risk is continuous, thresholds of 125 g/m^2 for men, and 110 g/m^2 for women are widely used for conservative estimates of LVH [60].

- **Blood vessels:** ***Carotid ultrasound:*** common carotid arteries are used for vascular hypertrophy, bifurcations and/or internal carotids are used for plaques (atherosclerosis) imaging. Carotid ultrasound examination may often detect vascular damage early and make risk stratification more precise [55]. *Low ankle-brachial BP index* of <0.9 signals advanced atherosclerosis [61]. *Carotid-femoral pulse wave* ***velocity*** provides a comprehensive non-invasive method of arterial stiffness, which is simple and accurate enough to be considered as a diagnostic procedure [41]. Although the relationship between aortic stiffness and events is continuous, a threshold > 12 m/s has been suggested as a conservative estimate of significant alterations of aortic function in middle age hypertensives. The invasiveness of *gluteal biopsies* which can demonstrate early alterations, makes this approach unsuitable for general use. *High resolution cardiac CT* for quantifying the increase in coronary calcium and *endothelial dysfunction* cannot be advocated as currently useful in the clinical evaluation of the hypertensive patient [1].
- **Kidney:** Renal insufficiency is now classified according to the eGFR calculated by the abbreviated *MDRD formula* [62]. Values of eGFR below 60 ml/min/1.73 m^2 indicate chronic renal disease (CRD) stage 3, while values below 30 and 15 ml/min/1.73 m^2 indicate CRD stages 4 and 5, respectively [63]. *Cockcroft-Gault formula* is valid in the range > 60 ml/min, but it overestimates creatinine clearance in CRD stage 3 to 5 [63]. Both formulae help to detect mild impaired renal function in face of serum creatinine values that are still in the normal range [63]. A reduction in GFR and an increase in CVD risk may also be inferred from the increased serum levels of *cystatin C* [64].
- **Fundoscopy:** ***Grade 1*** (arteriolar narrowing) and ***2*** (arterio-venous nipping) retinal changes are frequent and of milder degrees and their use for prognosis has been questioned [65]. These changes are largely non specific arteriolar alterations, except in young patients in whom deviation from an entirely normal retina should rise concern. In contrast, *grade 3* (haemorrhages and exudates) and ***4*** (papilloedema) retinal changes are associated with an increased risk of CVD events [66, 67].
- **Brain:** Cranial *CT* is only useful for prompt recognition of intracranial haemorrhage; otherwise *MRI* replaced CT in imaging silent brain infarcts, lacunar infarctions, microbleeds and white matter lesions whose prevalance increases with age and HT, and is associated with an increased risk of stroke, cognitive decline and dementia [68]. Silent brain infarcts imaging, in all hypertensive patients with neural disturbance, particularly memory loss is superior to availability and cost. Hypertension-related cognitive disturbances are rare in elderly patients, so cognitive tests may help to detect initial brain deterioration [69].

TREATMENT BENEFITS

As late as the 1950s and 1960s, some physicians believed that an elevated BP was necessary to provide an adequate blood supply to vital organs as people aged. There is little doubt from randomized placebo controlled trials that elderly patients benefit from antihypertensive treatment in terms of reduced cardiovascular morbidity and mortality, whether they have systolic-diastolic HT or ISH, including patients over 75-80 years of age (Table 1) [70].

Randomized Placebo Controlled Trials

The larger randomized controlled trials that have shown the benefit of antihypertensive treatment versus placebo or no treatment in elderly patients with systolic-diastolic HT used either a diuretic or a β-blocker as first-line therapy [71, 72, 73, 74]. A meta-analysis has pointed out that in the elderly β-blockers may have a less pronounced preventive effect on cardiovascular events than diuretics, but in many of these patients diuretics and β-blockers were used together [75].

In trials of ISH first-line drugs comprised a diuretic [13] or a dihydropyridine calcium antagonist (CA) [76]. Treatment was initiated with dihydropyridine CA also in two Chinese trials, one in systolic-diastolic HT [77] and the other in ISH [78], in which alternate rather than random allocation was used. In all these trials active therapy was superior to placebo or no treatment.

The landmark trial of Systolic Hypertension in the Elderly Program (SHEP) involving 4736 hypertensive individuals over age 60 with pretreatment SBP > 160 and DBP < 90 mmHg, first proved the benefit on cardiovascular morbidity and mortality with chlorthalidone (with the option of adding atenolol or reserpine). Non-fatal stroke was reduced by 37%, non-fatal myocardial infarction (MI) by 33%, congestive heart failure (HF) by 54% and overall CVD by 32% as compared with the placebo group. There were strong trends to decrease in transient ischemic attacks (25%), and in total (13%), cardiovascular (20%), cerebrovascular (29%) and coronary (20%) mortality [13]. This trial also pointed out that serum uric acid independently predicts CVD events in patients with ISH. These patients experienced the same benefit from diuretic-based treatment as those with low-baseline serum uric acid levels [79].

Using a similar design and sample size (4695 patients with ISH), the Systolic Hypertension in Europe (Syst-EUR) study compared a regimen based on longer-acting CA nitrendipine (with optional add-on enalapril and/or hydrochlorothiazide) to placebo and found a significant reduction in total strokes (42%) as well as overall CVD events (31%) [76]. In the Syst-Eur trial the rate of vascular dementia was also reduced by 50% [80], while it was not changed by the chlorthalidone-based therapy in the SHEP study, therefore a specific neuroprotective effect of dihydropyridine-type CA, nitrendipine was hypothesized.

The Syst-China trial confirmed the beneficial effect of nitrendipine in patients with ISH as it reduced total strokes by 38%, stroke mortality by 58%, all-cause mortality by 39%, cardiovascular mortality by 39%, fatal and non-fatal cardiovascular events by 37% [78].

Table 1. Effects of therapy in older hypertensive patients

CLINICAL TRIAL NAME								
	Australian	EWPHE	C & W	STOP	MRC	SHEP	HDFP	Syst Eur
Number of patients	582	840	884	1627	4396	4736	2374	4695
Age (years)	60-69	> 60	60-79	70-84	65-74	60≥80	60-69	> 60
Mean BP at entry, mmHg	165/101	182/101	197/100	195/102	185/91	170/77	170/101	174/86
Percent Reductions of Events in Treated Compared to Controls								
Stroke	33	36	42*	47*	25*	33*	44*	42*
CAD	18	20	+.03	13**	19	27*	15*	30
CHF	-	22	32	51	-	55*	-	29
CVD	31	29*	24*	40*	17*	32*	16*	31*

EWPHE: European Working Party on High Blood Pressure in the Elderly
C&W: Coope and Warrender
STOP: Swedish Trial in Older Patients with Hypertension
MRC: Medical Research Council Study
SHEP: Systolic Hypertension in the Elderly Program
HDFP: Hypertension Detection and Follow-up Program
Syst Eur: Systolic Hypertension in Europe Multicentre Trial
CAD: Coronary artery disease, CHF: Congestive heart failure, CVD: cerebrovascular disease
*: Statistically significant
**: Myocardial infarction only; sudden deaths decreased from 13 to 4.

A meta-analysis of eight placebo-controlled trials in 15,693 elderly patients followed for 4 years found that active antihypertensive treatment reduced coronary events (23%), strokes (30%), cardiovascular deaths (18%), and total deaths (13%), with the benefit particularly great in those older than 70 years. The absolute benefit was larger in men, in patients aged 70 years or more and in those with previous cardiovascular complications or wider PP. Treatment prevented strokes more effectively than coronary events [29]. Benefits of therapy have been demonstrated even in individuals over 80 years of age [71].

These findings summarized implies: 1) antihypertensive medications lead to significant reductions of CVD morbidity and mortality while having less significant effect on all cause mortality; 2) the benefit can also be seen at older ages, including patients with ISH; 3) the CVD risk reduction is similar in men and women and the beneficial effect is present across various ethnic groups; and 4) with regard to cause-specific events the risk of fatal or non-fatal stroke is reduced by about 30-40%, but, CVD events are reduced as well, though to a lesser degree by 20%. Finally, treatment appears to cause a large reduction in the incidence of HF.

Comparative Trials

The demonstration of the beneficial effects of BP lowering has made it ethically unacceptable to perform placebo controlled trials with an untreated group. For this reason in more recent trials the drug under investigation was compared with placebo in groups of patients already treated with other antihypertensive agents. This has provided additional evidence on the beneficial effect of various antihypertensive drugs also documenting that the benefit may be sustantial even when BP reductions are small and the initial BP is below the traditional cutoff defining HT. Some of these trials are as follows:

Subgroup analysis of the INSIGHT trial showed that patients with ISH were slightly more responsive than ordinary HT to treatment by long-acting nifedipine-GITS as significantly less patients required addition of a second drug. An important result from this study showed that patients with ISH whose DBP significantly decreased with increasing therapy were smokers with existing evidence of atherosclerosis [81, 82].

The STOP-2 trial found that the incidence of cardiovascular events was similar in elderly hypertensives randomized to a CA, an angiotensin converting enzyme inhibitor (ACEi), or conventional treatment with a diuretic or a β-blocker [83].

ALLHAT showed that a diuretic, a CA and an ACEi influenced cardiovascular events to the same extent also in the subgroup of patients older than 65 years [84].

In about more than 9000, 55 to 80 year old hypertensive patients with evidence of LVH, the LIFE trial showed a clear benefit of the angiotensin receptor antagonist (ARB) losartan in reducing cardiovascular events, particularly stroke, over the β-blocker atenolol [85]. The losartan benefits were particularly expressed in two pre-specified subgroups of patients; those with diabetes [86] and those with ISH [87].

In the SCOPE study in hypertensive patients aged 70 years or older the ARB candesartan (often administered on top of a diuretic), reduced BP modestly more than placebo (also frequently administered on top of diuretic-based conventional therapy) with a significant concomitant reduction in non-fatal stroke [88]. A subgroup analysis of SCOPE patients with ISH showed a significant 42% reduction of stroke in candesartan-treated patients [89].

In the VALUE trial the ARB valsartan and the CA amlodipine prevented the primary cardiac endpoint to the same extent, although BP remained higher on valsartan [90]. The VALUE findings strongly suggest that BP should be controlled to a level below 140/90 mm Hg within 3-6 months to prevent new or worsening cardiovascular disease [91].

The ASCOT study showed that treatment with the combination of amlodipine plus the ACEi perindopril was associated with reduced mortality and fewer cardiovascular endpoints than was treatment with atenolol combined with bendroflumethiazide, but the BP was slightly higher in the latter treatment arm [92]. However, in the ACCOMPLISH trial a fixed amlodipine-ACEi combination was superior to diuretic-ACEi in reduction of endpoints irrespective of age despite little BP difference between the treatment arms [93].

The Hypertension Optimal Treatment (HOT) study aimed to investigate the relationship between three levels of target DBP ($\leq$ 90, 85, and 80 mm Hg) and a low dose (75 mg daily) of acetylsalicylic acid to cardiovascular morbidity and mortality in hypertensive patients [94]. Felodipine was given as baseline therapy with the addition of other agents to a large group of 5987 elderly patients above 65 years of age with 54% of women [95]. Intensive lowering of BP was associated with a low rate of cardiovascular events without differences for the BP target groups. Acetylsalicylic acid significantly reduced major cardiovascular events with the greatest benefit seen in all MI. There was no effect on the incidence of stroke or fatal bleeds, but non-fatal major bleeds were twice as common. Likewise, the effect of atorvastatin was at least as strong in the elderly patients as in the younger patients in the lipid-lowering arm of the ASCOT study [96].

Comparative randomized trials show that for similar BP reductions, differences in the incidence of CVD morbidity and mortality between different drug classes are small, thus their benefit largely depend on BP lowering per se. All recent meta-regression analyses [97, 98, 99] underline the important role of BP lowering for all cause-specific events, with the exception of HF: whenever SBP is reduced by 10 mm Hg, independent of the agent used, both stroke and coronary events are markedly reduced [98, 99]. They also suggest that some antihypertensive agents may exert some cause-specific beneficial effects that are BP independent, i.e., an outcome reduction at no BP difference, CA on stroke, and ACEi on coronary events. This effect, however, is definitively smaller (5-10%) than the dominant protective effect exerted by lowering BP. They [97, 100] reported less protection of new onset HF with CA compared with 4 other drug classes, independent of possible differences in BP between treatments. New onset HF is often a difficult diagnosis. The diagnosis may be confounded by ankle oedema due to administration of CA. Furthermore, diuretics may mask HF symptoms. Therefore, some trials [90] considered only hospitalization for HF as a suitable endpoint. Even under this circumstance BP lowering probably remains of paramount importance because in the hypertensive coronary patients of the ACTION trial a BP reduction of 14.6/7.6 mm Hg in the group randomized to slow-release nifedipine was associated with a 38% reduction in the incidence of hospitalized HF compared with placebo [101].

THERAPEUTIC APPROACH

Lifestyle modifications as nonpharmacologic therapy are widely recognized to lower BP or CVD risk which are as follows [1]:

- smoking cessation
- weight reduction in obese patients
- reduction of excessive alcohol intake
- physical exercise
- reduction of salt intake
- increase in fruit and vegetable intake and decrease in saturated and total fat intake

In the Trial of Nonpharmacologic Interventions in the Elderly (TONE), reducing sodium to 80 mmol (2 grams) per day reduced BP over 30 months, and about 40% of those on the low-salt diet were able to discontinue their antihypertensive medications [102]. When weight loss was combined with salt reduction, an additional BP decrease was seen. Older persons should also be encouraged to avoid excessive alcohol intake and to remain as physically active as is feasible. Lifestyle modifications should be advised in all patients with the purpose to lower BP, to control other risk factors and to reduce the number of doses of antihypertensive drugs. Lifestyle modifications may fail to reach the target due to low long-term compliance [1].

Both, the level of SBP and DBP, and the profile and intensity of total cardiovascular risk are needed for starting antihypertensive treatment [1]. Quantification of total cardiovascular risk must include a search for subclinical organ damage (SOD) which is common in HT and has independent prognostic significance [103]. SOD should be assessed at screening and during treatment. Urinary protein excretion (including microalbuminuria), eGFR (MDRD formula), and ECG are suitable for routine use, but cardiac and vascular ultrasounds' use can be encouraged. In patients with HT the presence of SOD usually brings cardiovascular risk into the high range which is not possible in normotensive patients, although this may occur with multiple organ damage and metabolic syndrome.

Initiation of hypertensive treatment in elderly patients should follow the general guidelines.

In the elderly, antihypertensive treatment is highly beneficial, and the proportional benefit in patients aged more than 65 years is no less than that in younger patients. The choice of the drugs should thus not be guided by age. Thiazide diuretic, ACEi, CA, ARB, and β-blocker can be considered for initiation and maintenance of treatment also in the elderly. In no trial in which a benefit was shown, achieved SBP averaged less than 140 mm Hg. When SBP is higher than 140 mm Hg, also in the elderly drug treatment can be initiated and can be brought to below 140 mm Hg, provided treatment is conducted with particular attention to adverse responses, potentially more frequent in the elderly [103].

Evidence is now available from an outcome trial that antihypertensive treatment has benefits also in patients aged 80 years or more [104], starting with monotherapy and adding a second drug if needed. Due to patients' good conditions in this study data extrapolation to more fragile octogenarians is uncertain.

Older patients more frequently have other risk factors, target organ damage, and associated cardiovascular and non cardiovascular clinical conditions than younger ones. This means that the choice of the first drug often needs to be precisely tailored to individual characteristics. Furthermore, many patients will need two or more drugs to control BP, since in the elderly it is often particularly difficult to lower SBP to below 140 mm Hg [15, 105]. In routine practice, if the systolic goal is achieved, the diastolic goal will almost be reduced as well. The possible addition of lipid-lowering and antiplatelet agents should also be considered [1].

BP should always be measured both in the sitting and standing position in the elderly, because their higher risk of postural hypotension may be enhanced by antihypertenisve drugs [106].

A significant number of elderly individuals have widely variable BP with exaggerated high and low extremes. Such individuals deserve consideration for a slow titration approach as do individuals with a history of medication side effects and those with OH. Attention should be given to subjects with a very pronounced reduction in night-time BP, i.e., > 20%, so-called extreme dippers, because of the possibility that this leads to brain under-perfusion, particularly if a further BP fall is produced by treatment [107]. HBPM and ABPM make also possible to study how suitable and consistent an antihypertensive effect is between two drug doses by indices such as the trough-to-peak ratio and the smoothness index [32, 108].

Although differences between individual patients may exist, the risk of underperfusion of vital organs is very low, except in episodes of postural hypotension that should be avoided, particularly in the elderly and diabetic. The existence of a J-shaped curve relating outcomes to achieved BP is not an unknown entity since physicians began to investigate whether the lower the BP the better the prognosis [109]. SHEP investigators looked at the role of the on-treatment DBP in patients with ISH and concluded that an achieved DBP of less than 70 mm Hg, especially below 60 mm Hg identifies a high-risk group with poorer outcome due to possible overtreatment [110]. However, without a history of CHD at baseline, there was no evidence of harm down to a DBP of 55 mm Hg in the Syst-Eur trial [111]. Below 55 mm Hg there were insufficient data, and a low DBP was associated with higher non-cardiovascular mortality also in the placebo group demonstrating that the cause was not overtreatment. A higher mortality for SBP below 120 mm Hg and DBP below 60 mm Hg has been reported in a meta-analysis of several thousand patients [112]. This project points to reverse casualty, with other words that an initially high risk may be responsible for an excessive BP reduction during treatment and not vice versa.

One last point deserves greater attention when making recommendations for medical practice.

Remodeling of large arteries, small arteries, and cardiac structure associated with a BP elevation takes a long time, thus regression of organ damage has a slow time course. As randomized trials can only run for a few years, extrapolation of the results to the much longer life expectancy of patients is not without limitations because the benefit of antihypertensive treatment may become progressively more evident with time [113]. In the Syst-EUR and SHEP trials, the beneficial effects remained evident years after termination of the double-blind phase of the trial, despite the fact that antihypertensive treatment was started also in the placebo group [114, 115]. This ''legacy effect'' has also been reported for diabetic patients in Steno 2 trial and in the UKPDS trial [116, 117].

References

[1] Mancia G, De Backer G, Dominiczak A, et al. 2007 Guidelines for the Management of Arterial Hypertension. The Task Force for the Management of Arterial Hypertension of the European Society of Hypertension (ESH) and of the European Society of Cardiology (ESC). *J Hypertens* 2007; 25: 1105-1187.

[2] Chobanian AV, Bakris GL, Black HR, et al. The Seventh Report of the Joint National Committee on Prevention, Detection, Evaluation, and Treatment of High Blood Pressure: the JNC 7 report. *JAMA* 2003; 289: 2560-2572.

[3] D'Agostino RBS, Grundy S, Sullivan LM, Wilson P. Validation of the Framingham coronary heart disease prediction scores: results of the multiple ethnic groups investigation. *JAMA* 2001; 286: 180-187.

[4] Conroy RM, Pyorala K, Fitzgerald AP, et al. Estimation of ten-year risk of fatal cardiovascular disease in Europa: the Systemic Coronary Risk Evaluation (SCORE) project. *Eur Heart J* 2003; 24: 987-1003.

[5] Kannel WB, Gordon T, Schwartz MJ. Systolic versus diastolic blood pressure and risk of coronary heart disease. The Framingham study. *Am J Cardiol* 1971; 27: 335-346.

[6] Stamler J, Stamler R, Neaton JD. Blood pressure, systolic and diastolic and cardiovascular risks. *Arch Intern Med* 1993; 153: 598-615.

[7] Klag MJ, Brancati FL, Whelton PK, et al. Blood pressure and end stage renal disease in men. *N Egl J Med* 1996; 334: 13-18.

[8] Lewington S, Clarke R, Qizilbash N, Peto R, Collins R. Age-specific relevance of usual blood pressure to vascular mortality: A meta-analysis of individual data for one million adults in 61 prospective studies. Prospective Studies Collaboration. *Lancet* 2002; 360: 1903-1913.

[9] Franklin SS, Gustin WG, Wong ND, et al. Hemodynamic pattern of age-related changes in blood pressure: The Framingham Heart Study. *Circulation* 1997; 96: 308-315.

[10] Franklin SS, Jacobs MJ, Wong ND, L'Italien GJ, Lapuerta P. Predominance of isolated systolic hypertension among middle-aged and elderly US hypertensives: Analysis based on National Health and Nutrition Examination Survey (NHANES) III. *Hypertension* 2001; 37: 869-874.

[11] Vasan RS, Beiser A, Seshadri S, et al. Residual lifetime risk for devoloping hypertension in middle-aged women and men: The Framingham Heart Study. *JAMA* 2002; 287: 1003-1010.

[12] Izzo JL Jr, Levy D, Black HR. Clinical Advisory Statement. Importance of systolic blood pressure in older Americans. *Hypertension* 2000; 35: 1021-1024.

[13] SHEP Cooperative Research Group. Prevention of stroke by antihypertensive drug treatment in older persons with isolated systolic hypertension. Final results of the Systolic Hypertension in the Elderly Program (SHEP). *JAMA* 1991; 265: 3255-3264.

[14] Koch-Weser J. The therapeutic challenge of systolic hypertension. *N Engl J Med* 1973; 289: 481-483.

[15] Burt VL, Cutler JA, Higgins M, et al. Trends in the prevalance, awareness, treatment, and control of hypertension in the adult US population. Data from the health examination surveys, 1960 to 1991. Erratum in: Hypertension 1996 May; 27 (5): 1192. *Hypertension* 1995; 26: 60-69.

[16] Messerli FH, Ventura HO, Glade LB, et al. Essential hypertension in the elderly: haemodynamics, intravascular volume, plasma renin activity, and circulating catecholamine levels. *Lancet* 1983; 2: 983-986.

[17] Grassi G, Seravalle G, Bertinieri G, et al. Sympathetic and reflex alterations in systo-diastolic and systolic hypertension of the elderly. *J Hypertens* 2000; 18: 587-593.

[18] Pickering TG. Reflections in Hypertension: JNC 7.5. *J Clin Hypertens* 2007; 9: 901-904.

[19] Mancia G, Ferrari A, Gregorini L, et al. Blood pressure and heart rate variabilities in normotensive and hypertensive human beings. *Circ Res* 1983; 53: 96-104.

[20] O'Brien E, Asmar R, Beilin L, et al. Practice guidelines of the European Society of Hypertension for clinic, ambulatory and self blood pressure measurement. *J Hypertens* 2005; 23: 697-701.

[21] Björklund K, Lind L, Zethelius B, Berglund L, Lithell H. Prognostic significance of 24-h ambulatory blood pressure characteristics for cardiovascular morbidity in a population of elderly men. *J Hypertens* 2004; 22: 1691-1697.

[22] Staessen J, Lutgarde T, Fagard R, et al. Predicting cardiovascular risk using conventional vs ambulatory blood pressure in older patients with systolic hypertension. *JAMA* 1999; 282: 539-546.

[23] Stenehjem AE, Os I. Reproducibility of blood pressure variability, white coat effect and dipping pattern in untreated, uncomplicated and newly diagnosed essential hypertension. *Blood Press* 2004;13: 214-224.

[24] Bertineri G, Grass G, Rossi P, et al. 24 hour blood pressure profile in centenarians. *J Hypertens* 2002; 20: 1765-1769.

[25] O'Sullivan C, Duggan J, Atkins N, O'Brien E. Twenty-four ambulatory blood pressure in community-dwelling elderly men and women aged 60-102 years. *J Hypertens* 2003; 21: 1641-1647.

[26] Okhubo T, Asayama K, Kikuya M, et al. How many times should blood pressure be measured at home for better prediction of stroke risk? Ten year follow–up results from the Ohasama study. *J Hypertens* 2004; 22: 1099-1104.

[27] Parati G, Stergiou GS, Asmar R, et al. European Society of Hypertension guidelines for blood pressure monitoring at home: a summary report of the Second International Consensus Conference on Home Blood Pressure Monitoring. *J Hypertens* 2008; 26: 1505-1530.

[28] Parati G, Asmar R, Stergiou GS. Self blood pressure monitoring at home by wrist devices: a reliable approach? *J Hypertens* 2002; 20: 573-578.

[29] Staessen JA, Gasowski J, Wang JG, et al. Risks of untreated and treated isolated systolic hypertension in the elderly: meta-analysis of outcome trials. *Lancet* 2000; 355: 865-872.

[30] Pringle E, Phillips C, Thijs L, et al. Systolic blood pressure variability as a risk factor for stroke and cardiovascular mortality in the elderly hypertensive population. *J Hypertens* 2003; 21: 2251-2257.

[31] Kario K, Pickering TG, Umeda Y, et al. Morning surge in blood pressure as a predictor of silent and clinical cerebrovascular disease in elderly hypertensives: a prospective study. *Circulation* 2003; 107: 1401-1406.

[32] Menard J, Chatellier G, Day M, et al. Self-measurement of blood pressure at home to evaluate drug effects by the trough: peak ratio. *J Hypertens Suppl* 1994; 12: S21-S25.

[33] Masaki KH, Schatz IJ, Burchfiel CM, et al. Orthostatic hypotension predicts mortality in elderly men: The Honolulu Heart Program. *Circulation* 1998; 98: 2290-2295.

[34] Mukai S, Lipsitz LA. Orthostatic hypotension. *Clin Geriatr Med* 2002; 18: 253-268.

[35] Ooi WL, Hossain M, Lipsitz LA. The association between orthostatic hypotension and recurrent falls in nursing home residents. *Am J Med* 2000; 108: 106-111.

[36] Jonsson PV, Lipsitz LA, Kelley M, Koestner J. Hypotensive responses to common daily activities in institutionalized elderly. A potential risk for recurrent falls. *Arch Intern Med* 1990; 150: 1518-1524.

[37] Kelley GA, Kelley KS. Progressive resistance exercise and resting blood pressure: A meta-analysis of randomized controlled trials. *Hypertension* 2000; 35: 838-843.

[38] Zweifler AJ, Tariq Shahab S. Pseudohypertension: a new assesment. *J Hypertens* 1993; 11: 1-6.

[39] Hla K, Samsa G, Stoneking H, et al. Observer variability of Osler's maneuver in detection of pseudohypertension. *J Clin Epidemiol* 1991; 44: 513-518.

[40] Nally J, Jr. Management of renovascular hypertension. In Izzo J, Jr, Black H (editors): Hypertension Primer: The essentials of High Blood Pressure: Basic Science, Population Science, and Clinical Management. Philadelphia, PA: *Lippincott Williams & Wilkins;* 2003. pp 500-502.

[41] Laurent S, Cockcroft J, Van Bortel L, et al. on behalf of the European Network for Non-invasive Investigation of Large Arteries. Expert consensus document on arterial stiffness: methodological issues and clinical applications. *Eur Heart J* 2006; 27: 2588-2605.

[42] O'Rourke MF. Principles and definitions of arterial stiffness, wave reflections and pulse pressure amplification. In Safar ME, O'Rourke MF (editors), Arterial stiffness in hypertension. Handbook of Hypertension. *Elsevier;* 2006. Vol 23. pp 3-19.

[43] Morgan T, Lauri J, Bertram D, Anderson A. Effect of different antihypertensive drug classes on central aortic pressure. *Am J Hypertens* 2004; 17: 118-123.

[44] Chen CH, Nevo E, Fetics B, et al. Estimation of central aortic pressure waveform by mathematical transformation of radial tonometry pressure. Validation of generalized transfer function. *Circulation* 1997; 95: 1827-1836.

[45] Hope SA, Tay DB, Meredith IT, Cameron JD. Use of arterial transfer functions for the derivation of aortic waveform characteristics. *J Hypertens* 2003; 21: 1299-1305.

[46] Williams B, Lacy PS, Thom SM et al. The CAFE Investigators, for the Anglo-Scandinavian Cardiac Outcome Trial (ASCOT) Investigators. Differential Impact of Blood-Pressure-Lowering Drugs on Central Aortic Pressure and Clinical Outcomes: Principal Results of the Conduit Artery Function Evaluation (CAFE) Study. *Circulation;* 2006; 113: 1213-1225.

[47] Dhakam Z, McEniery CM, Yasmin, Cockcroft JR, Brown MJ, Wilkinson IB. Atenolol and eprosartan: differential effects on central blood pressure and aortic pulse wave velocity. *Am J Hypertens* 2006; 19: 214-219.

[48] Ridker PM. High-sensitivity C-reactive protein: potential adjunct for global risk assessment in the primary prevention of cardiovascular disease. *Circulation* 2001; 103: 1813-1818.

[49] Wang TJ, Gona P, Larson MG, et al. Multiple biomarkers for the prediction of first major cardiovascular events and death. *N Engl J Med* 2006; 355: 2631-2639.

[50] Ridker PM, Buring JE, Cook NR, Rifai N. C-reactive protein, the metabolic syndrome, and risk of incident cardiovascular events: a 8-year follow-up of 14719 initially healthy American women. *Circulation* 2003; 107: 391-397.

[51] Olsen MH, Wachtell K, Tuxen C, et al. N-terminal pro-brain natriuretic peptide predicts cardiovascular events in patients with hypertension and left ventricular hypertrophy: a LIFE study. *J Hypertens* 2004; 22: 1597-1604.

[52] Luft FC. Molecular genetics of human hypertension. *J Hypertens* 1998; 16: 1871-1878.

[53] Melander O. Genetic factors in hypertension-what is known and what does it mean? *Blood Press* 2001; 10: 254-270.

[54] Lifton RP, Gharavi AG, Geller DS. Molecular mechanisms of human hypertension. *Cell* 2001; 104: 545-556.

[55] Cuspidi C, Ambrosioni E, Mancia G, et al. Role of echocardiography and carotid ultrasonography in stratifying risk in patients with essential hypertension: the Assessment of Prognostic Risk Observational Survey. *J Hypertens* 2002; 20: 1307-1314.

[56] Okin PM, Devereux RB, Jern S, et al. LIFE Study Investigators. Regression of electrocardiographic left ventricular hypertrophy during antihypertensive treatment and prediction of major cardiovascular events. *JAMA* 2004; 292: 2343-2349.

[57] Devereux RB, Wachtell K, Gerdts E, et al. Prognostic significance of left ventricular mass change during treatment of hypertension. *JAMA* 2004; 292: 2350-2356.

[58] Olsen MH, Wachtell K, Ibsen H, et al. LIFE Study Investigators. Reductions in albuminuria and in electrocardiographic left ventricular hypertrophy independently improve prognosis in hypertension: the LIFE study. *J Hypertens* 2006; 24: 775-781.

[59] Verdecchia P, Angeli F, Borgioni C, et al. Changes in cardiovascular risk by reduction of left ventricular mass in hypertension: a meta-analysis. *Am J Hypertens* 2003; 16: 895-899.

[60] Devereux RB, Alonso DR, Lutas EM, et al. Echocardiographic assessment of left ventricular hypertrophy: comparison to necropsy findings. *Am J Cardiol* 1986; 57: 450-458.

[61] Feringa HH, Bax JJ, van Waning, et al. The long-term prognostic value of the resting and postexercise ankle-brachial index. *Arch Intern Med* 2006; 166: 529-535.

[62] Hallan S, Asberg A, Lindberg M, Johnsen H. Validation of the Modification of Diet in Renal Disease formula for estimating GFR with special emphasis on calibration of the serum creatinine assay. *Am J Kidney Dis* 2004; 44: 84-93.

[63] Moe S, Drueke T, Cunningham J, et al. Kidney Disease: Improving Global Outcomes (KDIGO). Definition and classification of chronic kidney disease: a position statement from Kidney Disease: Improving Global Outcomes (KDIGO). *Kidney Int* 2005; 67: 2089-2100.

[64] Shlipak MG, Katz R, Sarnak MJ, et al. Cystatin C and prognosis for cardiovascular and kidney outcomes in elderly persons without chronic kidney disease. *Ann Intern Med* 2006; 145: 237-246.

[65] Dimmitt SB, West JN, Eames SM, Gibson JM, Gosling P, Littler WA. Usefulness of ophthalmoscopy in mild to moderate hypertension. *Lancet* 1989; 1: 1103-1106.

[66] Wong TY, Klein R, Sharrett AR, et al. Retinal arteriolar narrowing and risk of coronary heart disease in men and women. The Atherosclerosis Risk in Communities Study. *JAMA* 2002; 287: 1153-1159.

[67] Wong TY, Klein R, Sharrett AR, et al. ARIC Investigators. Retinal microvascular abnormalities and incident stroke. The Atherosclerosis Risk in Communities Study. *Lancet* 2001; 358: 1134-1140.

[68] Vermeer SE, Hollander M, van Dijk EJ, et al. Silent brain infarcts and white matter lesions increase stroke risk in the general population: The Rotterdam Scan Study. *Stroke* 2000; 34: 1126-1129.

[69] Kilander L, Nyman H, Boberg M, Hansson L, Lithell H. Hypertension is related to cognitive impairment: A 20-year folow-up of 999 men. *Hypertension* 1998; 31: 780-786.

[70] Moser M (editor). Clinical Management of Hypertension. Professional Communications, Inc, 1999, fourth edition. p 198.

[71] Dahlöf B, Lindholm LH, Hansson L, et al. Morbidity and mortality in the Swedish Trial in Old Patients with Hypertension (STOP-Hypertension). *Lancet* 1991; 338: 1281-1285.

[72] Amery A, Birkenhager W, Brixko P, et al. Mortality and morbidity results from the European Working Party on High Blood Pressure in the Elderly trial. *Lancet* 1985; 1: 1349-1354.

[73] Coope J, Warrender TS. Randomized trial of treatment of hypertension in elderly patients in primary care. *Br Med J* 1986; 293: 1145-1151.

[74] MRC Working Party. Medical Research Council trial of treatment of hypertension in older adults: principal results. *Br Med J* 1992; 304: 405-412.

[75] Messerli FH, Grossman E, Goldbourt U. Are beta-blockers efficacious as first-line therapy for hypertension in the elderly? A systematic review. *JAMA* 1998; 279: 1903-1907.

[76] Staessen JA, Fagard R, Thijs L, et al. for the Systolic Hypertension in Europe (Syst-Eur) Trial Investigators. Randomized double-blind comparison of placebo and active treatment for older patients with isolated systolic hypertension. *Lancet* 1997; 350: 757-764.

[77] Gong L, Zhang W, Zhu Y, et al. Shanghai trial of nitrendipine in the elderly (STONE). *J Hypertens* 1996; 16: 1237-1245.

[78] Liu L, Wang JG, Gong L, et al. for the Syst-China Collaborative Group. Comparision of active treatment and placebo in older Chinese patients with isolated systolic hypertension. *J Hypertens* 1998; 16: 1823-1829.

[79] Franse LV, Pahor M, Di Bari M, et al. Serum uric acid, diuretic treatment and risk of cardiovascular events in the Systolic Hypertension in the Elderly Program (SHEP). *J Hypertens* 2000; 18: 1149-1154.

[80] Forette F, Seux ML, Staessen JA, et al. Prevention of dementia in randomized double-blind placebo-controlled Systolic Hypertension in Europe (Syst-Eur) trial. *Lancet* 1998; 352: 1347-1351.

[81] The INSIGHT Group. Morbidity and mortality in patients randomized to double-blind treatment with a long-acting calcium channel blocker or diuretic in the International Nifedipine GITS study: Intervention as a Goal in Hypertension Treatment (INSIGHT). *Lancet* 2000; 356: 366-372.

[82] Brown MJ, Castaigne A, de Leeuw Pw, et al. Influence of diabetes and type of hypertension on response to antihypertensive treatment. *Hypertension* 2000; 35: 1038-1042.

[83] Hansson L, Lindholm LH, Ekbom T, et al. Randomized trial of old and new antihypertensive drugs in elderly patients: cardiovascular mortality and morbidity in the Swedish Trial in Old Patients with Hypertension-2 study. *Lancet* 1999; 354: 1751-1756.

[84] The ALLHAT Officers and Coordinators for the ALLHAT Collaborative Research Group. Major outcomes in high risk hypertensive patients randomized to angiotensin converting enzyme inhibitor or calcium channel blocker vs diuretic: The Antihypertensive and Lipid-Lowering treatment to prevent Heart Attack Trial (ALLHAT). *JAMA* 2002; 288: 2981-2997.

[85] Dahlöf B, Devereux RB, Kjeldsen SE et al. Cardiovascular morbidity and mortality in the Losartan Intervention For Endpoint reduction in hypertension study (LIFE): a randomized trial against atenolol. *Lancet* 2002; 359: 995-1003.

[86] Lindholm LH, Ibsen H, Dahlöf B, et al. for the LIFE Study Group. Cardiovascular morbidity and mortality in patients with diabetes in the Losartan Intervention For Endpoint reduction in hypertension study (LIFE): a randomized trial against atenolol. *Lancet* 2002; 358: 1004-1010.

[87] Kjeldsen SE, Dahlöf B, Devereux RB, et al. Effects of losartan on cardiovascular morbidity and mortality in patients with isolated systolic hypertension and left ventricular hypertrophy: a Losartan Intervention For Endpoint reduction (LIFE) substudy. *JAMA* 2002; 288: 1491-1498.

[88] Lithell H, Hansson L, Skoog I et al. for the SCOPE study group. The Study on Cognition and Prognosis in the Elderly (SCOPE). Principal results of a randomized double-blind intervention trial. *J Hypertens* 2003; 21: 875-886.

[89] Papademetriou V, Farsang C, Elmfeldt D, et al. for the SCOPE study group. Stroke prevention with the angiotensin II type 1-receptor blocker candesartan in elderly

patients with isolated systolic hypertension: the Study on Cognition and Prognosis in the Elderly (SCOPE). *J Am Coll Cardiol* 2004; 44:1175-1180.
[90] Julius S, Kjeldsen SE, Weber M, et al. Cardiac events, stroke and mortality in high-risk hypertensives treated with valsartan or amlodipine: main outcomes of the VALUE trial. *Lancet* 2004; 363: 2022-2031.
[91] Weber M, Julius S, Kjeldsen SE, et al. Blood pressure dependent and independent effects of antihypertensive treatment on clinical events in the VALUE trial. *Lancet* 2004; 363: 2049-2051.
[92] Dahlöf B, Sever PS, Poulter NR, et al. Prevention of cardiovascular events with antihypertensive regimen of amlodipine adding perindopril as required versus atenolol adding bendroflumethiazide as required, in the Anglo-Scandinavian Cardiac Outcomes Trial-Blood Pressure Lowering Arm (ASCOT-BPLA): a multicentre randomized controlled trial. *Lancet* 2005; 366: 89-906.
[93] Jamerson K, Weber MA, Bakris GL, et al. for the ACCOMPLISH trial investigators. Benazepril plus amlodipine or hydrochlorothiazide for hypertension in high-risk patients. *N Engl J Med* 2008; 359: 2417-2428.
[94] Hansson L, Zanchetti A, Carruthers SG, et al. Effects of intensive blood pressure lowering and low dose aspirin in patients with hypertension: principal results of the Hypertension Optimal Treatment (HOT) randomized trial. *Lancet* 1998; 351: 1755-1762.
[95] Kjeldsen SE, Kolloch RE, Leonetti G, et al. Influence of gender and age on preventing cardiovascular disease by antihypertensive treatment and acetylsalicylic acid. The HOT study. *J Hypertens* 2000; 18: 629-642.
[96] Sever PS, Dahlöf B, Paulter NR, et al. for the ASCOT investigators. Prevention of coronary and stroke events with atorvastatin in hypertensive patients who have average or lower then average cholesterol concentrations in the Anglo Scandinavian Cardiac Outcomes Lipid Lowering Arm (ASCOT-LLA): a multicenter randomized controlled trial. *Lancet* 2003; 361: 1149-1158.
[97] Blood Pressure Lowering Treatment Trialists' Collaboration. Effects of different blood-pressure-lowering regimens on major cardiovascular events: results of prospectively-designed overviews updated until 1 March 2003. *J Hypertens* 2003; 362: 1527-1535.
[98] Verdecchia P, Reboldi G, Angeli F, et al. Angiotensin-converting enzyme inhibitors and calcium channel blockers for coronary heart disease and stroke prevention. *Hypertension* 2005; 46: 386-392.
[99] Blood Pressure Lowering Treatment Trialists' Collaboration. Blood pressure dependent and independent effects of agents that inhibit the renin-angiotensin system. *J Hypertens* 2007; 25: 951-958.
[100] Blood Pressure Lowering Treatment Trialists' Collaboration. Effects of different blood-pressure-lowering regimens on major cardiovascular events in individuals with and without diabetes mellitus. Results of prospectively-designed overviews of randomized trials. *Arch Intern Med* 2005; 165: 1410-1419.
[101] Lubsen J, Wagener G, Kirwan BA, et al. ACTION (A Coronary disease Trial Investigating Outcome with Nifedipine GITS) investigators. Effect of long-acting nifedipine on mortality and cardiovascular morbidity in patients with symptomatic stable angina and hypertension: the ACTION trial. *J Hypertens* 2005; 23: 641-648.

[102] Appel LJ, Espeland MA, Easter L, Wilson AC, Folmar S, Lacy CR. Effects of reduced sodium intake on hypertension control in older individuals: results from the Trial of Nonpharmacologic Interventions in the Elderly (TONE). *Arch Intern Med* 2001; 161: 685-693.

[103] Mancia G, Laurent S, Agabiti-Rosei E, et al. Reappraisal of European guidelines on hypertension management: a European Society of Hypertension Task Force document. *J Hypertens* 2009; 27: 2121-2158.

[104] Beckett NS, Peters R, Flecther AE, et al. for the HYVET Study Group. Treatment of hypertension in patients 80 years of age and older. *N Engl J Med* 2008; 158: 1887-1898.

[105] Mancia G, Grassi G. Systolic and diastolic blood pressure control in antihypertensive drug trials. *J Hypertens* 2002; 20: 1461-1464.

[106] Lakatta EG. Deficient neuroendocrine regulatin of the cardiovascular system with advancing age in healthy humans. *Circulation* 1993; 87: 631-636.

[107] Mancia G, Parati G, Henning M, et al. Relation between blood pressure variability and carotid artery damage in hypertension: baseline data from the European lacidipine Study on Atherosclerosis (ELSA). *J Hypertens* 2001; 19: 1981-1989.

[108] Parati G, Omboni S, Rizzoni D, Agabiti Rosei E, Mancia G. The smoothness index: a new reproducible and clinically relevant measure of the homogeneity of the blood pressure reduction with treatment for hypertension. *J Hypertens* 1998; 16: 1685-1691.

[109] Cruickshank JM, Thorp JM, Zacharias FJ. Benefit and potential harm of lowering high blood pressure. *Lancet* 1987; 329: 581-584.

[110] Somes GW, Pahor M, Shorr RI, Cushman WC, Applegate WB. The role of diastolic blood pressure when treating isolated systolic hypertension. *Arch Intern Med* 1999; 159: 2004-2009.

[111] Fagard RH, Staessen JA, Thijs L, et al. On-treatment diastolic blood pressure and prognosis in systolic Hypertension. *Arch Intern Med* 2007; 167: 1884-1891.

[112] Boutitic F, Gueyffier F, Pocock S, et al. INdividual Data ANalysis of Antihypertensive (INDANA) intervention. J-shaped relationship between blood pressure and mortality in hypertensive patients: new insights from a meta-analysis of individual-patient data. *Ann Intern Med* 2002; 136: 438-448.

[113] Laurent S, Briet M, Boutouyrie P. Large/small artery cross talk and recent morbidity-mortality trials in hypertension. *J Hypertens* 2009; 54: 388-392.

[114] Staessen JA, Thijs L, Fagard R, et al. for the Syst-EUR trial investigators. Effects of immediate versus delayed antihypertensive therapy on outcome in the Systolic Hypertension in Europe Trial. *J Hypertens* 2004; 22: 847-857.

[115] Kostis JB, Wilson AC, Freudenberger RS, et al. SHEP Collaborative Research Group. Long-term effect of diuretic-based therapy on fatal outcomes in subjects with isolated systolic hypertension with and without diabetes. *Am J Cardiol* 2005; 95: 29-35.

[116] Gaede P, Lund-Andersen H, Parving HH, Pederson O. Effect of a multifactorial intervention on mortality in type 2 diabetes. *N Engl J Med* 2008; 358: 580-591.

Holman RR, Paul SK, Bethel MA, Matthews DR, Neil HA. 10-years follow-up of intensive glucose control in type 2 diabetes. *N Engl J Med* 2008; 359: 1577-1589.

In: New Horizons in Geriatric Medicine. Volume 1
Editors: Ahmet Turan Isik, M. Refik Mas et al.
ISBN: 978-1-62808-972-1

Chapter 11

INSULIN RESISTANCE, DIABETES MELLITUS

Mahmut Yazici, M.D. and Mehmet Refik Mas, M.D.

SUMMARY

When considering changes in endocrine function of the elderly, it is important to distinguish between the effects of aging per se on the physiology of the endocrine system and those caused by age-related diseases, given the high prevalence of disorders both symptomatic and asymptomatic in the elderly. Moreover, the distinction between age and disease related to the change does not necessarily determine the therapeutic intervention.

The action of certain hormones decrease with age, the secretion of growth hormone may or may not offset these reductions in the responsiveness of the tissue.

- The appropriate goal for hemoglobin A1C (HbA1c) in elderly patients who have a life expectancy of more than ten years should be similar to those developed for younger adults (<7.0 percent). The aim should be slightly higher (≤ 8.0 percent) in frail elderly with multiple medical comorbidities and functional and those whose life expectancy is less than ten years. Individual goals for the very elderly may be even greater and should include efforts to preserve the quality of life and prevent hypoglycemia and complications.
- The risk of hypoglycemia, which can lead to a deterioration of cognitive functions and is significantly higher in the elderly. Therefore, avoiding hypoglycemia is an important consideration in the choice of therapeutic agents in the elderly.
- Elderly patients with diabetes should receive individualized advice on lifestyle changes, including medical nutrition assessment. The prescription of nutrition for the elderly with diabetes based on medical, lifestyle and personal factors.
- In the absence of specific indications-cons, suggested metformin as initial therapy for elderly patients with diabetes (Grade 2B). In patients with against-indications and / or intolerance to metformin, a sulfonylurea short-acting (e.g., glipizide) is an alternative option.

- In patients who can not tolerate or are not candidates for metformin or sulfonylureas, repaglinide is a reasonable alternative, especially in a patient with chronic renal failure with risk of hypoglycemia.
- • If glycemic targets are not met a single agent, the elderly patient should be evaluated by the contributing causes, such as difficulty adhering to medication side effects, or a misunderstanding of the terms of nutrition.

Indications for a second officer and the treatment options for patients who fail initial treatment with a lifestyle intervention and metformin or a sulfonylurea were similar in elderly and younger.

INTRODUCTION

Since the 19th century there were sporadic attempts to attribute changes of aging or another endocrine deficit and efforts to reverse these changes with a variety of endocrine therapies. This search for a hormonal "fountain of youth" continues today with, for example, the widespread use of dehydroepiandrosterone (DHEA) as a "nutritional supplement". The clinical significance of the greater is the growing practice of "off-label" prescribing human growth hormone (hGH) and potent androgenic steroids age-related decrease in GH / IGF-I and testosterone, respectively called "somatopause" and “andropause”. Proof of age-related changes in endocrine function and its clinical consequences are examined here, the change-related diseases are discussed briefly.

Physiology of Aging

The complexity of the aging process precludes simplistic formulations that equate aging hormone deficiency. Biological aging is characterized by progressive loss and largely predictable coordination cell and tissue function, so that the body becomes less able to reproduce and survive. The speed of this process is species-specific and changes occur in several organs and systems. Dysfunction is heterogeneous among systems and individuals and is first detected as a loss of reserve capacity and the ability to restore homeostasis, stress, and later by altered function at rest.

The basic mechanisms of aging are unknown. The best available evidence is consistent with the accumulation of a variety of (unrepaired) biochemical alterations that impair the function of nucleic acids, proteins and lipids in membranes. These alterations probably include oxidation by free radicals [1], but also non-enzymatic glycosylation [2], and epigenetic changes like DNA methylation and histone acetylation [3]. The extent to which differentiated cells are affected by aging determines physiological function, while the extent to which stem cells are affected determines the capacity to replace damaged cells and tissue repair [4].

A well-described phenomenon of aging is the deterioration of the wide distribution of the efficiency of signal transduction. Examples include a reduction in the endothelial vasodilator response to estrogen, possibly related to the progressive methylation of the estrogen receptor gene [an epigenetic modification] [5], and decreased response of Leydig cells to stimulation of gonadotropins (probably because of altered cell membrane biochemistry) [6, 7].

Endocrine Changes

In considering changes in endocrine function in the elderly is important to distinguish between the effects of aging per se on endocrine physiology and those caused by diseases related to age, given the high prevalence of asymptomatic symptomatic disorders in the elderly. The distinction is a simple concept, but not in practice.

As a practical approach, a change of the endocrine system that occurs in a significant proportion of the elderly, especially if they can document unidentified persons in serious chronic disease, is likely to be due to aging. On the other hand, when a change occurs in a small minority of older people is likely to be related to the disease.

The distinction between what is related to age and what is related to the disease is difficult because of the difficulty of defining the study populations free of age-related diseases "normal." People who each year at the same rate for a population unusually healthy elderly may be biased towards people who are biologically "younger" than their chronological age.

The distinction between age and disease related changes are not necessarily determine the therapeutic intervention, for example, can provide treatment for the hormonal changes of menopause, but not for subclinical hypothyroidism. It is currently unclear whether the treatment of many endocrine changes associated with age is beneficial [8].

Several general observations on the changes with the aging of the endocrine system are relevant:

- The endocrine system just to change a well-defined, abrupt and universal function of age is the hypothalamic-pituitary-gonadal females.
- The role of growth hormone insulin-like growth factor 1 (IGF-1) system, the hypothalamic-pituitary-gonadal men, and a portion (zona reticularis) of the adrenal cortex synthesizes all less gradually with dehydroepiandrosterone age in most people. Age-adjusted ranges of normal values of IGF-1, total and free testosterone or bioavailable concentrations of dehydroepiandrosterone can be defined, but if these values are physiologically optimum is unknown.
- The secretion of other hormones is also altered with age, but the changes are much less predictable, and it is not clear, age-adjusted normal values.
- The action of certain hormones decrease with age, the secretion of growth hormone may or may not offset the reductions in the reactivity of the tissue.

Regulatory Changes Fuels

There are several age-related changes in the regulation of glucose metabolism and appetite.

Insulin Regulation of Glucose Metabolism

The elderly are less sensitive to insulin than younger patients, as evidenced by hyperinsulinemia [9], a slight decrease in glucose tolerance and a 50 percent sensitivity to insulin [10]. These changes persist even when the data are corrected for body fat and fitness, two determinants of glucose utilization [11]. Insulin resistance is partly due to a decrease in protein content of muscle glucose transporter, GLUT-4 [12].

A decrease in insulin secretion may also contribute to glucose tolerance in the elderly with low and decreased insulin sensitivity. Not all elderly patients have hyperinsulinemia[10, 13], some of them hyperproinsulinemia rather than hyperinsulinemia [14], and some older subjects in response to insulin in the management of serum glucose is slow [13].

After all, the decrease in glucose clearance with age is mainly due to decreased tissue responsiveness to insulin with a lesser contribution of a slight change in the secretion of insulin. These changes are similar to those that often precede the development of type 2 diabetes in middle age, and, in fact, the incidence of type 2 diabetes is higher among younger adults.

Leptin

Leptin, a hormone produced by adipose tissue in proportion to fat mass, decreased appetite. Serum concentrations of leptin decrease with age [15], although some find that it is only in women [16]. The slight decrease in serum leptin with age may contribute to increased adiposity in the elderly.

Adiponectin

Adiponectin is a protein hormone secreted by adipocytes recently described. Reduced insulin resistance is associated with a reduced risk of atherosclerosis and has anti-inflammatory. Higher levels of adiponectin are associated with a reduced risk of diabetes in older men and women [17], but as this hormone is an indicator of the reduction of abdominal visceral fat content or mediator of the sensitivity insulin when drains visceral fat is still uncertain.

In a study of 58 women and 67 men aged 20 to 93 years analyzed by age group (<50, 50-70 and> 70 years), plasma adiponectin did not change significantly with the age in women but were higher for men over 70 years compared to younger men [18]. Higher levels of adiponectin observed in older men may reflect a change in the longitudinal aging or simply to improve the survival of men with more of the adipokines. Further studies are needed to elucidate this issue.

INSULIN RESISTANCE SPECTRUM AND THE CLINICAL DEFINITION

Introduction

Insulin resistance is a condition that is associated with a given concentration of insulin with a lower response than normal glucose (19). The first term began to be used for several years after the introduction of insulin therapy in 1922 to describe occasional diabetic patients who require increasing doses of insulin to control hyperglycemia. Most of these patients developed insulin resistance secondary to therapy against insulin antibodies at that time was unclean and from non-human species (20). Insulin antibodies are rare in patients treated with recombinant human insulin, and clinical disorders in which insulin resistance plays a major role have changed markedly. Insulin resistance, rather than being a rare complication of diabetes is now recognized as a component of several disorders, including the following (Table 1):

Table 1. Major causes of insulin resistance

Inherited states of target cell resistance
Leprechaunism (insulin-receptor mutations)
Rabson-Mendenhall syndrome (insulin-receptor mutations)
Type A syndrome of insulin resistance (insulin-receptor mutations in some, unknown signalling defect in most)
Some lipodystrophies
Secondary insulin resistance
Obesity (free fatty acids and adipocytokines may contribute)
Excess counterregulatory hormones (glucocorticoids, catecholamines, growth hormone, placental lactogen)
Type 2 diabetes mellitus (secondary to obesity and other factors)
Inactivity
Stress, infection (counterregulatory hormones)
Pregnancy (placental lactogen)
Immune mediated (anti-insulin antibodies, anti-insulin receptor antibodies in type B syndrome)
Miscellaneous (starvation, uremia, cirrhosis, ketoacidosis)
Multifactorial etiology of insulin resistance
Hypertension
Polycystic ovary syndrome
Metabolic syndrome
Most cases of type 2 diabetes mellitus

- extreme insulin resistance syndromes, syndrome type B with antibodies against the insulin receptor and rare inherited disorders [21], such as elf with mutations in the insulin receptor (22), and the lipodystrophic states [23]
- Most patients with type 2 diabetes
- Obesity, stress, infection, uremia, acromegaly, glucocorticoid excess, and pregnancy, which cause insulin resistance secondary

- disorders such as heart disease, hypertension, polycystic ovary syndrome, ovarian hyperthecosis and metabolic syndrome, in which the mechanism associated hyperinsulinemia is unknown

DEFINITION AND QUANTIFICATION

Insulin resistance can be defined as a response to insulin in normal, both endogenous and exogenous.

Resistance to Endogenous Insulin

Resistance to endogenous insulin is defined by high serum concentrations of insulin in combination with concentrations of glucose in the blood are normal or high. In practice, we measure serum insulin only in the evaluation of patients with clinical signs of extreme insulin resistance.

To confirm the diagnosis, it is also necessary to determine the structure and biological activity of insulin the patient is normal. There are rare cases of mutations in the insulin gene resulting in the production of insulin that has subnormal bioactivity but normal immunoactivity. These insulins circulate at high concentrations, simulating insulin resistance, but the response to exogenous insulin is normal [24].

RESISTANCE TO EXOGENOUS INSULIN

A decrease in response to exogenous insulin is evident in patients treated with insulin for diabetics who need higher doses to prevent hyperglycemia, although the dose of insulin in a given patient is an imperfect way to measure the degree of insulin resistance. However, most patients with insulin resistance (e.g., those with obesity) are not treated with insulin. In them, the resistance to exogenous insulin can be assessed and quantified by techniques such as tolerance test insulin clamp or intravenous technique euglycemic insulin. With the latter, glucose uptake induced by insulin is measured while the blood glucose concentration is maintained at a constant concentration (via a glucose infusion) to avoid the effects of hormones against confounding such as adrenaline and glucagon [25] (Figure 1).

Biochemical Markers

There is no consensus on when and how to assess patients insulin resistance possible. In a clinical setting would be useful to identify obese patients who are insulin resistant and at greatest risk of developing type 2 diabetes and cardiovascular disease. In a research setting, intravenous tolerance test, insulin suppression test or the euglycemic clamp technique was used insulin and is considered the gold standard. However, these techniques are impractical for routine clinical use. In a study of 258 nondiabetic, normotensive overweight, serum triglycerides, the proportion of lipoprotein triglycerides (HDL) and fasting insulin concentration were useful markers to identify insulin resistant subjects (measured by an insulin suppression test) [26]. Optimal cut points were identified as being 130 mg /dL (1.47 mmol / L), 3.0 (SI 1.8) and 109 pmol / L for triglycerides, HDL triglycerides and insulin , respectively. The sensitivity and specificity of cutoff points was 67, 64 and 57 percent and 71 percent, 68 and 85 respectively.

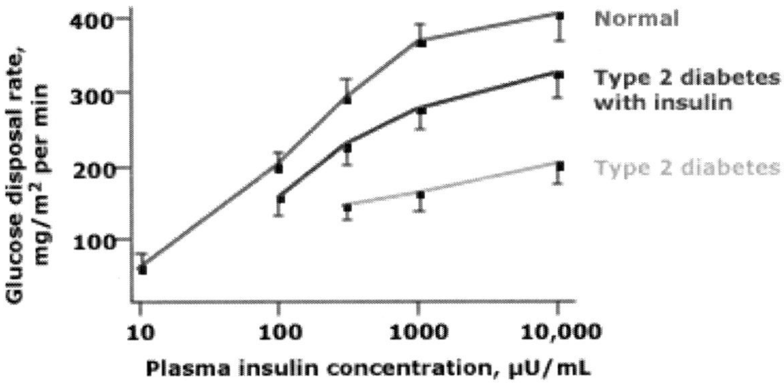

Data from Scarlett, JA, Gray, RS, Griffin, J, et al., *Diabetes Care* 1982; 5:353.

Figure 1. Euglycemic insulin clamp in type 2 diabetes. Insulin dose-response curves during euglycemic clamp studies in normal subjects (upper curve), patients with type 2 diabetes (lower curve), and patients with type 2 diabetes who had been aggressively treated with insulin (middle curve). Patients with type 2 diabetes have marked insulin resistance as evidenced by a much lower rate of glucose disposal at any insulin concentration. There was partial improvement in insulin responsiveness after aggressive insulin therapy. To convert plasma insulin values to pmol/L multiply by 6.0.

Clinical Spectrum

Insulin resistance can occur in a variety of ways. Hyperglycemia despite high doses of insulin is the classic, but many patients with extreme insulin resistance is not overt hyperglycaemia. However, most of these patients have one or more clinical features suggestive of severe insulin resistance (Table 2). These features include acanthosis nigricans, ovarian hyperandrogenism (PCOS), lipodystrophy, accelerated linear growth or problems, autoimmunity and muscle cramps. The presence of these characteristics should lead to the measurement of insulin in serum. One conclusion of hyperinsulinemia should encourage further studies to assess the presence of circulating anti-insulin receptor and other disorders listed in the table (Table 1).

In most cases, the precise basis for the relationship between insulin resistance and clinical outcomes are not yet defined. It is likely that high concentrations of insulin in stimulating specific serum insulin-responsive pathways are less affected than affecting glucose transport. This can occur through the activation of growth factor insulin-like 1 (IGF-1), receptors or receptor hybrids formed by covalent receptor subunit homologues of insulin and IGF -1 (Figure 2).

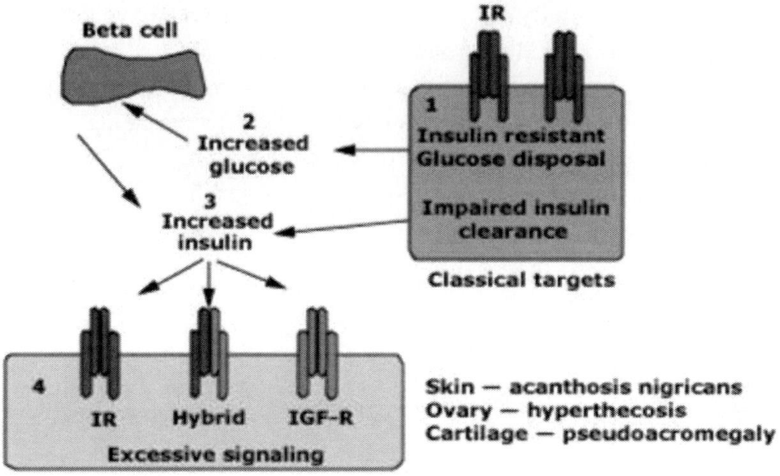

Adapted from Mantzoros, CS, Flier, JS, *Adv Endocrinol Metab* 1995; 6:193.

Figure 2. Possible mechanisms by which insulin resistance leads to the clinical manifestations of the polycystic ovary syndrome. Insulin resistance in muscle and adipose tissue leads to hyperglycemia and thus increased insulin secretion from the pancreatic beta cells. This insulin can cause changes in the skin, ovary, and cartilage via activation of insulin-like growth factor-1 (IGF-1) receptors or hybrid receptors formed by covalent linkage of subunits of the homologous receptors for insulin (IR) and IGF-1 (IGF-R).

ABNORMAL GLUCOSE METABOLISM

Glucose homeostasis varies extremely abnormal (diabetes or hypoglycemia) to normal. At one end of the spectrum are insulin-treated diabetic patients who require high doses of insulin to control hyperglycemia. Insulin resistance in these patients can be induced by the production of insulin antibodies or autoantibodies against the insulin receptor. Next on the spectrum are patients with diabetes not receiving insulin, as with most patients with type 2 diabetes in which there is also a component of the pancreatic beta cell damage.

However, many patients with insulin resistance, blood glucose concentrations normal or slightly elevated. Included in this group are the most obese patients, many patients with hypertension and hyperandrogenism, and those with inherited syndromes of severe insulin resistance, such as the type of syndrome. Some patients with insulin resistance due to antibodies against the insulin receptor have hypoglycemia [27].

Skin

Acanthosis nigricans and skin tags are commonly associated with primary insulin resistance, regardless of its molecular cause. Acanthosis nigricans is a skin lesion characterized by dark, velvety patches, hyperkeratotic. The lesions are usually found in the back of the neck, armpits [Figure 1], groin, and elbows, but can cover the entire surface of the skin, sparing the palms and soles. The lesions may be papillomatous. Histological features include hyperkeratosis, epidermal papillomatosis, and an increased number of melanocytes.

The common denominator in all cases of acanthosis nigricans, with the possible exception of a tumor-induced injury is resistance to insulin [28]. It can vary in severity and can be inherited or acquired.

Hyperandrogenism and Reproductive Abnormalities

Men with insulin resistance are not known to have reproductive problems. In contrast, women with insulin resistance commonly present with reproductive abnormalities [29].

For example, most women with severe tissue resistance to insulin, regardless of the cause, marked hyperandrogenism. This association has been described in women with type B syndrome [caused by insulin receptor antibodies] [30] or Type A syndrome [caused by genetic defects in the system of insulin signaling, as mutations insulin receptor gene] [21, 31, 32]. Women with virilization may have opened or hirsutism, amenorrhea and infertility. The ovary shows the histological changes hyperthecosis [33].

Most women with ovarian hyperandrogenism have a tissue resistance to insulin is identified by hyperinsulinaemia clamp studies, fasting or euglycemic [34]. The molecular basis of tissue resistance to insulin in these women is unknown. Studies in cultured skin fibroblasts suggest that about 50 percent of them have a defect in the phosphorylation of the insulin receptor [35].

The basis of the association between insulin resistance and ovarian hyperandrogenism is unknown, and there is no clear correlation between the severity of these disorders [35]. While the excess of androgens can cause a modest reduction in sensitivity to insulin [36], the primary abnormality is probably insulin resistance, making it somehow the fault of the ovary. Insulin receptors and receptors closely related IGF-1 are present in the cells of the ovary and stimulation of these receptors increases the production of androgens [37].

Reducing insulin resistance with metformin or thiazolidinediones low free testosterone levels in serum and reduced the cytochrome P450c17 [17-hydroxylase] activity in the ovaries [38, 39].

Linear and Acral Growth

Linear growth is normal in most patients with insulin resistance. There are, however, two pediatric disorders with severe insulin resistance, Rabson-Mendenhall and Leprechaun syndrome, in which growth is affected [40, 41]. Leprechaunism is due to complete or almost complete lack of function of insulin receptor and [42] is associated with a very linear growth retardation and developmental delay.

Pseudoacromegaly, however, is a syndrome that is associated with severe insulin resistance with a linear growth accelerated [43]. In these patients, hyperinsulinemia may promote growth of skeletal linear receptor activation of IGF-1.

Musculoskeletal Changes

Some patients with insulin resistance of tissues have severe muscle cramps related to exercise [44]. The severity of pain can sometimes be reduced by phenytoin [45].

Adipose Tissue

The quantity and distribution of adipose tissue is normal in most patients with insulin resistance, but some just abdominal obesity. High serum concentrations of free fatty acids [46] and increased release of tumor necrosis factor [TNF-alpha] extended the fat cells [47] have been implicated in the pathogenesis of obesity in these patients.

The lipodystrophy syndrome is a diverse group of clinical disorders characterized by an unusual amount and distribution of adipose tissue. Patients often have severe tissue resistance to insulin and perhaps some of the other clinical features of insulin resistance and acanthosis nigricans. Syndromes can be congenital or acquired, and atrophy of adipose tissue may be total or partial.

The lipodystrophy syndrome has been associated with highly active therapy (HAART), including antiretroviral therapy with protease inhibitors in patients infected with HIV. These patients have insulin resistance and hyperglycemia and hyperlipidemia earlier and more frequently than patients infected with HIV who are treated with other treatments [23].

Leptin-deficient patients with lipodystrophy, a decrease in leptin production in adipose tissue may also be involved in the pathogenesis of insulin resistance. The administration of leptin to these questions in the context of clinical trials, improved many of their metabolic disorders [48, 49].

In addition, patients with lipodystrophy and / or insulin resistance may also have low levels of adiponectin, another adipocyte hormone that acts as an endogenous insulin sensitizer [50]. Adiponectin is reduced with the accumulation of abdominal fat, while the models of a healthy diet and exercise to increase its circulating levels [51-53]. Peroxisome proliferator-activated receptor gamma activators, including the thiazolidinediones increase adiponectin levels in humans.

Autoimmunity

Some patients have severe insulin resistance as a result of autoantibodies directed against insulin receptor (type B syndrome of insulin resistance) [21]. These patients may have insulin resistance, diabetes or hypoglycemia, depending on the properties of antireceptor antibodies. Many also have other autoimmune diseases such as lupus erythematosus or scleroderma [54].

Metabolic Syndrome - There is an apparent link between abdominal obesity, insulin resistance, and a variety of abnormalities that affect the cardiovascular system, type 2 diabetes, hypertension, an atherogenic lipid profile, including hypertriglyceridemia and Serum lipoprotein cholesterol to high density and heart disease. This constellation of findings is called the metabolic syndrome (or syndrome of insulin resistance or syndrome X).

Treatment of Type 2 Diabetes Mellitus in the Elderly

Introduction

The prevalence of type 2 diabetes continues to increase steadily as more people live longer and become heavier. 2005-2006 Health and Nutrition Examination Survey National community-dwelling adults, the prevalence of diabetes increases with age and the age of 60 to 74 years (prevalence of 17.6 percent crude) [55]. From 1995 to 2004, the overall prevalence of type 2 diabetes in nursing homes 16 to 23 percent [56].

Older people with diabetes are at risk of developing a similar spectrum of macrovascular and microvascular complications, such as their younger counterparts with diabetes. However, the absolute risk of cardiovascular disease is much higher than younger adults. Older people with diabetes have excess morbidity and mortality compared to older people without diabetes [57]. They are also at high risk for polypharmacy, functional disabilities and common geriatric syndromes that include cognitive impairment, depression, urinary incontinence, falls and persistent pain [58].

This topic will review diabetes management in elderly patients and how management priorities and treatment options may differ between older and younger patients. The general management of type 2 diabetes are discussed separately.

Individualizing Management

Older adults with diabetes are a heterogeneous population that includes persons residing independently in communities, care centers or nursing homes. Thus, older people with diabetes can be fit and healthy or frail with many co-morbidity and functional disability.

The overall goals of diabetes in the elderly are similar to those of younger adults, including management of hyperglycemia and factors of risk. However, in frail elderly people with diabetes, prevention of hypoglycemia, hypotension, and drug interactions due to polypharmacy are even more worrying in young patients with diabetes. In addition, the management of co-existence of medical conditions is important because it affects their ability to self-management.

Glycemic Targets

There are few data that specifically address the objectives of optimal blood glucose in patients of advanced age. Hyperglycemia increases dehydration and decreased vision and knowledge [59], all of which contribute to functional decline and increased risk of falls in older people with diabetes. On the other hand, elderly patients tolerate relatively high levels of glucose in the blood before they manifest an osmotic diuresis due to the decline in glomerular filtration rate and lower the load of glucose in the delivery tubes resorption. In addition, the side effects of diabetes, particularly hypoglycemia, can lead to bad results, such as falls and traumatic exacerbation of comorbidities. Targets for glycemic control and management of risk factors should be based on the general health of the individual and the expected duration of survival, because the risk of complications depends on the duration.

The appropriate goal for hemoglobin A1C (HbA1c) in elderly patients who have a life expectancy of more than ten years should be similar to those developed for younger adults (<7.0 percent). The results suggest that the ACCORD study HbA1c from 7.0 to 7.9 percent (an average of 7.5 per cent) can be sure that lowering the target for patients with long diabetes 2 who are at high risk of cardiovascular disease [60]. Therefore, the aim should be slightly higher (≤ 8.0 percent) among the frail elderly with medical comorbidities and functional and where life expectancy is less than ten years. Individual goals for the very elderly may be even greater and must include efforts to preserve the quality of life and avoid hypoglycemia and its complications. These objectives are in line with the American Geriatrics Society, American Diabetes Association and European Diabetes Working Party [58, 61, 62].

Avoiding Hypoglycemia

The risk of hypoglycemia, which can lead to cognitive impairment and function, is significantly higher in the elderly. In addition, seniors may have neuroglycopenic manifestations of hypoglycemia (dizziness, weakness, delirium, confusion), against the adrenergic manifestations (tremor, sweating). These symptoms may be lost or badly as the primary neurological disease (e.g., transient ischemic attack), leading to inadequate communication of hypoglycemia in patients.

Episodes of hypoglycemia in the elderly may also increase the risk of adverse cardiovascular and cardiac autonomic dysfunction [63]. Moreover, severe hypoglycemia requiring hospitalization was associated with an increased risk of developing dementia is higher in patients with recurrent, although the direction of causality, if any, is unknown [64].

Even a mild episode of hypoglycemia can lead to adverse outcomes in the elderly frail. For example, episodes of dizziness or weakness increases the risk of falls and fractures that lead to placement in nursing home.

Given the risks, prevention of hypoglycemia is an important consideration in the choice of therapeutic agents and targets for blood glucose levels in the elderly. Insulin secretagogues such as sulfonylureas and meglitinides and all types of insulin should be used with caution in the frail elderly [65].

MODIFICATION OF LIFESTYLE

Food, weight reduction and exercise can be used to improve glycemic control, although most elderly patients with type 2 diabetes need medication on their diabetes.

Medical nutrition therapy (MNT) is the process by which suits the requirement of nutrition for people with diabetes based on medical, lifestyle and personal factors and is an integral component of diabetes management and the diabetes self-management education. In a randomized trial of medical nutrition intervention in adults ≥ 65 years, patients in the intervention group had significant improvements in fasting plasma glucose (-18.9 against -1.4

mg / dl) and HbA1c (- 0.5 percentage points compared to no change) than control patients [66].

In addition, the older group in the Programme for the prevention of diabetes (> 60 years at baseline) had a greater improvement in blood glucose over time, partly due to better adherence to the style of life program, compared to younger age groups [67, 68]. These data suggest that older people can respond well to lifestyle programs. Therefore, all patients with diabetes should receive medical nutrition assessment.

The choice of food has important clinical considerations:

- Older adults obese with diabetes can benefit from caloric restriction and increased physical activity with weight loss target of about 5 percent of body weight [58, 69].
- The elderly are most at risk of malnutrition and obesity. Weight loss increases the risk of morbidity and mortality in the elderly [70]. Therefore, unintentional weight loss should be addressed in the evaluation of medical nutrition.

Drug Therapy

There are few data specific to drug treatment in elderly patients [71]. However, most trials of diabetes medicine includes a wide range of patients, including those of 65> years. All types of oral hypoglycemic agents and insulin is safe for elderly patients, although each has its limitations. Drug treatment should be individualized based on the capabilities of the patient and comorbidities. "Start low and slow" is a good rule to follow when starting any new medicine in the elderly.

The following recommendations are based on tests conducted in the general population and clinical experience. Are compatible with the American Geriatrics Society, American Diabetes Association and the European Union directives Diabetes Working Party [58, 61, 62].

For patients without cons-indications to metformin (e.g., impairment, heart failure or kidney disease), we prefer to start treatment with metformin. However, in patients with cons-indications and / or intolerance to metformin, a short-acting sulfonylurea (e.g., glipizide) is an alternative option. In a patient with chronic kidney disease who are intolerant of sulfonylureas, repaglinide can be considered as initial therapy.

After a successful initial response to oral therapy, many patients fail to maintain target levels of HbA1c. If glycemic targets are not met a single agent, the elderly patient should be evaluated by the contributing causes, such as difficulty adhering to medication side effects or a misunderstanding of the terms of nutrition [58]. Elderly patients requiring more than one agent, distributors dose of pills can help improve compliance. Alternatively, family members or caregivers may be needed to help administer medications.

Indications for a second agent and the treatment options for patients who fail initial therapy with lifestyle intervention and metformin or a sulfonylurea were similar in patients older and younger (Table 1). This is discussed separately.

Metformin

Metformin is an attractive agent for use in the elderly due to a low risk of hypoglycemia. However, caution must be exercised in patients with diabetes because of the risk of lactic acidosis. Elderly patients often have impaired renal function despite a serum creatinine of normal appearance. They are also more at risk of developing other conditions that reduce renal function more or cause lactic acidosis (e.g., myocardial infarction, stroke, heart failure, pneumonia). A calculation (or estimated) GFR> 30 ml / min has been suggested as a safe level of renal function during the use of metformin.

Weight loss and gastrointestinal side effects may be limiting factors in older people taking metformin. Therefore, metformin should be used with caution in elderly patients. Cons-indications for use are discussed elsewhere.

Any elderly patient treated with metformin should be advised to stop taking the drug immediately if they fall ill for any reason, or if they have to undergo a procedure that requires the use of iodinated contrast.

Sulfonylureas

Sulfonylureas drugs are generally well tolerated. Hypoglycemia is the most common side effect and is more common with long-acting sulfonylureas (e.g., chlorpropamide, glibenclamide, glimepiride y). Therefore, avoid using long-acting sulfonylureas in older adults. We prefer to use a short-acting sulfonylureas such as glipizide.

The reported incidence of sulfonylurea-related hypoglycemia in the elderly is variable. In an observational study, the incidence in patients over 65 treated with glyburide or chlorpropamide was similar (16.6 episodes per 1000 person-years) [72]. In contrast, another study of 52 patients treated with glyburide or glipizide gastrointestinal therapeutic system (GITS), there were no episodes of hypoglycemia during fasting for 23 hours [73].

Drug-induced hypoglycemia is more likely to occur in the following cases in elderly patients and may be a limiting factor for the use of these drugs in the elderly:

- After the meal period or missed
- When you eat poorly or alcohol abuse
- When you have kidney or heart failure or intercurrent illness, gastrointestinal
- During treatment with salicylates, sulfonamides, fibrates (like gemfibrozil) and warfarin [74]
- After being in the hospital [72]

These problems can occur when a change in the overall health of older people with diabetes. In patients taking sulfonylureas, the presence and frequency of hypoglycemia should be assessed at each visit.

Thiazolidinediones

The thiazolidinediones (rosiglitazone and pioglitazone) improve insulin resistance. They also increase insulin secretion in response to glucose, at least in patients with impaired glucose tolerance.

Thiazolidinediones may be considered for some elderly patients, especially those with lower initial HbA1c, if no-indication against specific sulfonylureas or are unable or unwilling to consider insulin. This can be used in patients with renal failure, are well tolerated in older adults, and does not cause hypoglycemia. However, thiazolidinediones should not be used in patients with Class IIII or IV heart failure. In addition, limited experience, the high cost and concerns about fluid retention, congestive heart failure, myocardial infarction and rupture limit its usefulness, especially in the elderly. If a thiazolidinedione to be used as therapy, pioglitazone is preferred because of growing concerns about the atherogenic lipid profile and increased risk of cardiovascular events with rosiglitazone.

Meglitinides

Repaglinide and nateglinide are short-term glucose-lowering drugs that work similarly to sulfonylureas and have similar efficacy and less for lower blood glucose. Meglitinides are pharmacologically distinct from sulfonylureas and can be used in patients who are allergic to sulfa drugs. They have a similar risk of weight gain than sulfonylureas, but perhaps with less risk of hypoglycemia [75]. Unlike nateglinide, repaglinide is metabolized by the liver, with less than 10 percent excreted by the kidneys. Dose adjustments with this agent does not seem necessary in patients with renal failure. In addition, repaglinide is more effective in reducing HbA1c of nateglinide. Therefore, repaglinide may be considered as initial therapy in patients with chronic kidney disease who can not tolerate metformin and sulfonylureas.

Inhibitors of Alpha-Glucosidase

Acarbose and miglitol inhibit alpha-glucosidase GI tract that convert food starch and other complex carbohydrates into monosaccharides, which slows glucose absorption, resulting in a greater increase slow concentration of post-prandial glucose in the blood. These drugs may be used alone or in combination with insulin, sulfonylurea and metformin.

Acarbose and miglitol has not been widely tested in elderly patients with diabetes, but is likely to be very safe and effective. The main side effects that limit their use are flatulence and diarrhea are common.

DPP-IV

Dipeptidyl peptidase IV (DPP-IV) is a ubiquitous enzyme that inactivates a variety of other bioactive peptides, including the insulinotropic glucagon-like peptide-1 (GLP-1) and glucose-dependent polypeptide (GIP), so its inhibition may affect the regulation of blood glucose through multiple effects. DPP-IV have been shown to be moderately effective as monotherapy or in combination with metformin, sulfonylureas or thiazolidinediones.

DPP-IV have no risk of hypoglycemia and weight neutral when used as monotherapy, and can therefore be interesting to use agents in the elderly. However, the long-term safety with this class of drugs has not been established, and are relatively expensive. The dose of DPP-IV should be adjusted in patients with renal failure.

GLP-1 Therapy

The role of gastrointestinal peptides on glucose homeostasis is illustrated by the incretin effect in the oral glucose has a stimulating effect on the secretion of more insulin than intravenous glucose. This effect is mediated by several gastrointestinal peptides, particularly GLP-1. Exenatide and liraglutide are GLP-1 analog agents available for use as an adjunct to diet and exercise alone or in combination with oral agents in adults with type 2 diabetes. Exenatide is administered twice daily and liraglutide once daily by subcutaneous injection.

There is no risk of hypoglycemia with the use of GLP-1 analogues alone. Both drugs are sometimes associated with a significant reduction in weight. The most frequent adverse events are nausea, vomiting and diarrhea in 10 to 40 percent of treated patients. There have been postmarketing reports of acute pancreatitis and the deterioration of renal function in patients taking therapies GLP-1. However, there are enough data to know if there is a causal relationship. Because of concerns about renal toxicity, exenatide should not be used in patients with a creatinine clearance below 30 mL / min.

Pramlintide

Pramlintide is a synthetic analogue of amylin, which is administered by subcutaneous injection with prandial insulin. It is available for the treatment of type 1 and insulin treatment of type 2 diabetes. Requires multiple subcutaneous injections, and therefore its role in the treatment of diabetes in the elderly is limited.

Insulin

Insulin is often underutilized in the elderly because of fear (for the doctor, the patient or family) that is too complicated or dangerous. With the availability of long-acting insulins, it has become easier to use once-daily long-acting insulin or insulin monotherapy once daily oral hypoglycemic medications in patients who have control optimal glycemic. Patients may assume that the symptoms of fatigue due to "old age" rather than hyperglycemia. However, in many patients, the quality of life is significantly improved when taken once or twice daily intermediate-acting insulin or long.

Before insulin therapy, it is important to assess whether the patient is physically and mentally able to use an insulin pen or develop and administer the correct dose of insulin (syringes and vials) blood glucose monitoring, and recognize and treat hypoglycemia. For patients taking a fixed dose of insulin per day and are able to give insulin injections, but not its production, a family member or pharmacist can prepare for a week of insulin syringes and leave in the refrigerator. The plan could allow an elderly patient to continue living independently in their homes.

Insulin metabolism is altered in patients with chronic renal failure, so that less insulin is needed when the glomerular filtration rate below 50 ml / min.

Monitor Blood Glucose

Monitoring is usually necessary to achieve glycemic targets. A1C control usually twice a year in patients who achieve treatment goals and have stable glycemic control and quarterly in patients whose treatment has changed or not meeting glycemic targets.

The concentrations of glucose in the blood can also be controlled at home by the patient or caregiver. The effectiveness of self-monitoring of blood glucose (SMBG) in improving glycemic control in patients with type 2 diabetes is less clear than for type 1 diabetes.

AGS can be useful in patients with type 2 diabetes who take medications that can cause hypoglycemia (e.g., insulin). AMG can also be useful for some patients to take action to change eating habits or exercise, and the willingness to intensify drug therapy, based on the results of the AMG. However, self-glucose monitoring may not be necessary at all or only in exceptional circumstances, for elderly patients with type 2 diabetes who are treated with diet or are treated with oral agents are not associated with hypoglycemia.

Therefore, the AMG can be seen in some patients, depending on the medication and cognitive and functional abilities [58].

Detection of Microvascular Complications

Problems retinopathy, nephropathy and foot are important complications of diabetes mellitus in elderly patients. Follow the recommendations for elderly patients with diabetes are similar to those of younger patients (Table 2).

Retinopathy

The prevalence of retinopathy increases with increasing duration of diabetes (Figure 1).

Regular eye exams are extremely important for elderly patients with diabetes as poor vision can lead to social isolation, increased risk of accidents and impaired ability to measure blood glucose and the development of doses insulin. A comprehensive review should be performed by a qualified ophthalmologist or optometrist at diagnosis and at least once a year thereafter. The intention is that the screen is not only to diabetic retinopathy, but also for cataracts and glaucoma, which are more common in diabetic patients compared to elderly non-diabetic subjects. Cataracts are twice as common in people over 65 with diabetes compared to non-diabetic subjects of similar age (38.4 percent against 16.6 percent), while glaucoma is almost three times more common (11.2 percent against 3.8 percent) [76].

Table 2. Clinical manifestations of insulin resistance

Glucose homeostasis
Variable, including overt diabetes, impaired glucose tolerance, normal, and hypoglycemia
Cutaneous
Acanthosis nigricans
Skin tags
Alopecia
Reproductive
Amenorrhea
Hirsutism
Virilization
Infertility (in women)
Linear growth
Variable, including normal, impaired, increased
Adipose tissue
Variable, including normal, lipoatrophy, lipohypertrophy, obesity
Musculoskeletal
Variable, including normal, cramps, muscle hypertrophy, pseudoacromegaly
Lipid metabolism
Normal or hypertriglyceridemia
Autoimmunity
Type B syndrome with variety of immune phenotypes

Nephropathy

The availability of effective treatments for diabetic nephropathy, angiotensin converting enzyme [ACE] inhibitors led to the recommendation that all diabetic patients screened for microalbuminuria annually.

However, the prevalence of microalbuminuria increases in the population for reasons other than diabetic nephropathy. For patients already taking an ACE inhibitor or an antagonist of ACE may not be necessary or useful to continue testing for microalbuminuria annually.

Foot Problems

Foot problems are a major cause of morbidity in patients with diabetes and the risk is much higher in elderly patients. Vascular and neurological diseases contribute to injuries of the foot. It is estimated, for example, the prevalence of diabetic neuropathy in patients with type 2 diabetes is 32 percent overall and 50 percent in patients over 60 years [77, 78].

In addition to the increasing prevalence of neuropathy with age, over 30 percent of older patients with diabetes can not see or reach their feet, and can thus be unable to perform routine inspections of the foot.

It is recommended that elderly patients with diabetes have their feet checked at each visit, the review should include an assessment of the patient's ability to see and get to his feet, and research on family members or friends who could be trained to do routine inspections of the foot. Visits to the podiatrist on a regular basis should also be considered. Careful neurological examination and assessment of peripheral arterial disease should be performed at least once a year. It is also important that the advice on preventive foot care is given to any patient whose feet are at high risk.

Cardiovascular risk reduction - diabetes and age are major risk factors for coronary heart disease. Therefore, it is not surprising that heart disease is by far the leading cause of death in elderly patients with diabetes, and the effect of most interventions is more pronounced in them.

Risk reduction should focus on the following areas:

- Stop smoking
- Treatment of Hypertension
- Treatment of dyslipidemia
- Aspirin therapy
- Exercise

Stop Smoking

Smoking among patients with diabetes mellitus is an independent risk factor for all-cause mortality, mainly due to cardiovascular disease. Therefore, smoking cessation should be vigorously encouraged.

Treatment of Hypertension

Treatment of hypertension in elderly patients is clearly beneficial, even in patients older than 80 years. The recommended treatment goals and options of medications for diabetic patients and the elderly are discussed in detail elsewhere.

Treatment of Dyslipidaemia

Multiple abnormalities in lipid metabolism may contribute to increased atherosclerosis associated with diabetes. The beneficial effects of lipid-lowering therapy may be present in as little as six months [79]. In addition, the relative reduction in cardiovascular disease with the reduction of serum LDL is similar in older and younger patients with diabetes [80, 81].

The use of statins [except against-indication] to lower cholesterol in people with diabetes older with LDL cholesterol values persisting above 100 mg / dl [2.6 mmol / L], with the aim of lowering the LDL below 100 mg / dl [2.6 mmol / L]. Diabetic patients who already have cardiovascular disease, an LDL goal of 70 to 80 mg / dl [1.8 to 2.1 mmol / L] is justified, particularly in patients at high risk. They also recommend drug therapy in patients with serum HDL cholesterol below 35 mg / dL [0.9 mmol / L] or marked hypertriglyceridemia [$\geq$ 400 mg

/ dl [4.5 mmol / L]]. More detailed information on the use of lipid-lowering drugs in secondary prevention of coronary heart disease is elsewhere.

As with the goal of glycemic control, the objectives for the management of risk factors [hypertension, hyperlipidemia] should be adjusted life expectancy of elderly patients, comorbidity, cognitive status and personal preferences.

Aspirin

The value of aspirin daily in patients with known macrovascular disease [secondary prevention] is widely accepted. A meta-analysis of a large number of secondary prevention trials showed that the absolute benefit of aspirin is greater in people over 65 with diabetes and diastolic hypertension [82].

The role of aspirin in primary prevention of cardiovascular events in patients with diabetes is less certain. These tests and recommendations for aspirin therapy are discussed elsewhere.

Exercise

Exercise is beneficial to help maintain physical function, reduce the risk of heart disease and improve insulin sensitivity in patients with diabetes. In older people, exercise also improves body composition and the pain of arthritis, reduce falls and depression, increases strength and balance, improves quality of life and improves survival [83-86]. Studies on the frail have shown that weight training should also include aerobic exercise [87]. Patients with poor fitness in the risk of falls should be referred to an exercise physiologist and / or physical therapist to strengthen muscles and balance training in a safe environment.

Common Geriatric Syndromes Associated with Diabetes

Cognitive Disorders

Diabetes is associated with an increased risk of dementia. Many elderly patients with dementia are not diagnosed, especially in the early stages. Elderly patients with diabetes and cognitive dysfunction may have difficulty performing self-management and following complex regimens. Cognitive function should be assessed in diabetic patients aged when there is:

- Non-adherence
- frequent episodes of hypoglycaemia
- The deterioration of glycemic control, no obvious explanation.

Depression

Depression occurs at a higher rate in patients with diabetes compared to age matched controls [88, 89]. Depression is often undiagnosed and untreated in this population at high risk [90].

Depression has been associated with poor glycemic control and the rate of acceleration of coronary artery disease in diabetic patients [91]. Early identification of an assessment tool for short-term [e.g., Geriatric Depression Scale] and treatment can help to achieve better glycemic control [92].

Polypharmacy

The use of multiple drugs is common in older adults. The control of hyperglycemia and its associated risk factors often increase the number of drugs, even in elderly patients with diabetes. Side effects may worsen the co-morbidity and impair the patient's ability to manage his / her diabetes. Therefore, the list of drugs must be maintained and reviewed at each visit [58].

Falls

The increased risk of falls in older people with diabetes is multifactorial. Peripheral neuropathy and / or autonomous, reduced kidney function, muscle weakness, functional disability, vision loss, polypharmacy, co-morbidities such as osteoarthritis and mild hypoglycemia may even contribute to falls in elderly fragile.

While a good glycemic control prevents the progression of certain diabetic complications and may reduce the risk of falls, low blood sugar that occurs after an intensive glycemic control may increase the risk of falls. In a prospective observational study of 446 older adults with diabetes (average age 74 years), intensive blood glucose control (HbA1c $\leq$ 6 vs.> 8 percent) was associated with an increased risk of falls among users of the insulin (OR 4, 4, 95% CI 1.3 -14.5), but not in those treated with oral antidiabetic agents (OR 1.3, 95% CI: 0.7 to 2.5) [93]. Possible reasons for the gap include increasing the duration or severity of diabetes or more episodes of hypoglycemia in patients treated with oral insulin cons, the opportunities have not been explored rigorously in this observational study.

However, the benefits of glycemic control to reduce the complications of diabetes (and reduce the risk of falls) must be balanced with the possible increased risk of falls, with intensive insulin therapy. These results support the use of less stringent glycemic goals in the elderly. Furthermore, identification of causes of falls and the onset of exercise programs can reduce the risk of falls in these individuals.

Urinary Incontinence

Diabetes increases the risk of a woman developing urinary incontinence. Risk factors include urinary tract infections, vaginal infections, autonomic neuropathy (which causes all the neurogenic bladder or fecal impaction) and polyuria due to hyperglycemia. Although no direct evidence to suggest adverse effects of incontinence in people with diabetes, the identification and treatment is recommended to improve the quality of life of women.

A Nursing Home Patients

There are few studies and guidelines for the care of older people with diabetes living in nursing homes. Life expectancy, quality of life, severe functional impairment and other co-existing conditions mentioned above affect the definition of objectives and management plans. Exercise as tolerated, in any form is always important for all patients. Normal diet, no sweets concentrate can improve the quality of life and prevent weight loss.

Regimens should be chosen to achieve glycemic control possible with an emphasis on prevention and control of symptoms of hypoglycemia hyperglycemia.

REFERENCES

[1] Bokov A, Chaudhuri A, Richardson A. The role of oxidative damage and stress in aging. *Mech Ageing Dev* 2004; 125:811.

[2] Suji G, Sivakami S. Glucose, glycation and aging. *Biogerontology* 2004; 5:365.

[3] Egger G, Liang G, Aparicio A, Jones PA. Epigenetics in human disease and prospects for epigenetic therapy. *Nature* 2004; 429:457.

[4] Conboy IM, Conboy MJ, Wagers AJ, et al. Rejuvenation of aged progenitor cells by exposure to a young systemic environment. *Nature* 2005; 433:760.

[5] Post WS, Goldschmidt-Clermont PJ, Wilhide CC, et al. Methylation of the estrogen receptor gene is associated with aging and atherosclerosis in the cardiovascular system. *Cardiovasc Res* 1999; 43:985.

[6] Harman SM, Tsitouras PD. Reproductive hormones in aging men. I. Measurement of sex steroids, basal luteinizing hormone, and Leydig cell response to human chorionic gonadotropin. *J Clin Endocrinol Metab* 1980; 51:35.

[7] Mulligan T, Iranmanesh A, Kerzner R, et al. Two-week pulsatile gonadotropin releasing hormone infusion unmasks dual (hypothalamic and Leydig cell) defects in the healthy aging male gonadotropic axis. *Eur J Endocrinol* 1999; 141:257.

[8] Lamberts SW, van den Beld AW, van der Lely AJ. The endocrinology of aging. Science 1997; 278:419.

[9] Gumbiner B, Polonsky KS, Beltz WF, et al. Effects of aging on insulin secretion. *Diabetes* 1989; 38:1549.

[10] Røder ME, Schwartz RS, Prigeon RL, Kahn SE. Reduced pancreatic B cell compensation to the insulin resistance of aging: impact on proinsulin and insulin levels. *J Clin Endocrinol Metab* 2000; 85:2275.

[11] Shimokata H, Muller DC, Fleg JL, et al. Age as independent determinant of glucose tolerance. *Diabetes* 1991; 40:44.

[12] Houmard JA, Weidner MD, Dolan PL, et al. Skeletal muscle GLUT4 protein concentration and aging in humans. *Diabetes* 1995; 44:555.

[13] Chen M, Bergman RN, Pacini G, Porte D Jr. Pathogenesis of age-related glucose intolerance in man: insulin resistance and decreased beta-cell function. *J Clin Endocrinol Metab* 1985; 60:13.

[14] Gama R, Medina-Layachi N, Ranganath L, et al. Hyperproinsulinaemia in elderly subjects: evidence for age-related pancreatic beta-cell dysfunction. *Ann Clin Biochem* 2000; 37 (Pt 3):367.

[15] Isidori AM, Strollo F, Morè M, et al. Leptin and aging: correlation with endocrine changes in male and female healthy adult populations of different body weights. *J Clin Endocrinol Metab* 2000; 85:1954.

[16] Neuhäuser-Berthold M, Herbert BM, Lührmann PM, et al. Resting metabolic rate, body composition, and serum leptin concentrations in a free-living elderly population. *Eur J Endocrinol* 2000; 142:486.

[17] Kanaya AM, Harris T, Goodpaster BH, et al. Adipocytokines attenuate the association between visceral adiposity and diabetes in older adults. *Diabetes Care* 2004; 27:1375.

[18] Adamczak M, Rzepka E, Chudek J, Wiecek A. Ageing and plasma adiponectin concentration in apparently healthy males and females. *Clin Endocrinol* (Oxf) 2005; 62:114.

[19] Moller DE, Flier JS. Insulin resistance--mechanisms, syndromes, and implications. *N Engl J Med* 1991; 325:938.

[20] Kahn CR, Rosenthal AS. Immunologic reactions to insulin: insulin allergy, insulin resistance, and the autoimmune insulin syndrome. *Diabetes Care* 1979; 2:283.

[21] Kahn CR, Flier JS, Bar RS, et al. The syndromes of insulin resistance and acanthosis nigricans. Insulin-receptor disorders in man. *N Engl J Med* 1976; 294:739.

[22] Musso C, Cochran E, Moran SA, et al. Clinical course of genetic diseases of the insulin receptor (type A and Rabson-Mendenhall syndromes): a 30-year prospective. *Medicine* (Baltimore) 2004; 83:209.

[23] Tsiodras S, Mantzoros C, Hammer S, Samore M. Effects of protease inhibitors on hyperglycemia, hyperlipidemia, and lipodystrophy: a 5-year cohort study. *Arch Intern Med* 2000; 160:2050.

[24] Steiner DF, Tager HS, Chan SJ, et al. Lessons learned from molecular biology of insulin-gene mutations. *Diabetes Care* 1990; 13:600.

[25] Bergman RN, Finegood DT, Ader M. Assessment of insulin sensitivity in vivo. *Endocr Rev* 1985; 6:45.

[26] McLaughlin T, Abbasi F, Cheal K, et al. Use of metabolic markers to identify overweight individuals who are insulin resistant. *Ann Intern Med* 2003; 139:802.

[27] Taylor SI, Grunberger G, Marcus-Samuels B, et al. Hypoglycemia associated with antibodies to the insulin receptor. *N Engl J Med* 1982; 307:1422.

[28] Rogers DL. Acanthosis nigricans. *Semin Dermatol* 1991; 10:160.

[29] Poretsky L, Piper B. Insulin resistance, hypersecretion of LH, and a dual-defect hypothesis for the pathogenesis of polycystic ovary syndrome. *Obstet Gynecol* 1994; 84:613.

[30] Taylor SI, Dons RF, Hernandez E, et al. Insulin resistance associated with androgen excess in women with autoantibodies to the insulin receptor. *Ann Intern Med* 1982; 97:851.

[31] Taylor SI, Cama A, Accili D, et al. Mutations in the insulin receptor gene. *Endocr Rev* 1992; 13:566.

[32] Moller DE, Cohen O, Yamaguchi Y, et al. Prevalence of mutations in the insulin receptor gene in subjects with features of the type A syndrome of insulin resistance. *Diabetes* 1994; 43:247.
[33] Dunaif A, Hoffman AR, Scully RE, et al. Clinical, biochemical, and ovarian morphologic features in women with acanthosis nigricans and masculinization. *Obstet Gynecol* 1985; 66:545.
[34] Dunaif A, Segal KR, Shelley DR, et al. Evidence for distinctive and intrinsic defects in insulin action in polycystic ovary syndrome. *Diabetes* 1992; 41:1257.
[35] Dunaif A, Xia J, Book CB, et al. Excessive insulin receptor serine phosphorylation in cultured fibroblasts and in skeletal muscle. A potential mechanism for insulin resistance in the polycystic ovary syndrome. *J Clin Invest* 1995; 96:801.
[36] Cohen JC, Hickman R. Insulin resistance and diminished glucose tolerance in powerlifters ingesting anabolic steroids. *J Clin Endocrinol Metab* 1987; 64:960.
[37] Barbieri RL, Smith S, Ryan KJ. The role of hyperinsulinemia in the pathogenesis of ovarian hyperandrogenism. *Fertil Steril* 1988; 50:197.
[38] Nestler JE, Jakubowicz DJ. Decreases in ovarian cytochrome P450c17 alpha activity and serum free testosterone after reduction of insulin secretion in polycystic ovary syndrome. *N Engl J Med* 1996; 335:617.
[39] Dunaif A, Scott D, Finegood D, et al. The insulin-sensitizing agent troglitazone improves metabolic and reproductive abnormalities in the polycystic ovary syndrome. *J Clin Endocrinol Metab* 1996; 81:3299.
[40] Elders MJ, Schedewie HK, Olefsky J, et al. Endocrine-metabolic relationships in patients with leprechaunism. *J Natl Med Assoc* 1982; 74:1195.
[41] Rabson SM, Mendenhall EN. Familial hypertrophy of pineal body, hyperplasia of adrenal cortex and diabetes mellitus; report of 3 cases. *Am J Clin Pathol* 1956; 26:283.
[42] Taylor SI. Lilly Lecture: molecular mechanisms of insulin resistance. Lessons from patients with mutations in the insulin-receptor gene. *Diabetes* 1992; 41:1473.
[43] Flier JS, Moller DE, Moses AC, et al. Insulin-mediated pseudoacromegaly: clinical and biochemical characterization of a syndrome of selective insulin resistance. *J Clin Endocrinol Metab* 1993; 76:1533.
[44] Flier JS, Young JB, Landsberg L. Familial insulin resistance with acanthosis nigricans, acral hypertrophy, and muscle cramps. *N Engl J Med 1980*; 303:970.
[45] Minaker KL, Flier JS, Landsberg L, et al. Phenytoin-induced improvement in muscle cramping and insulin action in three patients with the syndrome of insulin resistance, acanthosis nigricans, and acral hypertrophy. *Arch Neurol* 1989; 46:981.
[46] Björntorp P. "Portal" adipose tissue as a generator of risk factors for cardiovascular disease and diabetes. *Arteriosclerosis* 1990; 10:493.
[47] Hotamisligil GS, Shargill NS, Spiegelman BM. Adipose expression of tumor necrosis factor-alpha: direct role in obesity-linked insulin resistance. *Science* 1993; 259:87.
[48] Oral EA, Simha V, Ruiz E, et al. Leptin-replacement therapy for lipodystrophy. *N Engl J Med* 2002; 346:570.
[49] Mantzoros CS. Whither recombinant human leptin treatment for HIV-associated lipoatrophy and the metabolic syndrome? *J Clin Endocrinol Metab* 2009; 94:1089.
[50] Brennan AM, Mantzoros CS. Leptin and adiponectin: their role in diabetes. *Curr Diab Rep* 2007; 7:1.

[51] Gavrila A, Chan JL, Yiannakouris N, et al. Serum adiponectin levels are inversely associated with overall and central fat distribution but are not directly regulated by acute fasting or leptin administration in humans: cross-sectional and interventional studies. *J Clin Endocrinol Metab* 2003; 88:4823.

[52] Fargnoli JL, Fung TT, Olenczuk DM, et al. Adherence to healthy eating patterns is associated with higher circulating total and high-molecular-weight adiponectin and lower resistin concentrations in women from the Nurses' Health Study. *Am J Clin Nutr* 2008; 88:1213.

[53] Blüher M, Williams CJ, Klöting N, et al. Gene expression of adiponectin receptors in human visceral and subcutaneous adipose tissue is related to insulin resistance and metabolic parameters and is altered in response to physical training. *Diabetes Care* 2007; 30:3110.

[54] Tsokos GC, Gorden P, Antonovych T, et al. Lupus nephritis and other autoimmune features in patients with diabetes mellitus due to autoantibody to insulin receptors. *Ann Intern Med* 1985; 102:176.

[55] Cowie CC, Rust KF, Ford ES, et al. Full accounting of diabetes and pre-diabetes in the U.S. population in 1988-1994 and 2005-2006. *Diabetes Care* 2009; 32:287.

[56] Zhang X, Decker FH, Luo H, et al. Trends in the prevalence and comorbidities of diabetes mellitus in nursing home residents in the United States: 1995-2004. *J Am Geriatr Soc* 2010; 58:724.

[57] Bethel MA, Sloan FA, Belsky D, Feinglos MN. Longitudinal incidence and prevalence of adverse outcomes of diabetes mellitus in elderly patients. *Arch Intern Med* 2007; 167:921.

[58] Brown AF, Mangione CM, Saliba D, et al. Guidelines for improving the care of the older person with diabetes mellitus. *J Am Geriatr Soc* 2003; 51:S265.

[59] Mooradian AD, Perryman K, Fitten J, et al. Cortical function in elderly non-insulin dependent diabetic patients. Behavioral and electrophysiologic studies. *Arch Intern Med* 1988; 148:2369.

[60] Action to Control Cardiovascular Risk in Diabetes Study Group, Gerstein HC, Miller ME, et al. Effects of intensive glucose lowering in type 2 diabetes. *N Engl J Med* 2008; 358:2545.

[61] Abbatecola AM, Paolisso G. Diabetes care targets in older persons. *Diabetes Res Clin Pract* 2009; 86 Suppl 1:S35.

[62] American Diabetes Association. Standards of medical care in diabetes--2011. *Diabetes Care* 2011; 34 Suppl 1:S11.

[63] Adler GK, Bonyhay I, Failing H, et al. Antecedent hypoglycemia impairs autonomic cardiovascular function: implications for rigorous glycemic control. *Diabetes* 2009; 58:360.

[64] Whitmer RA, Karter AJ, Yaffe K, et al. Hypoglycemic episodes and risk of dementia in older patients with type 2 diabetes mellitus. *JAMA* 2009; 301:1565.

[65] Matyka K, Evans M, Lomas J, et al. Altered hierarchy of protective responses against severe hypoglycemia in normal aging in healthy men. *Diabetes Care* 1997; 20:135.

[66] Miller CK, Edwards L, Kissling G, Sanville L. Nutrition education improves metabolic outcomes among older adults with diabetes mellitus: results from a randomized controlled trial. *Prev Med* 2002; 34:252.

[67] Knowler WC, Barrett-Connor E, Fowler SE, et al. Reduction in the incidence of type 2 diabetes with lifestyle intervention or metformin. *N Engl J Med* 2002; 346:393.

[68] Wing RR, Hamman RF, Bray GA, et al. Achieving weight and activity goals among diabetes prevention program lifestyle participants. *Obes Res* 2004; 12:1426.

[69] American Diabetes Association, Bantle JP, Wylie-Rosett J, et al. Nutrition recommendations and interventions for diabetes: a position statement of the American Diabetes Association. *Diabetes Care* 2008; 31 Suppl 1:S61.

[70] Wedick NM, Barrett-Connor E, Knoke JD, Wingard DL. The relationship between weight loss and all-cause mortality in older men and women with and without diabetes mellitus: the Rancho Bernardo study. *J Am Geriatr Soc* 2002; 50:1810.

[71] Neumiller JJ, Setter SM. Pharmacologic management of the older patient with type 2 diabetes mellitus. *Am J Geriatr Pharmacother* 2009; 7:324.

[72] Shorr RI, Ray WA, Daugherty JR, Griffin MR. Incidence and risk factors for serious hypoglycemia in older persons using insulin or sulfonylureas. *Arch Intern Med* 1997; 157:1681.

[73] Burge MR, Schmitz-Fiorentino K, Fischette C, et al. A prospective trial of risk factors for sulfonylurea-induced hypoglycemia in type 2 diabetes mellitus. JAMA 1998; 279:137.

[74] Bressler, P, DeFronzo, RA. Drugs and diabetes. *Diabetes Rev* 1994; 2:53.

[75] Papa G, Fedele V, Rizzo MR, et al. Safety of type 2 diabetes treatment with repaglinide compared with glibenclamide in elderly people: A randomized, open-label, two-period, cross-over trial. *Diabetes Care* 2006; 29:1918.

[76] Klein, R, Klein, BE. Vision disorders in diabetes. In: Diabetes in America. Harris, MI (Ed). NIH Publication No. 95-1468, 2nd Edition, 1995.

[77] Young MJ, Boulton AJ, MacLeod AF, et al. A multicentre study of the prevalence of diabetic peripheral neuropathy in the United Kingdom hospital clinic population. *Diabetologia* 1993; 36:150.

[78] Franklin GM, Kahn LB, Baxter J, et al. Sensory neuropathy in non-insulin-dependent diabetes mellitus. The San Luis Valley Diabetes Study. *Am J Epidemiol* 1990; 131:633.

[79] Randomised trial of cholesterol lowering in 4444 patients with coronary heart disease: the Scandinavian Simvastatin Survival Study (4S). *Lancet* 1994; 344:1383.

[80] Sacks FM, Tonkin AM, Craven T, et al. Coronary heart disease in patients with low LDL-cholesterol: benefit of pravastatin in diabetics and enhanced role for HDL-cholesterol and triglycerides as risk factors. *Circulation* 2002; 105:1424.

[81] Heart Protection Study Collaborative Group. MRC/BHF Heart Protection Study of cholesterol lowering with simvastatin in 20,536 high-risk individuals: a randomised placebo-controlled trial. *Lancet* 2002; 360:7.

[82] Collaborative overview of randomised trials of antiplatelet therapy--I: Prevention of death, myocardial infarction, and stroke by prolonged antiplatelet therapy in various categories of patients. Antiplatelet Trialists' Collaboration. *BMJ* 1994; 308:81.

[83] Christmas C, Andersen RA. Exercise and older patients: guidelines for the clinician. *J Am Geriatr Soc* 2000; 48:318.

[84] Karani R, McLaughlin MA, Cassel CK. Exercise in the healthy older adult. *Am J Geriatr Cardiol* 2001; 10:269.

[85] Morey MC, Pieper CF, Crowley GM, et al. Exercise adherence and 10-year mortality in chronically ill older adults. *J Am Geriatr Soc* 2002; 50:1929.

[86] Heath JM, Stuart MR. Prescribing exercise for frail elders. *J Am Board Fam Pract* 2002; 15:218.

[87] Fiatarone MA, O'Neill EF, Ryan ND, et al. Exercise training and nutritional supplementation for physical frailty in very elderly people. *N Engl J Med* 1994; 330:1769.

[88] Anderson RJ, Freedland KE, Clouse RE, Lustman PJ. The prevalence of comorbid depression in adults with diabetes: a meta-analysis. *Diabetes Care* 2001; 24:1069.

[89] Maraldi C, Volpato S, Penninx BW, et al. Diabetes mellitus, glycemic control, and incident depressive symptoms among 70- to 79-year-old persons: the health, aging, and body composition study. *Arch Intern Med* 2007; 167:1137.

[90] Newman SC, Hassan AI. Antidepressant use in the elderly population in Canada: results from a national survey. *J Gerontol A Biol Sci Med Sci* 1999; 54:M527.

[91] Lustman PJ, Clouse RE. Treatment of depression in diabetes: impact on mood and medical outcome. *J Psychosom Res* 2002; 53:917.

[92] Lustman PJ, Freedland KE, Griffith LS, Clouse RE. Predicting response to cognitive behavior therapy of depression in type 2 diabetes. *Gen Hosp Psychiatry* 1998; 20:302.

[93] Schwartz AV, Vittinghoff E, Sellmeyer DE, et al. Diabetes-related complications, glycemic control, and falls in older adults. *Diabetes Care* 2008; 31:391.

In: New Horizons in Geriatric Medicine. Volume 1
Editors: Ahmet Turan Isik, M. Refik Mas et al.
ISBN: 978-1-62808-972-1

Chapter 12

THYROID DISORDERS

Alper Sonmez and Omer Azal

ABSTRACT

This chapter will give insights for the diagnosis and treatment of thyroid disorders in the elderly. Thyroid disorders may cause significant morbidity if left untreated in the geriatric population. The diagnosis of the thyroid dysfunction in older patients is challenging since the presenting symptoms are sometimes atypical. Also the comorbidities and the confounders, common in this age group, may obscure the diagnosis. Therefore, it is always important to consider the possibility of thyroid disease in the elderly population. Serum TSH measurement should be performed as a screening test in the elderly. As the gland is often shrunken, the physical examination gives almost nothing in the elderly patient. The prudent physician should be patient while treating overt hypothyroidism. Low-dose levothyroxine should be implemented while starting the treatment and gradually increased within months. In treating hyperthyroidism, radioactive iodine rather than antithyroid medication seem to be definitive, well tolerated and effective. Surgical thyroid ablation is rarely necessary when the radioactive iodine therapy is not successful or in patients with multinodular goiter. Fine needle aspiration for cytology should be considered if the ultrasound findings are suspicious for malignancy.

INTRODUCTION

Despite the high prevalence of thyroid gland dysfunction and nodules in the aging population, the diagnosis and treatment of thyroid disorders may be challenging. The symptoms of thyroid dysfunction may be subtle which may cause the diagnosis to be overlooked or confused with coexisting illnesses. Even the symptoms may be attributed to normal aging. Therefore, a prudent doctor should always consider the possibility of thyroid disorder in an elderly, and appropriately order screening tests.

Due to the physiology of aging, a series of metabolic alterations may occur in thyroid hormone synthesis, secretion and catabolism [1]. However, these alterations do not seem to affect the serum levels of the stimulating hormone (TSH) and free thyroxine (FT4) in healthy elderly subjects [2]. But the issue of polypharmacy and the effects of comorbidities are the significant problems for an elderly patient with thyroid disorder [3]. Many drugs can interfere with the normal thyroid function while several others that contain iodine can mimic iodine action and lead to further problems with thyroid hormone synthesis [3-5] (Table-1). So, it is utmost important to take a look at the drug list of an elderly patient before starting to evaluate the laboratory tests.

Table 1. Drugs that interfere with the results of thyroid function tests

	TSH	FT4
Dopamine	↓	↓,→
Levodopa	↓	
Bromocriptine	↓	
Glucocorticoids	↓	↓,→
Octreotide	↓	
Amphetamines	↓	
Metoclopramide >1 mg/kg	↑	
Amiodarone	↑,↓,→	↑
Iodinated contrast media	↑	↑
Phenytoin		↓
Carbamazepine		↓
Furosemide (IV >80 mg/day)		↑
Nonsteroidal agents	↓,→	↑,→
IV heparin	↓,→	↑,→
Lithium	↑	
Sprinolacton	↑	

PRIMARY HYPOTHYROIDISM

Epidemiology

The prevalence of hypothyroidism is determined by several factors such as gender, ethnicity, and iodine intake. Also the estimates of the prevalence among the elderly vary depending on the populations studied and the criteria used to define the condition. "Overt hypothyroidism" which defines the cases of elevated TSH and low FT4 is seen in about 2-10% of the population over the age of sixty [6]. On the other hand, "Subclinical hypothyroidism", that is the elevation of TSH with normal FT4 levels is much more common, reaching to 20% over in the age of eighty [7, 8]. Both disorders are more frequent in women and steadily increase with age. According to different population surveys in different regions of the world, lack of sufficient dietary iodine content appears to have a protective effect on the development of hypothyroidism in the elderly [9].

Etiology

Chronic autoimmune thyroiditis (Hashimoto's disease) is the most common cause of hypothyroidism in iodine-sufficient areas [10]. On the other hand, iodine deficiency is the most common cause of hypothyroidism in especially mountainous regions of the world such as South East Asia, West Pacific and Africa. Antithyroid antibodies increase the risk of developing subclinical and overt hypothyroidism and they are elevated in the elderly population [8]. The other less common causes of hypothyroidism in the elderly are thyroid surgery, radiation therapy to the neck, previous radioactive iodine therapy for hyperthyroidism, or pituitary or hypothalamic disorders causing primary hypothyroidism. Finally, iodine containing medications, lithium and interferon alpha may precipitate hypothyroidism in susceptible elderly patients.

Clinical Manifestations

The signs and symptoms of hypothyroidism may not be clear in the elderly. Often there are few symptoms pointing to hypothyroidism. Therefore, a physician needs to be careful in diagnosing hypothyroidism in an elderly patient. For example, mental and physical slowing, often attributed to advancing age, may be the only symptoms of an elderly patient with hypothyroidism. Other symptoms of hypothyroidism such as cold intolerance, weight gain, dry skin, constipation, are also common features of the normal aging [11]. Furthermore, the specific findings may be exacerbated or masked by comorbid cardiovascular, neuropsychiatric, dermatologic, or rheumatologic conditions that are more common among the elderly [12, 13]. For example, an elderly with hypertension, congestive heart failure and atrial fibrillation may complaint of weakness, fatigue, constipation or weight gain which may likely occur due to the side effects of beta blocker, calcium antagonist or digitalis in his medications. Meanwhile, these symptoms may also be indicative of hypothyroidism for this patient. Hypothyroidism in the elderly can increase cholesterol levels and exacerbate atherosclerothic cardiovascular disorders, respiratory problems and sleep apnea. Hypothyroidism can also worsen depression and cognitive function. Neuropsychological testing of elderly patients with hypothyroidism has demonstrated that they score lower on Mini-Mental Status Tests, and other specific indices such as visual-spatial function, memory, word fluency, attention, and psychomotor function. On the other hand, it is not clear whether subclinical hypothyroidism has a significant clinical feature or not [14]. Although decreased quality of life, dyslipidemia, left ventricular dysfunction, neuropsychiatric problems have been reported in patients with subclinical hypothyroidism, levothyroxine (L-T4) treatment does not always improve these parameters [15].

Diagnosis

An elderly patient with physical or mental dysfunction or any finding suggestive of hypothyroidism should undergo testing for hypothyroidism [11]. Positive family history of thyroid disease, past treatment for hyperthyroidism, or a history of surgery or radiotherapy to the neck may be indicative of the presence of hypothyroidism. Measuring serum TSH level is the best screening test and hypothyroidism is the most likely diagnosis in a patient with an elevated levels. Rare cases with central hypothyroidism are presented with low or normal TSH levels. After the establishment of high TSH levels, a serum FT4 should be obtained to distinguish overt from subclinical hypothyroidism. This distinction is important, since overt hypothyroidism should be treated, while there is controversy over treating subclinical hypothyroidism [15]. In the later occasion it is advisable to repeat the TSH in a few months before diagnosing the patient as subclinical hypothyroidism. Because, factors such as recovery from illness, changes in medications, or various forms of thyroiditis may cause temporary elevations in TSH levels. In addition, mildly elevated serum TSH levels in older subjects may occasionally normalize in the follow up period. Thyroid antibody testing after establishing the diagnosis of hypothyroidism, is not useful in an elderly patient as positive results do not change the treatment decisions. The only benefit measuring anti-thyroid antibody levels is to confirm a suspected diagnosis of autoimmune thyroiditis as the underlying cause of primary hypothyroidism. If the thyroid is normal on examination no imaging is needed. If the gland is asymmetric or hard, or if a palpable nodule is present, further evaluation with thyroid ultrasound and tissue sampling may be necessary.

Management

The standard treatment in an elderly patient diagnosed with overt hypothyroidism is once daily L-T4, taken orally. Other forms of thyroid hormone, including thyroid extract or T3 preparations are not recommended. Randomized trial have not shown any benefit of this mode of treatment on the improvement of symptoms, mood, cognitive function, or quality of life [16, 17]. Moreover, they can precipitate angina and arrhythmias in the susceptible patients. Average L-T4 replacement doses are lower in older patients, compared to young patients. This is due to the decreased clearance of T4 with age. In order to allow the heart and central nervous system to adjust to increasing levels of thyroid hormone, L-T4 treatment is usually implemented with a partial weekly dose increases. The so called “start low, go very slow” approach is therefore instituted with an initial L-T4 dose of 25 to 50 micrograms daily. Older patients with no evidence of heart disease, stroke or dementia may be started on larger doses and proceed to full hormone replacement more quickly [18]. In patients who experience increased angina pectoris, symptoms of congestive heart failure, or mental changes such as confusion will need to have their dose of L-T4 decreased, then more gradually increased over several months’ time. The patient and family members must be aware of a possible increase in angina, shortness of breath, confusion and change in sleep habits, and notify the prescribing physician if these occur. Most patients require lifelong therapy with periodic measurement of serum TSH levels. Once a steady state of TSH levels has been achieved, patients should be monitored every 6 to 12 months for clinical response to the treatment, adherence to medication, and observation of drug interactions. Education of the patient and family is very important, since in many elderly individuals coexisting memory impairment may cause nonadherence to the therapy. Alternately, the inadequately treated hypothyroidism may precipitate mental impairment. Lastly, it is important to mention that there are differences in hormone potency and bioavailability in various batches of hormone.

Subclinical Hypothyroidism

Thyroid hormone replacement is the standard treatment in overt hypothyroidism with serum TSH levels over 10mIU/L. However, the benefits are much less clear in patients in subclinical hypothyroidism with TSH levels below 10mIU/L [14, 15]. Recent studies show that subclinical hypothyroidism does not significantly increase cardiovascular morbidity and mortality in subjects over the age of 65[19, 20]. So, it is not clear whether the TSH elevation in subclinical values is a normal aspect of aging or, an improper resetting of the normal range [9]. A decision to treat an elderly patient with a mildly elevated TSH level should depend on the presence of clinical findings of hypothyroidism. If TSH is below 10 U/ml, it is practical to repeat the test in 3-4 months and not starting thyroid hormone replacement unless there are substantial symptoms attributable to hypothyroidism.

Myxedema Coma

Myxedema Coma is a rare but fatal endocrine emergency which usually affects the eldest elderly group. A typical patient is referred to the emergency department in lethargy or coma which was precipitated due to a major physiologic stress such as trauma, systemic infection or surgery [21, 22]. Among the other precipitating factors are medications such as lithium, amiodarone or tranquilizers. Cold temperatures can also precipitate the clinical picture. The clinical features are severe mental deterioration, confusion, and disorientation as well as lethargy and psychosis. The skin is usually dry and scaly, the hair is sparse, and the voice is hoarse. Among the other findings are bradycardia, cardiomegaly, pericardial effusion, hypothermia and hyponatremia. Myxedema coma should be treated in an intensive care unit with supportive care, including critical care-level monitoring of vital signs, rewarming with heating blankets, correction of fluid and electrolyte imbalances, avoidance of hypnotics and sedatives, empiric treatment of suspected underlying infections, and mechanical ventilatory support as indicated. Treatment also involves the administration of a loading dose of 200-300 mcg of intravenous thyroxine, followed by 50 mcg daily administrations. Due to the theoretical risk of concomitant adrenal insufficiency, empiric treatment with glucocorticoids is also recommended [21, 22].

HYPERTHYROIDISM

Epidemiology

The prevalence of hyperthyroidism is determined by gender, age, iodine intake status and the cut-off value used to define a low TSH level. According to the Whickham Survey, the overall rate of hyperthyroidism is about 2-3% in the general population with subclinical hyperthyroidism (low TSH, normal F T4 /F T3 levels) higher than the overt cases (low TSH with high FT4 and F T3 levels) [8]. Although there is not much data, hyperthyroidism is thought to be less prevalent in the aging population. This is probably because of increased Graves's Disease rate in young women. There are however, substantial amount of iatrogenic hyperthyroidism cases in the geriatric population that occur due to overtreatment with L-T4. A slight increase in hyperthyroidism risk is present in over the age of 80, due to the increased prevalance of toxic multinodular guatr in these subjects. Although the numbers vary between the different studies, the overall prevalence of hyperthyroidism in the aging population is about 2% [23, 24].

Etiology

Toxic multinodular goiter and Graves disease are the most common causes of hyperthyroidism in the elderly population. The relative frequency of toxic nodular goiter is greater than the Graves disease occurring 50% of older patients with hyperthyroidism, especially in areas of low or borderline iodine intake [25]. Solitary toxic adenomas are rare in elderly patients. Subacute thyroiditis, a less common cause of transient hyperthyroidism, is rarely clinically significant as it is self-limited and resolves in a few weeks.

A number of medications can cause hyperthyroidism being the most common is thyroid hormone, as discussed above [3-5]. Failure to wait an appropriate amount of time before a dose increase may result in hyperthyroidism. Iodine-induced hyperthyroidism [Jod-Basedow disease] may be caused by increased iodine uptake from sources such as mucolytics or contrast media. Amiodarone-induced thyrotoxicosis is one of the most significant drug induced hyperthyroidism problems in the elderly patients with arrhythmias. Patients receiving amiodarone should be monitored at 6 month intervals for thyroid hormone levels to screen for the onset of amiodarone induced thyroid dysfunction [26].

Clinical Features

As with hypothyroidism, the clinical picture in hyperthyroidism can be insidious in the elderly patients. Palpitations, enlarged thyroid gland, tremor, restlessness and anxiety, and signs of thyroid eye disease are common in young patients with hyperthyroidism. Many of these findings are due to the hyperadrenergic state induced by hyperthyroidism and are less common in the elderly [27, 28]. Instead, only one of the above symptoms may present vaguely or there may be no symptoms at all. It is also likely that the symptoms of hyperthyroidism may be masked due to the medications for coexisting diseases. For example, the signs of thyrotoxicosis such as tachycardia and tremulousness may be masked in a patient taking a beta blocker for hypertension or angina. Hyperthyroidism without clear symptoms of thyrotoxicosis in an elderly was long ago described as "apathetic hyperthyroidism", and characterized by apathetic facies, muscular weakness, excessive weight loss, depression, lethargy, arrhythmias, normal thyroid gland or small goiter [29]. Agitation and confusion can also be the presenting symptoms. If not recognized early, apathetic hyperthyroidism can lead to an extensive and expensive evaluation for malignancy, gastrointestinal disorder, or cardiac disease. Therefore any clinical change in a previously stable elderly patient in the setting of vague or nonspecific symptoms should warrant thyroid evaluation. Atrial fibrillation is a well-documented presentation of hyperthyroidism in the elderly [30]. For this reason, elderly patients with atrial fibrillation should always have TSH measured to rule out occult hyperthyroidism. Due to the increased risk for cerebrovascular embolism and stroke, atrial fibrillation is a major reason to consider treatment of even subclinical hyperthyroidism in the elderly. Another recent area of concern is the possible link between subclinical hyperthyroidism and the development of dementia though the mechanism is not clear [31].

Diagnosis

The diagnosis of hyperthyroidism in the elderly is not always problematic. However, several issues should be considered in the interpretation of the laboratory tests. A normal TSH almost always rules out, but a low TSH does not necessarily prove the presence of hyperthytroidism. If an elderly patient has a low but detectable TSH level, a careful assessment and further laboratory testing are necessary to distinguish true hyperthyroidism from nonthyroidal illness or drug effects. Low levels of TSH along with elevated FT4 levels confirm the diagnosis of overt hyperthyroidism. But, FT4 level may be normal in a small group of patients despite low TSH levels. In this case, the serum FT3 should be measured to rule out T3 toxicosis, a common entity in the elderly hyperthyroid patients [33]. It usually occurs due to a nodule producing excessive T3 and suppressing serum TSH and FT4 levels. On the other hand, high FT4 with normal or low FT3 levels can also be seen in several clinical conditions. In amiodarone induced thyrotoxicosis, inhibition of the 5' deiodinase enzyme blocks the peripheral conversion of T4 to T3 and results in reduced FT3 and elevated FT4 levels [34]. If both the FT4 and FT3 levels are normal in a patient with a low TSH, the patient is likely to have subclinical hyperthyroidism. It is important to rule out nonthyroidal illness, since treatment may be indicated for subclinical hyperthyroidism, but not for nonthyroidal illness.

Physical examination of the thyroid gland is not usually helpful in the elderly. A diffusely enlarged, palpable gland is consistent with Graves's disease. The presence of thyroid autoantibodies is suggestive of the diagnosis. A large nodule or multiple large nodules would suggest hyperfunctioning multinodular thyroid disease. In this case a thyroid ultrasound along with a radioiodine scan is indicated to evaluate the anatomy and functionality of the thyroid nodules.

Management

Antithyroid medication, surgery and radioactive iodine (RAI) are the three treatment strategies for hyperthyroidism. The choice depends on several factors such as the etiology, the severity of the clinical picture, and the medical condition of the patient [35]. Surgery may pose higher risk due to age-related comorbidities and addition of antithyroid medications would be cumbersome as many elderly are taking multiple drugs. On the other hand, RAI is reliable, effective, and free of significant side effects. However, the probability of hypothyroidism in the long term is expected in the majority of the patients. Therefore, RAI is generally the preferred treatment in the elderly. However, many elderly patients are hesitated to have RAI and inclined to refuse this choice. It is advisable to implement thionamides for a few weeks before proceeding to RAI since it may cause temporary release of preformed thyroid hormone from the gland and lead to cardiac decompansation in the elderly. In order to allow the thyroid gland to sufficiently uptake iodine, thionamides should be withdrawn 3-7 days before RAI. They can be recommenced a week later if the elderly subject has severe disease, incomplete biochemical control or significant complications (e.g., atrial fibrillation). FT4 levels and clinical status should be evaluated every 4-6 weeks after the RAI. If high FT4 levels still persist 6 months after RAI, a second course may be used. Patients should be followed by FT4 and TSH levels in order to detect hypothyroidism during the course of disease. Hypothyroidism rates may be slightly lower in those with toxic nodules because of relative sparing of normal thyroid tissue through concentration of isotope in the autonomous nodules. Hypothyroidism after the RAI treatment is expected in many patients but the course may not be totally predictable.

The onset of action of thionamides is much faster than the RAI. Therefore, they are preferred as alternatives in cardiac patients with Graves Disease or toxic multinodular goiter. Methimazole is preferable to propylthiouracil as it is more potent, associated with fewer side effects [36]. A typical starting dose of methimazole is 20-30 mg per day as a single daily dose. In contrast, propylthiouracil is typically given in divided doses, with an equivalent dosage of 200mg for 20 mg of methymazole. The thionamides are usually discontinued after 12–18 months, to see if a remission has occurred in patients with Graves disease [35]. However, they must be given continuously for toxic multinodular goiters [37]. The major but rare [less than 0.5%] adverse reaction of thionamide treatment is agranulocytosis. It occurs early in the course of treatment and is more common with larger doses but reversible on discontinuation of therapy [38]. Agranulocytosis is usually sudden in onset and occasionally fatal. Baseline leukocyte count with repeat testing with the onset of sore throat, fever, or other signs of infection is recommended. Rash, arthralgia, and myalgia are other potential side effects.

Surgery is not the preferred treatment strategy in the elderly hyperthyroidism. Because elderly subjects generally have multiple chronic medical conditions, including cardiac problems and they have relatively higher risk of intraoperative complications of anesthetics and surgery. It may be an alternative in the presence of multinodular toxic goiter or a large single autonomous nodule to which RAI may not work fully [39]. Surgery may also be necessary in those patients who have dysphagia or tracheal compression or if there is suspicion of malignancy. If surgery is considered as an option, clinical and biochemical euthyroidism should be restored by thionamides. Occasionally, patients with amiodarone-induced thyrotoxicosis may proceed to thyroidectomy, if they have decompensated cardiac disease. Due to the large iodine load, RAI is usually ineffective in those patients and thionamides have unpredictable efficacy [34].

The treatment of subclinical hyperthyroidism is controversial. Asymptomatic patients with a mild decrease in serum TSH level should be monitored closely as the risk of atrial fibrillation is increased in these patients. Subclinical hyperthyroidism may also increase the risk of osteroporosis and dementia in postmenopausal women. The treatment decisions should be individualized for these cases. Consensus guidelines suggest that elderly subjects with atrial fibrillation or with other vascular risk factors should be considered for treatment [40]. Thionamides are better alternatives to RAI in normalizing the TSH values in these patients.

Several adjunctive medications are implemented during the course of treatment. Beta-blockers can be given to control tachycardia and tremors. If beta-blockers are contraindicated, non-dihyropiridine calcium channel blockers can be chosen as alternatives. Salicylates can be used for relief of local pain and tenderness in cases of subacute thyroiditis. Occasionally short-term glucocortocoids are required in more severe cases. Anticoagulation with warfarin is indicated in patients with atrial fibrillation [32, 35]. Psychotropic drugs are seldom necessary for the psychiatric problems which may occur during the course of hyperthyroidism. These are generally resolved after the patient becomes euthyroid.

Hyperthyroid Storm

Hyperthyroid storm is an emergency situation which requires intensive care and close supervision. Patients present with fever, delirium, tachycardia, hypotension, vomiting, diarrhea and jaundice, and abnormal liver function tests. Stress factors such as surgery, trauma or systemic infections may precipitate the clinical features. Patients with thyroid storm should be treated in an intensive care unit with close monitoring. The initial measures to stabilize the systemic decompansation are the supplementation of oxygen and intravenous fluids, correction of electrolyte abnormalities, specific treatment of arryhtmia and aggressive control of hyperthermia (by applying ice pacs, cooling blankets and acetaminophen). Along with emergency measures, high dose thionamides (propylthiouracil is preferred because of its early onset of action and inhibitory effect of T4 to T3 conversion) should be given. Iodine compounds (lugol iodine or potassium iodine) block the release of thyroid hormone from the gland. They can be given orally or via the nasogastric tube. The intravenous contrast agents such as ipodate can be used to block the T4 to T3 conversion. Glucocorticoids are also used to decrease the peripheral conversion of T4 and to prevent relative adrenal insufficiency [41].

Thyroid Nodules and Cancer

Thyroid nodules are common in the general population with a further increase in frequency in the elderly [42]. According to the imaging studies, nearly half of the subjects over the age of 65 years have thyroid nodules [43]. The prevalence is much higher in iodine deficient areas. The initial evaluation of a thyroid nodule in an elderly is not different from that of the young adults. Serum TSH is measured as a first step and if the TSH is suppressed, a radionuclide thyroid scan should be performed [44]. Most of these nodules are nonfunctional and small in diameter. Therefore no further evaluation is required in the majority of elderly patients. Rarely, suppressed TSH levels indicative of toxic nodular goiter can be found. High FT3 and normal FT4 concentrations along with suppressed TSH values are the common laboratory finding of toxic multinodular goiter. The approach to these patients is described in the hyperthyroidism section.

An established thyroid nodule can be a benign adenoma, cancer, cyst or inflammation. The size and ultrasound features of the nodule help the clinician to assess the risk of malignancy. Nodules having greater diameters than 1–1.5 cm or those with suspicious ultrasound features should undergo fine needle aspiration biopsy to rule out thyroid cancer [44]. Malignancy is not expected in the autonomous nodules, which are also called “functioning” or “hot” nodules by radioiodine scan. The risk of thyroid cancer in a palpable nodule is 5%, accounting for 1% of all the malignancies. The frequency of thyroid cancer is lower but the aggressiveness is higher in the elderly population; the higher the age at diagnosis, the poorer the prognosis of thyroid cancers. The steady decline in survival with age is valid in both well differentiated papillary or follicular cancers and poorly differentiated medullary or anaplastic cancers. Therefore, thyroid nodules in the elderly should be evaluated thoroughly unless the patient is extremely old or medically frail [45].

Papillary thyroid cancer is the most common type in the elderly as seen in the young adults. Nearly half of the elderly thyroid cancer cases are papillary cancers and women are affected more frequently than men. It is commonly presented as an asymptomatic thyroid nodule and less often with lymphadenopathy, hoarseness or dysphagia. Distant metastases involving the lungs, bones brain and soft tissues are not frequently seen [46, 47]. Follicular cancer cases are the second most frequent thyroid cancers which are also more common in women and in iodine deficient areas. Follicular cancer has a higher mortality rate than papillary cancers due to its higher tendency of metastasis and higher frequency of extraglandular recurrences [47]. Medullary thyroid cancers are neuroendocrine tumors which are more aggressive than the papillary or follicular cancers. The familial forms of medullary thyroid cancers are mostly seen in younger patients while the frequency of the sporadic cases is higher in the older patients. Most patients are presented with a palpable nodule while the systemic presentations are increased due to distant metastasis and due to the secretory products of tumor. Age and stage are also the most significant predictors of mortality in medullary thyroid cancers [48]. Anaplastic thyroid cancers consist only 1-2% of all the thyroid cancers but the majority of the cases occurs in the elderly with a peak incidence in the 7th decade. It usually presents with a rapidly growing mass and symptoms of compression. Most of the patients have distant metastases at time of diagnosis [49].

The treatment principles of thyroid cancers in the elderly are similar to those in the younger patients. Total thyroidectomy plus RAI ablation of the remaining tissue is the valid approach. For many times, doctors and the family members of the patients are not willing to perform surgery in elderly. It should be kept in mind that age itself is not a specific contraindication for surgery. As thyroid cancers have more aggressive prognosis in the elderly population, surgery should always be the primary choice. Especially aggressive thyroid cancers may be risky to leave alone, and the value of doing surgery generally outweighs the value of not doing it. It may only be better to do nothing in a frail elderly with a very low life expectancy, than to treat goiters that are not life-threatening [45].

CONCLUSION

Thyroid disorders are common in older individuals and often present with atypical symptoms, which are sometimes attributed to normal aging process or coexisting diseases. Therefore, physicians should always think of thyroid disorders in geriatric subjects with vague symptoms. The non-thyroidal illness and the effect of medications or co-morbidities may sometimes confound the laboratory tests. Serum TSH measurement should be performed as a screening test in the elderly. Measuring the FT4 and FT3 levels are the next steps in case of the suppressed TSH levels. When the TSH is elevated, the FT4 measurement will help to tell the overt from the subclinical hypothyroidism. Doctors should be watchful for the cardiac decompansation during the treatment of hypothyroidism. The dosages of the L-T4 should be low at the beginning and should carefully be increased in 4-6 week intervals. In treating hyperthyroidism, radioactive iodine rather than antithyroid medication seem to be definitive, well tolerated and effective. Close follow-up of all patients ever having received this therapy is needed to identify the development of hypothyroidism. Surgical thyroid ablation is rarely needed in elderly hyperthyroidism who fail to respond to radioactive iodine therapy and in patients with multinodular goiter. As in the young patients a thyroid nodule should always be evaluated for the probability of hyperthyroidism and malignancy. No further test is needed for the nodules smaller than 1cm in diameter and normal TSH values. Suspicious nodule should be evaluated hystologicaly. If there is a thyroid malignancy, surgery is the definitive treatment and it must not be deferred because of the age of the patients. Age is never a contraindication for a thyroidectomy.

REFERENCES

[1] Hershman JM, Hassani S, Samuels MH. Thyroid diseases. In: Hazard WR, et al., Eds. Principles of Geriatric Medicine and Gerontology. 6th ed. New York, NY: McGraw-Hill; 2008:1287-1304.

[2] Franklyn JA, Ramsden DB, Sheppard MC. The influence of age and sex on tests of thyroid function. *Ann Clin Biochem*. 1985; 22:502-5.

[3] Ananthakrishnan S, Pearce EN. Influence of drugs on thyroid function tests. In: G.A. Brent Eds. Thyroid Function Testing. New York, NY: Springer Science; 2010:251-268.

[4] Dong BJ. West J Med. 2000; 172(2): 102–106.

[5] Sarne D, Effects of the environment, chemicals and drugs on thyroid function. Chapter 5a, In; *Thyroidmanager.org* (Updated 21 December 2010).

[6] Samuels MH. Subclinical thyroid disease in the elderly. *Thyroid*. 1998;8: 803-813.

[7] Canaris GJ, Manowitz NR, Mayor G, Ridgway EC. The Colorado thyroid disease prevalence study. *Arch Intern Med*. 2000;160:526-534.

[8] Tunbridge WM, Evered DC, Hall R, Appleton D, Brewis M, Clark F, Evans JG, Young E, Bird T, Smith PA. The spectrum of thyroid disease in a community: the Whickham survey. *Clin Endocrinol* (Oxford). 1977;7:481-493.

[9] Kim KI. Hypothyroidism in the Elderly, Chapter 8. In: Hershmann Eds. Endocrinology of aging. *Endotext.org* (Last Revised: January 22, 2011).

[10] Szabolcs I, Podoba J, Feldkamp J, Dohan O, Farkas I, Sajgó M, Takáts KI, Góth M, Kovács L, Kressinszky K, Hnilica P, Szilágyi G.Comparative screening for thyroid disorders in old age in areas of iodine deficiency, long-term iodine prophylaxis and abundant iodine intake. *Clin Endocrinol* (Oxf), 1997; 47(1): 87-92.

[11] Stuck LM, McFarland KF. Hypothyroidism in the elderly. When symptoms are not a 'normal' part of aging. *Postgrad Med*. 1991;90(8):141-146.

[12] Trivalle C, Doucet J, Chassagne P, Landrin I, Kadri N, Menard JF, Bercoff E. Differences in the signs and symptoms of hyperthyroidism in older and younger patients. *J Am Geriatr Soc*. 1996 ;44(1):50-53.

[13] Doucet J, Trivalle C, Chassagne P, Perol MB, Vuillermet P, Manchon ND, Menard JF, Bercoff E. Does age play a role in clinical presentation of hypothyroidism? *J Am Geriatr Soc*. 1994;42:984-986.

[14] Ceresini G, Morganti S, Maggio M, Usberti E, Fiorino I, Artoni A, Teresi G, Belli S, Ridolfi V, Valenti G, Ceda GP. Subclinical thyroid disease in elderly subjects. *Acta Biomed*. 2010;81 Suppl 1:31-36.

[15] Fatourechi V. Subclinical hypothyroidism: an update for primary care physicians. *Mayo Clin Proc.* 2009;84(1):65-71.

[16] Escobar-Morreale HF, Botella-Carretero JI, Gómez-Bueno M, Galán JM, Barrios V, Sancho J. Thyroid hormone replacement therapy in primary hypothyroidism: a randomized trial comparing L-thyroxine plus liothyronine with L-thyroxine alone. *Ann Intern Med,* 2005;142(6): 412-24.

[17] Saravanan P, Simmons DJ, Greenwood R, Peters TJ, Dayan CM. Partial substitution of thyroxine (T4) with tri-iodothyronine in patients on T4 replacement therapy: results of a large community-based randomized controlled trial. *J Clin Endocrinol Metab*, 2005; 90(2): 805-812.

[18] Roos A, Linn-Rasker SP, van Domburg RT, Tijssen JP, Berghout A. The starting dose of levothyroxine in primary hypothyroidism treatment: a prospective, randomized, double-blind trial. *Arch Intern Med*, 2005; 165(15): 1714-1720.

[19] Cappola AR, Fried LP, Arnold AM, Danese MD, Kuller LH, Burke GL, Tracy RP, Ladenson PW. Thyroid status, cardiovascular risk, and mortality in older adults. *JAMA* 2006; 295(9):1033-1034.

[20] Park YJ, Lee EJ, Lee YJ, Choi SH, Park JH, Lee SB, Lim S, Lee WW, Jang HC, Cho BY, Woo JI, Kim KW Subclinical hypothyroidism (SCH) is not associated with metabolic derangement, cognitive impairment, depression or poor quality of life (QoL) in elderly subjects. *Arch Gerontol Geriatr.* 2010;50(3):e68-73.

[21] Jordan RM. Myxedema coma. Pathophysiology, therapy, and factors affecting prognosis. *Med Clin North Am.* 1995; 79(1): 185-194.

[22] Wall CR. Myxedema coma: Diagnosis and treatment. *Am Fam Physician.* 2000;62(11):2485-2490.

[23] Wilson S, Parle JV, Roberts LM, Roalfe AK, Hobbs FDR, Clark P, Sheppard MC, Gammage MD, Pattison HM, Franklyn JA. Prevalence of subclinical thyroid dysfunction in the elderly in England, the Birmingham Elderly Thyroid Study (BETS): a community based cross-sectional survey. *J Clin Endocrinol Metab.* 2006;91:4809-4816.

[24] Falkenberg M, Kagedal B, Norr A. Screening of an elderly female population for hypo- and hyperthyroidism by use of a thyroid hormone panel. *Acta Med Scand.* 1983;214:361-365.

[25] Díez JJ. Hyperthyroidism in patients older than 55 years: an analysis of the etiology and management. *Gerontology.* 2003;49(5):316-323.

[26] Bogazzi F, Bartalena L, Martino E. Approach to the patient with amiodarone-induced thyrotoxicosis. *J Clin Endocrinol Metab.* 2010;95(6):2529-2535.

[27] Bhattacharyya A, Wiles PG. Thyrotoxicosis in old age: a different clinical entity? *Hosp Med.* 1999;60(2):115-118.

[28] Nordyke RA, Gilbert FI, Harada ASM. Graves' Disease. Influence of age on clinical findings. *Arch Intern Med.* 1988;148:626-631.

[29] Lahey FH. Apathetic thyroidism. *Ann Surg.* 1931;93:1026.

[30] Patanè S, Marte F. Atrial fibrillation associated with subclinical hyperthyroidism. *Int J Cardiol.* 2009;134(3):e155-158.

[31] Kalmijn S, Mehta KM, Pols HA, Hofman A, Drexhage HA, Breteler MM.Subclinical hyperthyroidism and the risk of dementia. The Rotterdam study. *Clin Endocrinol* (Oxf). 2000;53(6):733-737.

[32] Franklyn J, Parle L. Hyperthyroidism in aging. In: *Endotext.com* (Updated: February 23, 2007

[33] Martino E, Pacchiarotti A, Aghini-Lombardi F, Grasso L, Bambini G, Baschieri L, Pinchera A. Acta Endocrinol (Copenh). 1985;110(3):354-359.

[34] Basaria S, Cooper DS. Amiodarone and the thyroid. *Am J Med.* 2005;118:706-714.

[35] Franklyn JA. The management of hyperthyroidism. *N Engl J Med.* 1994; 330: 1731-1738.

[36] Nakamura H, Noh JY, Itoh K, Fukata S, Miyauchi A, Hamada N. Comparison of methimazole and propylthiouracil in patients with hyperthyroidism caused by Graves' disease. *J Clin Endocrinol Metab.* 2007;92(6):2157-2162.

[37] Vitti P, Rago T, Tonacchera M, Pinchera A. Toxic multinodular goiter in the elderly. *J Endocrinol Invest.* 2002;25(10 Suppl):16-18.

[38] Meyer-Gessner M, Benker G, Lederbogen S, Olbricht T, Reinwein D. Antithyroid drug-induced agranulocytosis: clinical experience with ten patients treated at one institution and review of the literature. *J Endocrinol Invest.* 1994;17(1):29-36.

[39] Porterfield JR Jr, Thompson GB, Farley DR, Grant CS, Richards ML. Evidence-based management of toxic multinodular goiter (Plummer's Disease).*World J Surg.* 2008;32(7):1278-1284.

[40] Surks MI, Ortiz E, Daniels GH, Sawin CT, Col NF, Cobin RH, Franklyn JA, Hershman JM, Burman KD, Denke MA, Gorman C, Cooper RS, Weissman NJ. Evidence-based consensus guidelines for the diagnosis and management of subclinical thyroid disease. *JAMA* 2004;291:228-238.

[41] Nayak B, Burman K. Thyrotoxicosis and thyroid storm. *Endocrinol Metab Clin North Am.* 2006;35(4):663-686.

[42] Gupta KL. Neoplasm of the thyroid gland. *Clin Geriatr Med.* 1995;11:271-290.

[43] Mazzaferri E. Management of a solitary thyroid nodule. *NEJM* 1993; 328:553-559.

[44] Cooper DS, Doherty GM, Haugen BR, Kloos RT, Lee SL, Mandel SJ, Mazzaferri EL, McIver B, Pacini F, Schlumberger M, Sherman SI, Steward DL, Tuttle RM. Revised American Thyroid Association management guidelines for patients with thyroid nodules and differentiated thyroid cancer.American Thyroid Association (ATA) Guidelines Taskforce on Thyroid Nodules and Differentiated Thyroid Cancer. *Thyroid.* 2009;19(11):1167-1214.

[45] Crockett SS, Hershman JM. Thyroid Nodules and Cancer in the Elderly. In: Endotext. Org (Last Revised: May 6, 2009)

[46] Caron NR, Clark OH. Papillary thyroid cancer. *Curr Treat Options Oncol.* 2006;7(4):309-319.

[47] Mazzaferri EL, Kloos RT. Clinical review 128: Current approaches to primary therapy for papillary and follicular thyroid cancer. *J Clin Endocrinol Metab.* 2001;86(4):1447-1463.

[48] Ahmed SR, Ball DW. Clinical review: Incidentally discovered medullary thyroid cancer: diagnostic strategies and treatment. *J Clin Endocrinol Metab.* 2011;96(5):1237-1245.

[49] Dackiw AP. Anaplastic thyroid cancer. *Cancer Treat Res.* 2010;153:75-84.

In: New Horizons in Geriatric Medicine. Volume 1
Editors: Ahmet Turan Isik, M. Refik Mas et al.
ISBN: 978-1-62808-972-1

Chapter 13

OSTEOARTHRITIS

Nese Olmez

ABSTRACT

Osteoarthritis (OA) is one of the most common causes of chronic disability in elderly and is related with a reduced quality of life. OA is clearly associated with aging, but there are additional factors that contribute to the development of OA like systemic (genetics, diet, estrogen use, and bone density) and local factors (muscle weakness, obesity, injury, malalignment). OA occurs as a result of various biochemical, biomechanical, inflammatory, and immunologic factors, not solely from the wearing down of the joints.

Aging-related changes of joint tissues that occur at the cellular level are cell senescence, decreased anabolic response to growth factors, accumulation of oxidative damage to DNA and telomere shortening. Changes within the extracellular matrix are increased collagen crosslinking by advanced glycation endproducts (AGEs), accumulation of modified and degraded extracellular matrix components and increased calcification. Age-related changes also occur in muscle, bone, fat, and the nervous system in elderly people that suggests OA to be a complex disease. How these aging changes interact with etiological factors to cause OA is unknown. Advanced imaging methods, evidence from genetic and biomarker studies has led to better understanding of the natural course of OA, provides information for early diagnosis and understanding the basic mechanisms by which aging affects joint tissues.

Although OA is most common in the hands, involvement of the knees and hips is usually much more disabling. OA management should consist of a combination of nonpharmacologic and pharmacologic treatment options. Usually all OA guidelines agree on shared recommendations for treatment. A wide array of agents have been studied for disease modification in OA, but the existing pharmacologic agents have not been shown to have convincing disease- modifying efficacy. More research is needed to provide new targets for slowing or preventing the development of OA. In the elderly, the management of OA has to be individualized for each patient according to the severity of symptoms and joint damage, joints affected, comorbidities, drug interactions, prior treatments, patient wishes and illness perceptions. Difficulties for patients to access health professional services also has to be considered in the treatment plan.

There is a rapid increase in the prevalence of OA because of aging population. This places a tremendous burden on health care system and causes great impact on elderly people and society. Further studies are needed to provide the early diagnosis and interventions that can help reduce the impact of OA on health care.

Introduction

Osteoarthritis (OA) is the most common cause of chronic disability in older adults. Age is one of the strongest risk factors for OA [1, 2, 3]. OA prevalence increases with age [3] such that only a small percent of elderly people are free of radiographic osteoarthritis [4]. Aging is likely to play play a role in the development of osteoarthritis in existence of other risk factors [5]. Obesity, previous knee injury, female sex, and the presence of hand OA were investigated as other constant risk factors for OA in a recent metaanalysis [1].

Exposure to various risk factors and biologic changes accumulate with aging. Interaction between etiological factors and aging process in OA is not well known [3]. The connection between aging changes in cells and tissues and OA in older adults is an important subject of recent research studies. Age related changes of joint tissues includes cell senessence, mitochondrial dysfunction, altered growth factor signaling and changes in subchondral bone and synovium [5, 6]. Age-related changes also occur in muscle, bone, fat, and the nervous system in elderly people that a more general and systemic approach will be needed to better understand the link between aging and OA [5].

Treatment of OA includes both nonpharmacologic and pharmacologic options as mentioned in current OA treatment guidelines [7-11]. In elderly people there are several issues to be considered in the treatment of OA like comorbidities [12], drug interactions [13] and cognitive status [14].

This chapter while giving general information about OA, mainly will focus on several aspects and impacts of OA in the elderly population. Problems in the implementation of management strategies in the elderly will also be discussed.

Epidemiology

OA is the most common type of arthritis [2]. The prevalence of OA increases with age such that 30 to 50% of adults over the age of 65 years suffer from this condition [3, 15]. Lawrence et al. reviewed published analyses from available national surveys to estimate prevalence for each of the most commonly affected joints (knees, hips, and hands) as well as for overall OA. They estimated that 26.9 million adults age 25 and older have clinical OA of some joint (up from the estimate of 21 million for 1995). As there is a rapid increase in the prevalence of OA growing impact on health care and public health systems in the future is expected [3].

Prevalence

OA can be defined pathologically, radiographically, or clinically in epidemiologic studies [16]. Various studies gives different prevalence of OA according to the definition of OA, joints studied, and the characteristics of the study population [17-22]. Not all persons who have radiographic

OA have symptoms, and not all persons who have joint symptoms have radiographic OA [23]. Use of different clinical and radiographic criteria may give different prevalence of OA in studies which makes the estimation of the prevalence of OA difficult [3].

Results of the Framingham Osteoarthritis Study showed that the prevalence of radiographic knee OA in subjects aged >60 increased with each decade of life from 33% among those aged 60-70 to 43.7 % among those >80 years of age.

Prevalence of symptomatic knee OA in these subjects was 9.5 % and increased with age in women but not men [19]. In the Johnson Country Osteoarthritis cohort, the prevalence of radiographic knee OA was 26.2% in the 55-64 year range to nearly 50% in the patients aged >75. The prevalence of symptomatic knee OA increased from 16.3% to 32.8% in these age groups [21].

In this cohort prevalence of symptomatic hip OA was 5.9% in the 45-54 age group and 17% in the patients >75 years of age [22]. In survey of Zoetermeer, radiographic involvement of the distal interphalangeal joints in the hand was present in more than half of men over the age of 65 and more than half of women over the age of 55years [17]. In the Framingham Study 13% of men and 26% of women over the age of 70 were found to have symptomatic hand OA [20].

Disc degeneration of lumbar and cervical spine was found to be more often present than absent in both men and women aged >50 in survey of Zoetermeer [17]. The prevalence of radiological OA increased strongly with age and peak values for cervical spine (peak: men 84.8%, women 84.3%), lumbar spine (peak: 71.9%, women 67.3%), and distal interphalangeal joints of the hands (peak: men 64.4%, women 76%) were observed in older age groups [17].

Incidence

Because OA is a chronic disease occurring mostly among the elderly, risk or death from other diseases makes direct estimation of the cumulative incidence of OA difficult [16]. The age and sex standardized incidence rates of symptomatic hip, knee, and hand OA were 88, 240 and 100/ 100,000 person-years respectively and the incidence rates of symptomatic OA of either hand, or knee, or hip increase rapidly around age 50 and then reach the peak values after age 70 [24].

Etiology and Pathogenesis

Pathogenesis

OA occurs as a result of various biochemical, biomechanical, inflammatory, and immunologic factors, not solely from the wearing down of the joints [25] that can result in both structural and functional failure of synovial joints, which include loss of articular cartilage, meniscal degeneration, and osteophytes [26].

Aging and Osteoarthritis Pathogenesis

Aging does not cause OA alone but rather plays a role in the development of OA in the existence of other risk factors [5]. Obesity is one of the constant risk factors besides age as shown in a recent metaanalysis [1]. It is unclear, how obesity is associated with aging to result in OA [5]. Aged people lose muscle mass and gain fat mass which could contribute to progression of OA because of joint loading [27]. A long-term exercise and weight loss intervention resulted in reduced knee joint loads in older adults in a randomized clinical trial [28]. Also local or systemic production of adipokines and other inflammatory mediators in fat may negatively affect joint tissues [5]. The infrapatellar fat pad in the knee may be a source of production of these mediators and one study showed that age and size of infrapatellar pad are positively correlated in knee OA patients [29, 30].

Factors that are associated with the absence of OA were examined in a cohort study of 90-year-olds and reported that only 16% of people in that aged population were free of radiographic OA. Increased body mass index (BMI) was negatively associated with absence of OA [4].

Studies suggest that low grade chronic systemic inflammation may also play a role in the pathogenesis of age-related conditions including osteoarthritis [31]. Decline in muscle strength, loss of proprioception, degenerative changes in the meniscus and joint ligaments, increased bone turnover, as well as calcification of joint tissues are other age-related factors that may contribute to the development of OA [32-34]. Sarcopenia, which is age-related loss of muscle mass, strength, and functional decline, is the most characteristic feature of age-related changes in the neuromuscular system. Components of weakness are loss of muscle mass and other factors like changes at the level of the motor neuron and motor unit [35]. A more general and systemic approach will be needed to better understand the link between aging and OA as there is a variety of age-related changes in different systems [5].

Aging Changes in Joint Tissues

Aging-related changes of joint tissues can be divided into changes that occur at the cellular level like decreased anabolic response to growth factors, accumulation of oxidative damage to DNA and cellular proteins, telomere shortening, cell senescence and those that occur within the extracellular matrix such as increased collagen crosslinking by advanced glycation endproducts (AGEs), accumulation of modified and degraded extracellular matrix components, increased calcification, however changes within the cells and matrix can interact with eachother [36].

Cellular Changes

Cartilage

Cartilage in OA is characterized by an imbalance in matrix synthesis and matrix degradation [37]. Age-related reduction in the number of chondrocytes in cartilage has been reported in many studies [38, 39]. Apoptotic chondrocytes has been reported in OA cartilage [39]. Chondrocytes have been shown to exhibit telomere shortening a classic feature of cell senescence [40]. Cell senescence can also result in a phenotypic alteration of cells called the senescent secretory phenotype (SASP) [41, 42]. It is not known whether chondrocyte death is a cause or consequence of OA, though studies suggest that chondrocyte death is a key player in cartilage degeneration [43].

Senescence-Associated Secretory Phenotype (SASP)

Through the increased production of inflammatory cytokines and MMPs and a reduced response to growth factors, SASP contributes to the imbalance between anabolic and catabolic activity in the cartilage [6].

Cells exhibiting the SASP produce cytokines and matrix metalloproteinases (MMPs) including IL-1b, IL-6, IL-8, MMP-3 and MMP-13 which are very similar to those found in OA joint tissues [44].

The development of the SASP may be related to increased production of reactive oxygen species (ROS) from mitochondrial dysfunction and/or from activation of pro-inflammatory pathways induced as part of the aging stress response [45].

Altered Growth Factor Signaling in Aging and OA

Key matrix stimulating growth factors in cartilage include IGF-I, OP-1 (BMP-7), and TGF-β. There is substantial evidence for a decline in the chondrocyte response to IGF-I with aging [46, 47] and in chondrocytes isolated from OA cartilage [47, 48]. Age-related alterations in the TGF-β signaling pathway may also contribute to the development of OA [49].

Mitochondrial Dysfunction, Reactive Oxygen Species (ROS) and OA

Mitochondria are an important source of ROS. Oxidative damage in articular cartilage was shown by a study reporting increased nitrotyrosine (a measure of oxidative damage to proteins) with aging, as well as with OA [50]. An aging-related increase in ROS levels could play an important role in the development of OA [51]. The increase in levels of various inflammatory mediators in OA, including IL-1, IL-6, IL-8, TNF-α, and other cytokines can stimulate the production of ROS and ROS in turn can be involved in the increased production of MMPs [52]. Increased levels of ROS can result in DNA damage in OA cartilage [53], in mitochondrial DNA [54]. This can contribute to the SASP [55] and the decrease in response to growth factors reported in aging and OA chondrocytes [56].

Autophagy, Cell Death and OA

Autophagy is a protective mechanism in normal cartilage and its aging-related loss is linked with cell death and OA [57]. Hypoxia inducible factor-2α (HIF-2 α) has been suggested to suppress autophagy in chondrocytes [58]. Decline in levels of high-mobility group box protein 2 (HMGB2) which is expressed in superficial zone of chondrocytes with aging is another factor [59] that cause chondrocyte death and HMGB2 deficient mice were found to develop premature OA.

Extracellular Matrix Changes

Reduction in cartilage resiliency and hydration because of age-related changes in the size, structure, and sulfation of aggrecan is seen [60-63]. Accumulation of advanced glycation end-products (AGEs) results in increased cross-linking of collagen molecules [64, 65].

Degradation and loss of type II collagen has been noted in cartilage from hip joints of older individuals [66] and in normal appearing knee cartilage obtained at autopsy [67], however, it is not clear whether the collagen damage represents aging changes or early OA [36].

Subchondral Bone

In contrast to previous reports, recent studies found that the subchondral bone in OA was poorly mineralized and perhaps less stiff than normal bone [68, 69]. Inflammatory mediators produced by subchondral bone cells diffuse through the calcified cartilage zone and affect the overlying articular cartilage [70]. In areas of cartilage loss, localized areas of increased bone remodeling has been noted which has been shown to be associated with pain in OA [71]. In asymptomatic individuals, increasing age has been shown to be a risk factor for the development of bone marrow lesions [72].

Synovium

The degree of synovitis present in OA is variable [73]. Elevated serum levels of CRP [74] and cytokines including IL-6 [75] in people with OA indicate that inflammation plays a role in OA. The growth factor TGF-β may be responsible for the stimulation of synovial hypertrophy and osteophyte formation [76].

In older adults calcification and crystal formation within joint tissues may play a role in OA progression. Whether OA and CPPD are separate conditions or closely connected is unknown [77, 78].

Etiological Factors

Etiology of OA is not completely understood. OA has a multifactorial etiology. Systemic factors like genetics, diet, estrogen use, and bone density and local factors such as muscle weakness, obesity, injury, malalignment plays a role in the development of OA [2]. The relative importance of risk factors may vary for different joints, for different stages of the disease, and for the progression of disease, and for radiographic versus symptomatic disease. Risk factors may act differently according to individual radiographic features, such as osteophytes and joint space narrowing [16].

Risk Factors

Age

Age is one of the strongest risk factors for OA of all joints [1, 2, 3]. OA prevalence increases with age [3]. Biologic changes that occur with aging and cumulative exposure to risk factors may increase the prevalence and incidence of OA [16].

Gender and Hormones

OA is more prevalent and more severe in women [79]. Just after menopause incidence of OA in women rises which suggest that estrogen deficiency plays a role in OA. The role of estrogen in OA is complex, the results of studies about estrogen use and OA are conflicting [80-83].

Ethnicity

Racial differences in self-reported pain and function in OA varies in studies [84,85]. Pain and functional limitations in patients with knee OA are greater for African-Americans than Caucasians [86]. These differences may be explained by body mass index (BMI) and depressive symptoms, and differences in function may also be largely influenced by pain [87]. Biomarker studies suggest that biological and genetic factors may also play a role in ethnic variations [88].

Genetics

Twin and family studies have estimated the heritable component of OA to be between 50 and 65% with larger genetic influences for hand and hip OA than for knee OA and this inheritance may vary by joint site [89-91].There is a strong genetic predisposition for hand OA. The presence of osteophytes was the most sensitive biomarker for hand OA heritability [92].

Diet

Dietary factors are the subject of considerable interest in OA. There are studies about vitamin D [93], vitamin C [94], and other nutritional factors such as Vitamin E, K and Selenium and OA with conflicting results [95-97].

Bone Mineral Density (BMD)

Women with radiographically defined knee OA have greater BMD than do women without knee OA and are less likely to lose that higher level of BMD [98] which supports the role of elevated BMD in the pathogenesis of OA. High BMD and BMD gain decreased the risk of progression of radiographic knee OA, but may be associated with an increased risk of incident knee OA [99].

Obesity

Being overweight may both have a role in development of OA and also increases the risk for radiographic progression [100, 101]. Weight loss can reduce the risk for OA as shown in the Framingham Study [102] and decrease pain and disability in established knee OA [103, 104]. The relationship between overweight and hip OA is weaker than that with knee OA [105, 106].

Congenital/Developmental Conditions

Knee laxity [107], proprioception deficit [108], and knee malalignment [109] are found to be related to knee OA. Limb length inequality is another factor that can alter biomechanics at the knee and hip [110].

Congenital subluxation, Legg-Calvé- Perthes disease, and slipped capital femoral epiphysis have been associated with occurrence of hip OA in later life [111-113]. Abnormal center-edge angle or acetabular dysplasia were associated with an increased risk of incident hip OA in women [114].

Injury/Surgery

Meniscal tear requiring meniscectomy, a trans-articular fracture, or anterior cruciate ligament (ACL) injury, can result in an increased risk of OA [115, 116]. Incidental meniscal damage on MRI is quite common in the elderly [117]. Age-related changes in the meniscus may contribute to the development and progression of knee OA [118]. As shown in MRI studies, ACL disruption is common in older adults with knee OA, even without a known history of trauma [119].

Occupation

Repetitive use of joints at work is associated with an increased risk of OA. Farmers have a high prevalence of hip OA [120]. In the cotton mill workers the prevalence of Heberden's nodes was higher [121]. Workers whose jobs required repeated pincer grip had more OA at distal interphalangeal joints than did workers whose job required power grip [122]. Knee OA was more common in men whose jobs required both carrying and kneeling or squatting [123].

Physical Activity/Sports

Sports activities that demand high-intensity, acute, repetitive joint impact and twisting are at high risk of osteoarthritis, like in knees of U.S football and soccer players and elbows of baseball pitchers [124, 125]. Former elite long distance runners are at high risk for the development of knee and hip OA [126, 127]. Besides there are studies reporting that in the absence of acute injury, moderate long distance running and jogging did not appear to increase the risk of OA [128, 129].

Risk Factors for Symptomatic OA

Not all patients with radiographic OA have joint symptoms [2]. Women with radiographic knee OA were more likely to have symptoms than men [19] and African Americans reported more knee and hip symptoms than Whites [21]. Severe radiographic OA and joint space narrowing rather than osteophytes was more strongly associated with pain [130].

Muscle Strength

Quadriceps muscle weakness not only results from disuse in painful knee OA but also is a risk factor for structural damage to the joint [131]. In contrast, maximal force exerted on specific joints might influence development of OA. Greater quadriceps muscle strength in the existence of malalignment and laxity is associated with an increased risk of knee OA progression [132].

Diagnosis

There is no single test to be used to define OA, but a combination of the tests increases the chance of the diagnosis. American College of Rheumatology (ACR) proposed set of criteria combining both clinical and radiologic definitions for diagnosis of knee, hip and hand OA [133-135]. ACR Classification Criteria for knee and hip OA are shown in Table 1, ACR Classification Criteria for hand OA are shown in Table 2.

Table 1. ACR classification criteria for osteoarthritis of the knee and hip*

Classification Criteria for Osteoarthritis of the Hip
Traditional format
Hip pain plus at least two of the following:
ESR of less than 20 mm per hour
Femoral or acetabular osteophytes on radiographs
Joint space narrowing on radiographs
Classification-tree format
Hip pain plus femoral or acetabular osteophytes on radiographs
or
Hip pain plus joint space narrowing on radiographs and an erythrocyte sedimentation rate (ESR) of less than 20 mm per hour

Classification Criteria for Idiopathic Osteoarthritis of the Knee
Traditional format
Knee pain plus osteophytes on radiographs and at least one of the following:
Patient age older than 50 years
Morning stiffness lasting 30 minutes or less
Crepitus on motion
Classification-tree format
Knee pain and osteophytes on radiographs
or
Knee pain plus patient age of 40 years or older, morning stiffness lasting 30 minutes or less and crepitus on motion

* (References [133,134]).

Table 2. ACR classification criteria for osteoarthritis of the hand

Hand pain, aching or stiffness
plus
Hard tissue enlargement of two or more of 10 selected joints
plus
Fewer than three swollen metacarpophalangeal joints
plus
Hard tissue enlargement of two or more distal interphalangeal joints
or
Deformity of two or more of 10 selected joints
- 10 selected joints are the second and third distal interphalangeal joints, the second and third proximal interphalangeal joints and the first carpometacarpal joints (of both hands).

* (Reference [135]).

European League Against Rheumatism (EULAR) multidisciplinary guideline development Group developed ten key recommendations for the diagnosis of hand OA [136].

Researchers of the Translational Research in Europe Applied Technologies for Osteo-Arthritis (TREAT-OA) consortium recently gave recommendations for standardization of radiographic symptomatic OA. Radiographic knee OA was defined as "definite osteophytes and possible joint space narrowing". Radiographic hip OA was defined as "at least definite joint space narrowing", and no consensus was reached for the definition of radiographic hand OA. Since all studies defined symptomatic OA differently, it was also not possible to standardize symptomatic OA. The authors recommended including pain, clinical assessment of OA as well as radiographic data in this definition [137].

Clinical Features

Symptoms of OA include pain, crepitus, limited or reduced range of motion, and joint stiffness lasting < 30 minutes. Joint deformity like varus angulation, joint instability and leg shortening may result in later stages of disease. Joint effusion can be seen during an acute episode of the disease [138-140]. Use related pain is the most important and frequent symptom of OA [141]. Pain usually begins within a few minutes of start of joint use. Night pain is seen in patients with advanced OA, with overuse and an inflammatory episode of the disease [138].

Localization

Generalized OA

There are no validated criteria for generalized OA. Polyarticular OA, including the presence of Heberden's nodules as a marker of generalized OA has been studied in different populations [142, 143]. Generalized OA may be a distinct disease [142] in which systemic, genetic predisposition is more important than local mechanical factors [144].

Spesific Joint Localization

OA primarily affects hip, knee, spine and hand [138].

Hip OA

Superior migration of the femoral head which is seen in 78% of patients with hip OA, is the most common pattern. Besides, sclerosis, cysts, and osteophytes are seen. In 22% of patients medial pattern is seen. The axial migration pattern is rare in primary OA [145]. Destructive OA was clearly more common in the unilateral cases, whereas the mild, bilateral cases of OA were found to be mostly hypertrophic. Destructive and more severe OA was more frequent in in older age-groups [146]. The most used radiographic investigation of hip OA is an anteroposterior view of the pelvis with the patient in a standing position and internal rotation of the feet (15 to 20 degrees). An oblique view may be needed to observe posterior pole changes [147]. Generalized hip pain, pain in the lateral and anterior thigh or groin, pain with prolonged ambulation, antalgic gait, decreased range of motion, pain in internal rotation, and a positive Trendelenburg sign are symptoms and signs of hip OA [133,148].

Knee OA

Medial and lateral tibiofemoral and patellofemoral involvement is seen in knee OA. Medial tibiofemoral pattern is more homogeneous [138]. Knee OA is usually bilateral and affects more than one compartment. In one third of patients unicompartmental disease is seen. In approximately 30% of these patients with unicompartmental knee OA the medial compartment is affected, in 3% it is the lateral compartment and in 69% the disease predominantly involves the patello-femoral joint. Unilateral and isolated medial tibiofemoral OA were more common in men [149]. When evaluating the tibiofemoral compartment the patient should be in a standing position. The patellofemoral compartment is evaluated by performing a sky view. Because OA usually begins at the posterior part of the tibiofemoral compartment a view performed while the knees are flexed has been recommended. Schuss view is one of these techniques [150].

Hand OA

The most common areas of involvement in hand OA in decreasing frequency are the distal interphalangeal (DIP) joints, the base of the thumb, the proximal interphalangeal (PIP) joints, and the metacarpophalangeal (MCP) joints [151]. Clinically apparent bony nodules about the DIP joint are called Heberden's nodes; similar features about the PIP joints are called Bouchard's nodes [152,153]. Currently, conventional radiography (CR) is the method of choice for evaluation of hand OA, owing to high feasibility and low costs. CR provides a two-dimensional picture of bony changes, such as osteophytes, erosions, cysts, and sclerosis, and joint space narrowing which is as an indirect measure of cartilage loss [154]. Radiologic appearance is mostly hypertrophic type. Erosive hand OA has been proposed as a distinct entity [138]. Some authors stated that erosive OA is not a separate disease entity but an aggressive acute form of hand OA [155].

Spinal OA

OA of spinal joints is common. It often results from the degenerative changes in the intervertebral fibrocartilaginous discs, vertebral bodies or posterior apophyseal joints. Osteophytosis on the vertebral bodies is a prominent finding. Some classify degenerative changes of the apophyseal joints as true OA. Degenerative changes are most frequent in areas of maximal motion. Symptoms of spinal OA are localized pain, stiffness and radicular pain [156]. *Diffuse idiopathic skeletal hyperostosis (DISH)* is a common degenerative entesopathy. The most characteristic finding is calcification and ossification of anterior longitudinal ligament in the midthoracic spine but changes are also seen in the cervical and lumbar levels [157].

Etiology

One classification divides people with OA into those in whom the cause is known as secondary OA or those in whom the cause is unknown as primary OA [2, 158]. Articular diseases that are etiologic factors for secondary OA are septic arthritis, inflammatory joint disease, gout, pseudogout, Paget's disease, ochronosis, acromegaly, hemochromatosis, Wilson's disease and primary osteochondromatosis [159].

LABORATORY INVESTIGATIONS

No specific diagnostic laboratory abnormalities exist in primary OA. Routine blood count, erythrocycte sedimentation rate, biochemical analysis and urine analysis are used to rule out other diagnoses and secondary causes of OA [156]. Especially for elderly people or in those with other chronic illnesses, a blood count, creatinine concentration, and liver function tests before starting the patient on non-steroidal anti-inflammatory drugs (NSAIDS) has to be considered [160].

Sinovial fluid in OA is noninflammatory. Aspirated fluid has a high viscosity and a low cell count (leucocyte count<2000/mm^3) [156,161]. CPPD and apatite crystals can be seen in more severe OA [162].

Biomarkers

Biomarkers could play an important role in disease detection in early molecular stages, monitoring the disease progression and the response to treatment and selecting patients for recruitment to drug trials [163]. For pre-radiographic OA, no reliable soluble biochemical markers have been proposed. Post-radiographic serum and urinary OA soluble biomarkers are serum Hyaluronic Acid (sHA), serum Cartilage Oligomeric Matrix Protein (sCOMP), urinary C-telopeptide of type II collagen (uCTX-II) and serum and urine Coll2-1 and its nitrated form Coll2-1NO2 [164, 165]. These proteins can be measured in serum and/or urine by enzyme-linked immunosorbent assays (ELISA) or other biochemical and immunological techniques [166]. In a study by Golightly et al., serum COMP was found to be highly predictive of incident osteophytes, and both COMP and serum hyaluronan were predictive of incident joint space narrowing suggesting that osteophyte and joint space narrowing were detected by different biomarkers [167]. Biomarker levels may vary due to changes in the renal and hepatic function, food intake, physical activity and circadian rhythm [168, 169].

Radiographic Investigations

OA is no longer viewed as a passive, degenerative disorder, but rather an active disease process driven primarily by mechanical factors and should be considered as a disease of a whole joint organ. Therefore imaging of OA requires techniques which can visualize the whole joint organ. Advanced imaging methods has led to better understanding the natural course of OA, provides information for early diagnosis and monitoring of OA [138, 170].

Conventional Radiography (CR)

Traditionally, OA structural changes have been assessed with radiographs to establish the diagnosis of OA and to monitor the progression of the disease. The main shortcomings of radiography are its insensitivity to change and its lack of soft-tissue depiction [171]. Active research on CR focuses on measurements of joint space width and alignment of the knee joint [170]. The Kellgren and Lawrence system was the first standardized method for assessing knee OA on radiographs. This system uses a global score of radiologic features that are believed to be indicative of OA [172]. Bony features include marginal osteophytes, subchondral sclerosis, and subchondral cysts and provide an indirect estimate of cartilage thickness and meniscal integrity [171]. (Figure 1 shows relatively early conventional radiographic knee OA findings.)

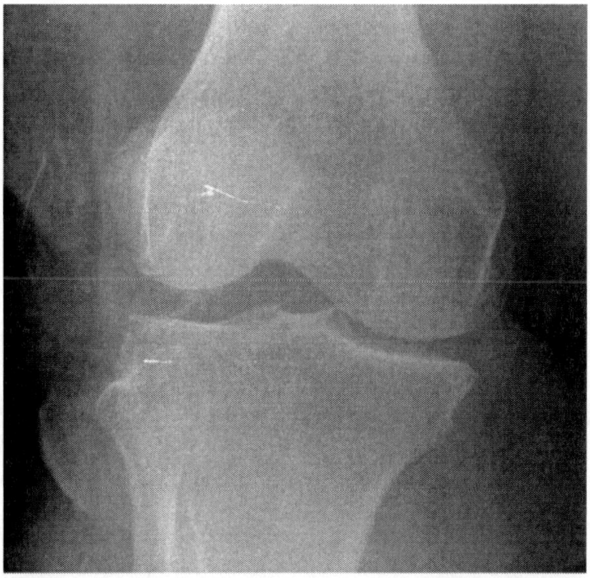

Figure 1. Knee OA findings in a 54 year-old female patient. Subchondral cyst and osteophyte formation, medial joint space narrowing.

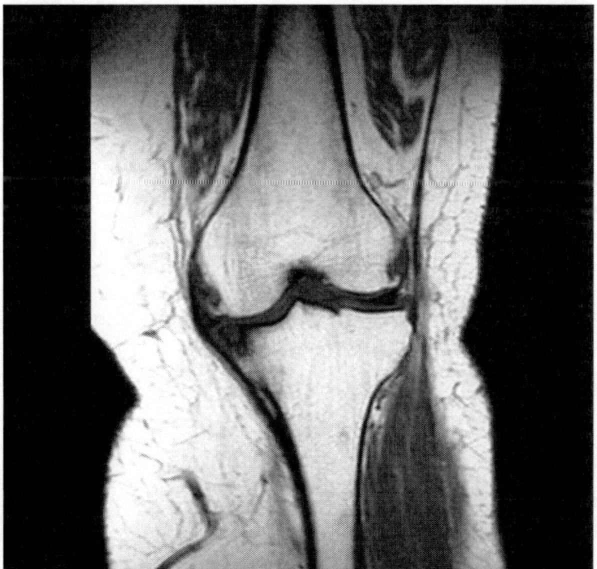

Figure 2. Spin echo coronal MR image of estoarthritic knee joint. Medial joint space narrowing, osteophytes and subchondral cysts are seen.

Magnetic Resonance Imaging (MRI)

Advanced MRI techniques, enabled direct visualization of cartilage. Pre-radiographic cartilage changes detected by MRI can be measured reliably by a semiquantitative or quantitative approach [173]. MRI findings of knee OA are shown in Figure 2 and MRI findings of advanced hip OA are shown in Figure 3.

Several methodologies have been studied and validated to assess many properties of articular cartilage using MRI.

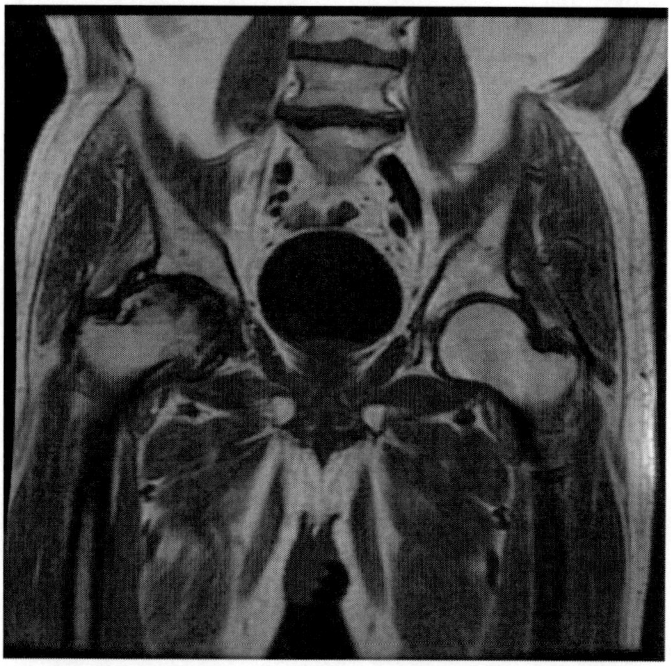

Figure 3. Magnetic resonance imaging findings of advances hip OA in a 81 year old male patient. Femoral head deformation, osteophytes and subchondral cystic degeneration on the femoral head and asetabulum prominent on the right hip.

A) Semiquantitative (SQ) Analysis

Several SQ scoring systems for knee OA are Whole Organ Magnetic Resonance Imaging Score (WORMS) [174], the Knee Osteoarthritis Scoring System (KOSS) [175] and the Boston-Leeds Osteoarthritis Knee Score (BLOKS) [176]. SQ analysis helps understanding of the pathophysiology and natural history of OA and the clinical implications of structural changes. These articular features include articular cartilage integrity, subarticular bone marrow abnormalities, subchondral cysts, subarticular bone attrition, marginal and central osteophytes, medial and lateral meniscal integrity, anterior and posterior cruciate ligament integrity, medial and lateral collateral ligament integrity, synovitis and effusion, and intraarticular loose bodies, periarticular cysts and bursitis [177].

B) Quantitative Approaches

Quantitative approaches assess cartilage tissue parameters such as volume, thickness, or other measures as continuous variables using 3D nature of MR imaging [178]. Several imaging protocols for quantitative analysis of cartilage morphology exist [179-182].

C) Compositional and Biochemical Analysis

These techniques attempt to selectively demonstrate the GAG components and/or the collagen fiber network of the extracellular matrix and are usually summarized as compositional imaging of cartilage [177]. Different techniques (DGEMRIC, Sodium 23 MR imaging, T2 mapping, T1ρ(rho) mapping, Diffusion-weighted MR imaging) for compositional MR imaging of cartilage exist [183-186] in literature but there is little uniformity in their diagnostic application [187].

Computed tomography (CT) scan and arthro- CT scan shows cartilage and bone abnormalities.

Contrast Enhanced Computed Tomography (CECT) can be used to monitor and quantify changes in the GAG content and biomechanical properties of articular cartilage [188, 189]. Helical computed tomography can provide a diagnosis of hip OA by showing cartilage lesions, which are usually located in the anterosuperior part of the acetabulum [190].

Ultrasonography (US)

US detects effusion and synovitis but gives less accurate information for cartilage abnormalities. US is used commonly in inflammatory diseases, however less frequently used in OA as an adjuvant modality, rather than a routine diagnostic test [191]. The benefits of US over radiography include the ability to image soft-tissue structures and the potential to detect small or early structural lesions [192, 193]. The pathologies examined in OA using US were most commonly effusion, synovial thickening or hypertrophy, cartilage parameters, vascularity, Baker's cysts, osteophytes, tendon and ligament abnormalities, meniscal changes, bursitis, erosions and panniculitis as shown in a review by Keen et al. [194]. US is emerging as a useful imaging technique, particularly in the field of hand OA research [170].

Treatment Options

The aims of management in OA are to educate patients about the disease and its management, to control pain and improve function, to prevent disease progression, minimize disability, and improve quality of life [140]. Severity of symptoms and joint damage, the number of joints affected, comorbidities, drug requirements, prior treatments, patient wishes and illness perceptions are to be evaluated before planning treatment. Local cost, availability, delivery, and patient acceptability are also important aspects to be considered besides efficacy and side-effects of treatments [195]. Several guidelines have been developed for the management of osteoarthritis [7-11]. Osteoarthritis management should consist of a combination of nonpharmacologic and pharmacologic treatment options. Usually all OA guidelines agree on shared recommendations.

Several aspects to be considered in the implementation of treatment guidelines in the elderly OA patients

- Factors other than severity of OA that may influence pain and disability should be evaluated. These factors are age, sex, marital and socioeconomic status, duration of arthritis, , chronic diseases, BMI, social support, psychosocial factors, differences in pain threshold and tendency to central sensitization and worse mental health [196-199].

- Older patients with OA are likely to have co-existent morbidities which can interact with each other and cause high levels of disability and management problems. Recognizing and treating comorbidity in older people with OA is crucial in the management of OA [12]. Multidisiplinary approach is needed to manage comorbidities. Most guidelines do not provide information on treatment of patients with comorbidities [200]. Almost half of patients with chronic diseases have more than one disease [201, 202].
- Difficulties for patients to access health professional service and poor integration of multidisciplinary services should be considered in the treatment plan [203].

Nonpharmacologic Treatment Options

Non-pharmacologic treatments were clearly underutilized [204, 205]. Combination of pharmacological and non-pharmacological treatments is frequently employed in clinical practise for the management of hip and/or knee OA [7-11].

Patient Education and Lifestyle Changes

All patients with hip and knee OA should be given information and education about the objectives of treatment and the importance of changes in lifestyle, exercise, weight reduction, and other measures to unload the damaged joints [10].

Weight Reduction

Patients with hip and knee OA, who are overweight, should be encouraged to lose weight and maintain their weight at a lower level [10]. A combined weight loss and exercise regimen results in a greater improvement in pain and physical function [103].

Physical Therapy Agents and Assistive Devices

Referral to a physical therapist for evaluation and instruction in appropriate exercises to reduce pain and improve functional capacity and to advice appropriate assistive devices is recommended in patients with symptomatic hip and knee OA [10].

Assistive Devices

Walking aids can reduce pain in patients with hip and knee OA. Patients should be informed of optimal use of a cane or crutch in the contralateral hand. For those with bilateral disease, frames or wheeled walkers are preferable [10]. Unloader braces appear more effective than neoprene sleeves in relieving symptoms in patients with varus gonarthrosis [206]. Therapeutic knee taping demonstrated a significant reduction in knee pain [207].

Thermal Modalities

Some thermal modalities may be effective for relieving symptoms in hip and knee OA [10]. Heat and cryotherapy are used very widely in the management of patients with OA with reported effects on pain, quadriceps strength and function [208-210].

Therapeutic Ultrasound (US)

Therapeutic US may be beneficial in terms of pain and function in patients with knee OA [211,212]. US treatment was found to increase the effectiveness of isokinetic exercise for functional improvement of knee OA, and pulsed US has a greater effect than continuous US [213].

Transcutaneous Electrical Nerve Stimulation (TENS)

TENS is a recommended treatment for relief of pain in existing guidelines for the management of knee OA [214]. Evidence for efficacy of TENS is reported in reviews [215, 216]. TENS does not have serious adverse effects. The short-term efficacy of TENS in providing clinically significant pain relief in patients with knee OA has been confirmed [217]. Rutjes et al. could not confirm that TENS is effective for pain relief. They concluded that study sample sizes were small and have questionable quality and appropriately designed trials of adequate power are warranted [218].

Acupuncture

Acupuncture may be of symptomatic benefit in patients with knee OA [219]. In a recent Cohrane review, sham-controlled trials showed statistically significant benefits of acupuncture in the treatment of OA; however, these benefits were small. Waiting list-controlled trials of acupuncture for peripheral joint OA suggest statistically significant and clinically relevant benefits may be due to expectation or placebo effects [220].

Exercise

Regular aerobic walking exercises and home-based quadriceps muscle strengthening exercises are recommended for knee OA patients. Both of these exercises reduce pain and disability from knee OA [221]. Adherence to exercise is a key predictor of response and patients should be encouraged to maintain exercise programmes [222]. For hip OA, exercise recommendation is largely based on clinical expertise [223]. Pain relief and improvement in stiffness in patients with symptomatic hip OA following exercise in water is reported [10]. For patients with hip and/or knee OA, aquatic exercise appears to have some beneficial short-term effects while no long-term effects have been documented [224].

The Board of Directors of the American Geriatrics Society (AGS) recommended that [225] exercise programs should be individualized for each patient. Controlling pain, increasing flexibility, and improving muscle strength and endurance should be the goal. Regular moderate-level exercise does not exacerbate OA pain or accelerate the pathological process of OA. Increasing the level of physical activity in OA patients reduces pain and morbidity, modifies risk factors for chronic diseases prevalent in the older population and improves psychologic health and functional status [226, 227].

Pharmacologic Treatment

Pharmacologic treatment considerations for older adults

-Adverse drug reactions are more frequent in older patients. Sensitivity to central nervous system active drugs, including opioid analgesics, increases with age [228, 229]. Age-associated differences in efficacy, sensitivity, and toxicity should also be expected [13, 228]. Physician should start with the lowest effective dose, monitor frequently on the basis of expected absorption and know pharmacokinetics of the agents, and titrate the dose according to steady-state blood levels and clinically demonstrated effects [13]. Frequent monitoring is important because drug-drug and drug-disease interactions is increased in elderly persons. Health care providers should be aware of all new drugs, over-the-counter medications, and herbal products added to the treatment and should taper and discontinue drugs that do not provide therapeutic outcome effects [13].

- Comorbid conditions

Concomitant medications must be considered when selecting pharmacotherapy for older adults because polypharmacy leads to the potential for many pharmacodynamic and pharmacokinetic drug interactions [13, 140].

- Increased risk of drug induced disease

Older patients are often at increased risk of drug-induced renal and hepatic toxicities. Renal function should be monitored in patients taking NSAIDs, and patients with renal insufficiencies should avoid use of NSAIDs [13,140].

Non-Opioid Analgesics

Asetominophen (Parasetamol)

Asetominophen (parasetamol) is the first choice for mild-to-moderate OA-related pain because of its safety and effectiveness [7-11]. The maximum recommended dose is 4 gr per day for patients with normal renal and hepatic function, and in those with no history of alcohol abuse.

Dose reduction is recommended in patients with renal or hepatic dysfunction or those with harmful alcohol use [230]. Recent recommendations by the Osteoarthritis Research Society International [231] draws attention to the increased risk of upper GI side effects, the mild loss of renal function and the increased risk of hypertension with high dose, long-term use especially in older adults. Acetaminophen is often associated with hepatotoxicity. A retrospective study found transient increases in alanine aminotransferase (ALT), which usually resolved or decreased with continued treatment; further, there were no cases of hepatotoxicity or hepatic failure [232]. Liver function tests (ALT) should be monitored at baseline and periodically when considering long-term use for older adults with OA [232].

Non-Steroidal Anti-Inflammatory Drugs (NSAIDS)

If asetominophen fails, NSAIDs should be given at the lowest effective dose and long-term use should be avoided if possible to reduce side effects [7-11]. Persistent use of traditional nonselective NSAIDs is associated with life-threatening gastrointestinal (GI) bleeding especially in older patients, with multiple-system disease [230]. The risk of peptic ulcers, perforations increases with age, concurrent use of other medications, and with longer duration of therapy [233]. Although the GI side effects are reduced with the concomitant administration of misoprostol or proton-pump inhibitors, misoprostol may not be well tolerated by elderly persons [234].

GI protection that is associated with the use of COX-2 selective agents is largely lost when low-dose aspirin is administered concurrently for CV prophylaxis [235]. History of GI bleeding or peptic ulcer disease would preclude use of traditional NSAIDs and COX-2–specific agents if the patient was also on prophylactic aspirin therapy [13, 140].

Current evidence supports the use of cyclooxygenase (COX)-2 selective agents in patients with no specific contraindications [236,237]. However, clinicians must stay informed about drug-drug and drug-disease interactions associated with COX-2 inhibitors [230]. In patients with cardiovascular (CV) risk factors, both non-selective and COX-2 selective agents should be used with caution [10].

In a systematic review selective COX 2 inhibitors were found to be associated with a moderate increase in the risk of vascular events, as are high dose regimens of ibuprofen and diclofenac, but high dose naproxen is not associated with such an excess [238]. In the USA all marketed prescription NSAIDs, both non-selective and COX-2 selective carry a boxed warning about their potential for causing CV events and GI bleeding. NSAIDs should be avoided in those at high risk of myocardial infarction or stroke. Patients using NSAIDs should be also monitored for increases in blood pressure, and patients with uncontrolled hypertension should avoid use [13, 140].

Opioids and Narcotic Analgesia

Where other pharmacological agents have been ineffective, or are contraindicated, the use of weak opioids and narcotic analgesics can be considered for the treatment of refractory pain in patients with hip or knee OA. Stronger opioids should only be used for the management of severe pain in exceptional circumstances. The chronic use of opioids for persistent pain or some other analgesic strategies may have fewer life-threatening risks than does the long-term daily use of high-dose nonselective NSAIDS [230].

Opioids of Particular Concern

Propoxyphene efficacy is similar to that of aspirin or acetaminophen alone, but drug accumulation, neuroexcitatory effects, and ataxia or dizziness may add morbidity in older patients. For patients with persistent mild to moderate pain, other analgesic strategies are more appropriate [239].

Tramadol acts centrally on the μ-opioid receptors and also inhibits the reuptake of norepinephrine and serotonin [240]. Tramadol is not associated with GI bleeding or cardiovascular events unlike NSAIDs. Despite this, tramadol should be used with caution due to potential renal or hepatic dysfunction and the lowest possible dose should be administered in older adults [240, 241]. Efficacy and safety of tramadol are reported to be similar to those of equianalgesic doses of codeine and hydrocodone, including potential for drowsiness and nausea. Tramadol should be used with caution in patients with a history of seizure disorder or those taking tricyclic or selective serotonin reuptake inhibitor antidepressants because of the threat of seizures [230].

Frequent side effects of opioids include nausea (30%), constipation (23%), dizziness (20%), somnolence (18%) and vomiting (13%). The withdrawal rate was 31% for strong opioids (oxymorphone, oxycodone, oxytrex, fentanyl, morphine sulphate) compared with a withdrawal rate of 19% for the weaker opioids (tramadol, tramadol/paracetamol, codeine and propoxyphene) [242]. Older adults may consider the use of laxatives and stool softeners to minimize constipation. Due to the high incidence of adverse effects, diminished mental capacity, and the potential risk of fractures because of falls in older adults, long-term use of opioids is questionable [228, 229].

Fentanyl transdermal patches provide continuous medication for 24 hours, an improvement in pain control, but are not to be used in opioid-naive patients. Adverse effects are similar to those experienced with other opioids; the patch is thought to be more tolerable due to fewer reports of constipation [243, 244].

Topical Analgesia

Topical NSAIDs and capsaicin can be effective as adjunctives and alternatives to oral analgesic/ anti-inflammatory agents in knee OA [10]. These topical agents may offer benefit for patients with contraindications to use of systemic agents and with a suboptimal response to conventional therapy [130]. Topical NSAIDs are safe with no more side effects than placebo [245]. Evidence for the efficacy of topical capsaicin in patients with knee OA is supported by a metaanalysis [246]. Lidocaine 5% patches may also offer a topical alternative for pain relief in some patients with OA [247]. Comparable effect with celecoxib 200 mg daily have been reported in knee OA patients [248].

Disease Modifying OA Drugs (DMOADs)

Primarily because OA was previously thought to be a cartilage-centric disease, the first substances that protected articular cartilage were termed as chondroprotective agents, these same agents were renamed as DMOADs [249]. DMOADs can cause slowing or complete halt in disease progression, regeneration of the target tissue and even prevent the disease development. A wide variety of DMOADs including glucosamine sulfate, chondroitin sulfate, sodium hyaluronan, doxycycline, matrix metalloproteinase (MMP) inhibitors, bisphosphonates, calcitonin, diacerein and avocado– soybean unsaponifiables (ASUS) are subjects of research studies [250-252]. Several other agents that are currently in the early stages of development are receptor activator of nuclear factor κb ligand (RANKL; also called tumor necrosis factor ligand superfamily member 11) [253], cathepsin K [254], proteoglycan 4 (lubricin) [255], metalloproteinase inhibitor 3 (TIMP-3) [256] and aggrecanase inhibitors [257].

There is no clear consensus on definition of clinically meaningful endpoint for structure modifying trials in OA [258]. Convincing disease-modifying efficacy have not been shown with the existing pharmacologic agents. Future therapeutic developments should aim both symptom and structure modification and consider the complexity of OA [259].

Glucosamine, Chondroitin and Diacerein

Data on efficacy of glucosamine and chondroitin are conflicting. The Glucosamine /Chondroitin Arthritis Intervention Trial (GAIT) [260] failed to demonstrate a significant reduction in overall pain after 24 weeks; however, a subgroup of patients with moderate pain did experience significant pain reduction. Another study of GAIT failed to demonstrate a reduction in joint width loss [261]. A systematic review found conflicting results based on glucosamine formulation [262] while another meta-analysis concluded that there is likely evidence of some degree of efficacy for these agents [263]. Neither glucosamine, chondroitin, nor their combination was effective for pain reduction or JSN in another meta-analysis [264]. In patients with mild-to-moderate knee OA, glucosamine sulfate and chondroitin sulfate may be used based on efficacy and a minimal side effect profile [140, 265].

Structure Modifying Effects of Glucosamin, Chondroitin, Diacerein

Glucosamine sulphate and chondroitin sulphate may have structure-modifying effects in patients with symptomatic knee OA, while diacerein may have structure-modifying effects in patients with symptomatic OA of the hip [10]. Structure-modifying effect with glucosamine sulphate 1500 mg/day in patients with knee OA is reported in various studies [262, 266, 267]. Symptomatic benefit data with chondroitin sulphate in knee OA patients are conflicting [267, 268]. Structure-modifying effect of chondroitin sulphate is supported by a metanalysis [269]. Diacerein has anti-inflammatory and analgesic properties when taken orally twice per day. Studies have shown it to be equally effective when compared with NSAIDs for pain control. The most common adverse effect of diacerein is diarrhea [270]. Diacerein may have structure-modifying effects in patients with hip OA [270, 271].

Other disease-Modifying Agents

Doxycycline has been studied and may slow the progression of OA. Due to adverse effects such as nausea, heartburn, and photosensitivity, withdrawals were more frequent in the doxycycline group [272, 273]. Monoclonal antibody tanezumab were recently discontinued due to subjects experiencing a worsening of OA and some requiring joint replacement in a clinical trial of knee OA. This adverse effect was not evident in patients without OA [274]. Anticytokine therapy, in particular interleukin-1 and tumor necrosis factor-α, have not been shown to be clinically effective in the treatment of OA [275].

Intra-articular Treatments

Intra-articular (IA) Hyaluronate Injections

Intra-articular injection of HA helps to improve elasticity and viscosity in the joints, provides a slight benefit in pain relief when compared with NSAIDs [276]. HA injections have similar clinical effects [277], slower onset and longer duration of action compared with corticosteroid injections. However, they are more costly [276]. These injections have to be performed by an experienced physician to reduce the risk of infection. The most common adverse effect of intra-articular injections is pain at the injection site [276, 277].

Intra-articular Glucocorticoid Injections

Intra-articular triamcinolone, betamethasone, or methylprednisolone injections are alternative treatments for patients experiencing acute local inflammation with effusion and as an adjunct with oral agents or as monotherapy if patients are not responding or unable to tolerate other treatment options [276]. The dose of the injection is dependent on the size of the joint being treated. These agents are useful for acute exacerbations of OA, but long-term pain relief has not been established [276, 278].

IA steroid injection in patients with OA hip is also studied [278, 279]. As compared with knee injection, hip injection is technically difficult, and use of fluoroscopy is necessary. Patients with hip OA that is symptomatic, unresponsive to maximum tolerated doses of analgesia and other medical treatments, and interferes with quality of life/function maybe referred to interventional radiologists for corticosteroid injection [279].

Potential side effects of IA corticosteroid include post-injection flares of pain, crystal synovitis, haemarthrosis, joint sepsis and para-articular tissue atrophy, as well as systemic corticosteroid effects such as fluid retention or aggravation of hypertension or diabetes mellitus. To maximise benefit and reduce the risk of fat necrosis and para-articular tissue atrophy, accurate placement of IA injections is essential. Repeat injections more than four times annually are generally not recommended [10, 280].

Surgery

Surgery should be reserved as a last-line management strategy for OA patients who are refractory to less invasive methods. Surgical interventions performed in OA of lower extremities include total joint arthroplasty, unicompartmental knee replacement, joint lavage and debridement, osteotomy and joint preserving surgical procedures and joint fusion [10].

Joint Lavage and Arthroscopic Debridement

Studies about these procedures have conflicting results. Some studies have demonstrated short-term symptom relief, others suggest that improvement in symptoms could be attributable to a placebo effect [281-284].

Arthroscopic debridement includes joint lavage, the removal of loose bodies, debris, mobile fragments of articular cartilage, torn menisci and impinging osteophytes; and joint lavage is currently recommended as useful treatment for patients with knee OA [10]. 50-80% of patients were typically recorded as having decreases in knee pain lasting from 1 to 5 years [281]. In medial compartment knee OA, one RCT compared articular debridement and lavage alone and found better results for debridment group compared to wash out group [282]. However a good quality, placebo- controlled RCT in which patients with knee OA were randomly assigned to receive arthroscopic debridement, arthroscopic lavage or placebo (sham) surgery with a skin incision and simulated arthroscopy showed no significant differences between the groups in the primary end point pain at 24 months, or in any of the other secondary outcome measures of pain and function at any time point [283]. This is one of only a very few placebo-controlled RCTs of surgical procedures in which sham surgery has been undertaken, though ethical and practical issues of this study is being criticised [284].

Total Joint Arthroplasty

In patients with hip and knee OA who are not obtaining adequate pain relief and functional improvement with a combination of pharmacological and non-pharmacological treatments, total hip arthroplasty (THA) and knee joint arthroplasty (TKA) should be considered [285-287]. THA is more effective than TKA in restoring patients with hip or knee OA to normal function and age is not an obstacle to effective surgery [287]. Predictors of poorer outcome following THA are higher age, more preoperative pain, musculoskeletal co-morbidities such as low back pain, and OA in the non-operated hip [288]. More severe pain, functional limitation, low mental health scores and medical co-morbidities are poorer outcome predictors following TKA [289].

After development of criteria for the appropriateness of indications for THA [290] and TKA [291], physical and social functions improved significantly greater following arthroplasty [292]. Prosthesis rejection and infection are among the serious complications [140]. Joint arthroplasty should not be delayed to preserve optimal restorative function [293].

Unicompartmental Knee Replacement (UKA)

UKA is effective in patients with unicompartmental knee OA. Knee pain and function were comparable 5 years after UKA and TKA [294].

Osteotomy and Joint Preserving Surgical Procedures

Intertrochanteric varus or valgus osteotomy has been used as a treatment for hip OA [295] and pelvic or femoral osteotomies are widely advocated to correct the biomechanics in young patients with hip dysplasias before the development of symptomatic hip OA [296].

High tibial osteotomy is being performed for realignment of the varus deformity and reduction of stress on the medial compartment of the knee and redistribution of the load from the medial compartment to the lateral compartment [297,298]. High tibial osteotomy may offer an alternative intervention that delays the need for joint replacement for the young and physically active patients with significant symptoms from unicompartmental knee OA [10, 299,300].

Joint Fusion

Joint fusion can be considered when joint replacement has failed in patients with knee OA [10]. Severe pain and instability in an unreconstructable knee following an infection at the site of a previous knee arthroplasty is the most common indication for knee arthrodesis in patients with knee OA [301]. Arthrodesis of the contralateral hip or knee and significant OA in the ipsilateral hip or ankle are contraindications to knee arthrodesis [302]. Complications include shortening of the leg., peroneal nerve palsy, pain associated with migration of the metal nail, thrombophlebitis and non-union [301].

Outcome Measures of OA

OMERACT III conference established a core set of outcome measures for future phase III clinical trials of knee, hip, and hand OA. 4 domains that were reported to be evaluated are pain, physical function, patient global assessment, and, for studies of one year or longer, joint imaging [303]. Pain is evaluated either with a single, general question or by specific questions included in Western Ontario and McMaster Universities (WOMAC) questionnaire pain subscale [138, 304, 305]. Functional impairment can be evaluated using WOMAC Functional Scale [304, 305] which is a questionnaire including daily activities or using Lequesne's algofunctional index [306] which is a composite index.

Impact of OA on Individuals and Society

OA is investigated as one of the major causes of disability in the elderly [307]. Higher direct medical costs were reported in patients with OA compared with non-arthritic controls [308]. OA disables about 10% of people who are older than 60 years, compromises the quality of life of more than 20 million Americans, and costs the United States economy more than $60 billion per year [309].

OA has detrimental effects on individuals physical function and quality of life, and places a tremendous burden on health care system [310-312]. It is important to identify factors that predict the use of OA-related health care in guiding health care providers and decision makers regarding future consumption of resources and services [313]. Women, older individuals, and nonwhites generally use greater levels of traditional medical care for arthritis [314] and women and nonwhites are less likely to undergo arthroplasty [315, 316].

There has been increasing interest in the utility of patients' self-reported health-related quality of life (HRQOL) as a predictor of health care utilization. In a study of OA patients, greater pain frequency was associated with increased physician visits, analgesic or antiinflammatory drug use, and increased arthroplasty rate and poorer general health was associated with increased analgesic or antiinflammatory use but decreased arthroplasty rate [317]. These HRQOL variables, especially pain frequency, can be valuable tools for estimating future health care use among older adults with OA [317] .

CONCLUSION

Age is a primary risk factor which makes the joint more susceptible to the development of OA in the existence of etiological factors. How aging changes contribute to the development of OA is not known. More information is needed to better understand the etiopathogenesis of OA. Management of OA in elderly people is more complex owing to comorbidities, drug interactions and diminished access to health care services. With the aging population, the prevalence of osteoarthritis increases. OA is a growing health problem and a major public health issue. Its consequences have significant impact on elderly population and society.

Osteoarthritis in elderly cause diminished functional independence, self care and quality of life and increased health care costs. In order to reduce the impact of OA on elderly population and society, establishment of early diagnosis and development of prevention strategies and effective treatment options are mandatory.

References

[1] Blagojevic M; Jinks C; Jeffery A; Jordan KP. Risk factors for onset of osteoarthritis of the knee in older adults: a systematic review and meta-analysis. *Osteoarthritis Cartilage*, 2010;18(1):24-33.

[2] Felson DT; Lawrence RC; Dieppe PA; Hirsch R; Helmick CG; Jordan JM, et al. Osteoarthritis: new insights. Part 1: the disease and its risk factors. *Ann. Intern. Med.*, 2000;133(8):635–46.

[3] Lawrence RC; Felson DT; Helmick CG; Arnold LM; Choi H; Deyo RA, et al. Estimates of the prevalence of arthritis and other rheumatic conditions in the United States: Part II. *Arthritis. Rheum.,* 2008;58(1):26–35.

[4] Goekoop RJ; Kloppenburg M; Kroon HM; Dirkse LE; Huizinga TW; Westendorp RG, et al. Determinants of absence of osteoarthritis in old age. *Scand. J. Rheumatol.*, 2011; 40:68–73.

[5] Loeser RF. *Aging and osteoarthritis Current Opinion in Rheumatology*, 2011; 23:492–496.

[6] Loeser RF. Age-Related Changes in the Musculoskeletal System and the Development of Osteoarthritis *Clin. Geriatr. Med.*, 2010; 26(3): 371–386.

[7] Zhang W; Doherty M; Leeb BF; Alekseeva L; Arden NK; Bijlsma JW, et al. EULAR evidence based recommendations for the diagnosis of hand osteoarthritis. *Ann. Rheum. Dis*, 2009;68:8-17.

[8] Zhang W; Doherty M; Peat G; Bierma-Zeinstra MA; Arden NK; Bresnihan B, et al. EULAR evidence based recommendations for the diagnosis of knee osteoarthritis. *Ann. Rheum. Dis.,* 2010;69:483-9.

[9] Jordan KM; Arden NK; Doherty M; Bannwarth B; Bijlsma JW; Dieppe P, et al. EULAR recommendations 2003: an evidence based approach to the management of knee osteoarthritis. *Ann. Rheum. Dis.*, 2003;62(12):1145-55.

[10] Zhang W; Moskowitz RW; Nuki G; Abramson S; Altman RD; Arden N, et al. OARSI recommendations for the management of hip and knee osteoarthritis. *Osteoarthritis Cartilage,* 2008; 16: 137-62.

[11] Zhang W; Doherty M; Arden N; Bannwarth B; Bijlsma J; Gunther KP, et al. EULAR evidence based recommendations for the management of hip osteoarthritis. *Ann. Rheum. Dis.,* 2005; 64: 669-681.

[12] Kadam U; Croft P. Clinical comorbidity in osteoarthritis: associations with physical function in older patients in family practice. *J. Rheum.,* 2007;34 (9):1899–904.

[13] AGS Panel on Chronic Pain in Older Persons. The management of chronic pain in older persons. American Geriatrics Society. *J. Am. Geriatr. Soc.*, 1998;46:635-651.

[14] Wise BL; Niu J; Zhang Y; Wang N; Jordan JM; Choy E, et al. Psychological factors and their relation to osteoarthritis pain. *Osteoarthritis Cartilage,* 2010;18:883–7.

[15] Murphy L; Schwartz TA; Helmick CG; Renner JB; Tudor G; Koch G, et al. Lifetime risk of symptomatic knee osteoarthritis. *Arthritis Rheum,* 2008;59(9):1207-1213.

[16] Zhang Y; Jordan JM. Epidemiology of osteoarthritis *Clin. Geriatr. Med.*, 2010 August; 26(3): 355–369.

[17] van Saase JL; van Romunde LK; Cats A; Vandenbroucke JP; Valkenburg HA. Epidemiology of osteoarthritis: Zoetermeer survey. Comparison of radiological osteoarthritis in a Dutch population with that in 10 other populations. *Ann. Rheum. Dis.,* 1989;48(4):271–280.

[18] Dillon CF; Rasch EK; Gu Q; Hirsch R. Prevalence of knee osteoarthritis in the United States: arthritis data from the third National Health and Nutrition Examination Survey 1991-1994. *J. Rheumatol.,* 2006;33:2271–9.

[19] Felson DT; Naimark A; Anderson J; Kazis L; Castelli W; Meenan RF. The prevalence of knee osteoarthritis in the elderly. The Framingham Osteoarthritis Study. *Arthritis. Rheum.,* 1987 Aug;30(8):914-8.

[20] Zhang Y; Niu J; Kelly-Hayes M; Chaisson CE; Aliabadi P; Felson DT. Prevalence of symptomatic hand osteoarthritis and its impact on functional status among elderly: the Framingham Study. *Am. J. Epidemiol.,* 2002;156:1021-7.

[21] Jordan JM; Helmick CG; Renner JB; Luta G; Dragomir AD; Woodard J. Prevalence of knee symptoms and radiographic and symptomatic knee osteoarthritis in African Americans and Caucasians: the Johnston County Osteoarthritis Project. *J. Rheumatol.,* 2007;34(1):172-80.

[22] Jordan JM; Helmick CG; Renner JB; Luta G; Dragomir AD; Woodard J, et al. Prevalence of hip symptoms and radiographic and symptomatic hip osteoarthritis in African Americans and Caucasians: the Johnston County Osteoarthritis Project. J. *Rheumatol.,* 2009;36(4):809–815.

[23] Hannan MT; Felson DT; Pincus T. Analysis of the discordance between radiographic changes and knee pain in osteoarthritis of the knee. *J. Rheumatol.,* 2000;27(6):1513–7.

[24] Oliveria SA; Felson DT; Reed JI; Cirillo PA; Walker AM. Incidence of symptomatic hand, hip and knee osteoarthritis among patients in a health maintenance organization. *Arthritis. Rheum.,* 1995;38(8):1134–1141.

[25] Lajeunesse D; Reboul P. Subchondral bone in osteoarthritis: a biologic link with articular cartilage leading to abnormal remodeling. *Curr. Opin. Rheumatol.,* 2003;15(5):628–633.

[26] Nuki G. Osteoarthritis: a problem of joint failure. Z Rheumatol, 1999;58(3):142–147.

[27] Delmonico MJ; Harris TB; Visser M; Park SW; Conroy MB; Velasquez-Mieyer P, et al. Longitudinal study of muscle strength; quality; and adipose tissue infiltration. *Am. J. Clin. Nutr.*, 2009; 90:1579–1585.

[28] Messier SP; Legault C; Loeser RF; Van Arsdale SJ; Davis C; Ettinger WH, et al. Does high weight loss in older adults with knee osteoarthritis affect bone-on-bone joint loads and muscle forces during walking? *Osteoarthritis Cartilage*, 2011;19:272–280.

[29] Distel E; Cadoudal T; Durant S; Poignard A; Chevalier X; Benelli C. The infrapatellar fat pad in knee osteoarthritis: an important source of interleukin-6 and its soluble receptor. *Arthritis. Rheum.,* 2009; 60:3374–3377.

[30] Chuckpaiwong B; Charles HC; Kraus VB; Guilak F; Nunley JA. Age-associated increases in the size of the infrapatellar fat pad in knee osteoarthritis as measured by 3T MRI. *J. Orthop. Res.*, 2010; 28:1149–1154.

[31] Goekoop RJ; Kloppenburg M; Kroon HM; Frölich M; Huizinga TW; Westendorp RG, et al. Low innate production of interleukin-1beta and interleukin-6 is associated with the absence of osteoarthritis in old age. *Osteoarthritis Cartilage,* 2010;18:942–947.

[32] Felson DT. Risk factors for osteoarthritis: understanding joint vulnerability. *Clin. Orthop. Relat. Res.,* 2004;(427 Suppl):16–21.

[33] Pai YC; Rymer WZ; Chang RW; Sharma L. Effect of age and osteoarthritis on knee proprioception. *Arthritis. Rheum.,* 1997;40(12):2260–2265.

[34] Rosenthal AK. Calcium crystal deposition and osteoarthritis. *Rheum. Dis. Clin. North. Am.,* 2006;32(2):401–412.

[35] Berger MJ; Doherty TJ. Sarcopenia: Prevalence, Mechanisms, and Functional Consequences. In: Mobbs CV, Hof PR (Eds). Body Composition and Aging. Interdiscipl Top Gerontol. Basel: *Karger*; 2010; vol 37: 94–114.

[36] Loeser RF; Shakoor N. Aging or osteoarthritis: which is the problem? *Rheum. Dis. Clin. N. Am.*, 2003; 29: 653–673.

[37] Goldring MB; Goldring SR. Osteoarthritis. *J. Cell. Physiol.,* 2007;213(3):626–634.

[38] Aigner T; Kim HA; Roach HI. Apoptosis in osteoarthritis. *Rheum. Dis. Clin. North Am.*, 2004;30(3): 639–653.

[39] Kuhn K; D'Lima DD; Hashimoto S; Lotz M. Cell death in cartilage. *Osteoarthritis Cartilage,* 2004;12(1):1–16.

[40] Martin JA; Buckwalter JA. Telomere erosion and senescence in human articular cartilage chondrocytes. *J. Gerontol. A. Biol. Sci. Med. Sci.*, 2001;56(4):B172–179.

[41] Campisi J. Senescent cells; tumor suppression; and organismal aging: good citizens; bad neighbors. *Cell,* 2005;120(4):513–522.

[42] Campisi J; d'Adda di Fagagna F. Cellular senescence: when bad things happen to good cells. *Nat. Rev. Mol. Cell Biol.*, 2007;8(9):729–740.

[43] Zamli Z; Sharif M. Chondrocyte apoptosis: a cause or consequence of osteoarthritis? *Int. J. Rheum. Dis.*, 2011; 14(2): 159–166.

[44] Freund A; Orjalo AV; Desprez PY; Campisi J. Inflammatory networks during cellular senescence: causes and consequences. *Trends Mol. Med.*, 2010;16:238–246.

[45] Haigis MC; Yankner BA. The aging stress response. *Mol Cell*, 2010; 40:333– 344.

[46] Martin JA; Ellerbroek SM; Buckwalter JA. Age-related decline in chondrocyte response to insulinlike growth factor-I: the role of growth factor binding proteins. *J. Orthop. Res.*, 1997;15(4):491–498.

[47] Loeser RF; Shanker G; Carlson CS; Gardin JF; Shelton BJ; Sonntag WE. Reduction in the chondrocyte response to insulin-like growth factor 1 in aging and osteoarthritis: studies in a non-human primate model of naturally occurring disease. *Arthritis. Rheum.,* 2000;43(9):2110–2120.

[48] Dore S; Pelletier JP; DiBattista JA; Tardif G; Brazeau P; Martel-Pelletier J. Human osteoarthritic chondrocytes possess an increased number of insulin-like growth factor 1

binding sites but are unresponsive to its stimulation. Possible role of IGF-1-binding proteins. *Arthritis. Rheum.*, 1994;37(2):253–263.

[49] van der Kraan PM; Blaney Davidson EN; van den Berg WB. A role for age-related changes in TGFbeta signaling in aberrant chondrocyte differentiation and osteoarthritis. *Arthritis. Res. Ther.*, 2010;12(1):201.

[50] Loeser RF; Carlson CS; Del Carlo M; Cole A. Detection of nitrotyrosine in aging and osteoarthritic cartilage: Correlation of oxidative damage with the presence of interleukin-1 beta and with chondrocyte resistance to insulin-like growth factor 1. *Arthritis. Rheum.*, 2002;46(9):2349–2357.

[51] Henrotin YE; Bruckner P; Pujol JP. The role of reactive oxygen species in homeostasis and degradation of cartilage. *Osteoarthritis Cartilage*, 2003;11(10):747–755.

[52] Nelson KK; Melendez JA. Mitochondrial redox control of matrix metalloproteinases. *Free Radic. Biol. Med.*, 2004;37(6):768–784.

[53] Davies CM; Guilak F; Weinberg JB; Fermor B. Reactive nitrogen and oxygen species in interleukin-1- mediated DNA damage associated with osteoarthritis. *Osteoarthritis Cartilage,* 2008;16(5):624– 630.

[54] Grishko VI; Ho R; Wilson GL; Pearsall AW 4th. Diminished mitochondrial DNA integrity and repair capacity in OA chondrocytes. *Osteoarthritis Cartilage*, 2009;17(1):107–113.

[55] Yudoh K; Nguyen T; Nakamura H; Hongo-Masuko K; Kato T; Nishioka K. Potential involvement of oxidative stress in cartilage senescence and development of osteoarthritis: oxidative stress induces chondrocyte telomere instability and downregulation of chondrocyte function. *Arthritis. Res. Ther.*, 2005;7(2): R380–391.

[56] Yin W; Park JI; Loeser RF. Oxidative stress inhibits insulin-like growth factor-I induction of chondrocyte proteoglycan synthesis through differential regulation of phosphatidylinositol 3- Kinase-Akt and MEK-ERK MAPK signaling pathways. *J. Biol. Chem.*, 2009;284(46):31972–31981.

[57] van den Berg WB. Osteoarthritis year 2010 in review: pathomechanisms. *Osteoarthritis Cartilage,* 2011; 19: 338-341.

[58] Bohensky J; Terkhorn SP; Freeman TA; Adams CS; Garcia JA; Shapiro IM, et al. Regulation of autophagy in human and murine cartilage: hypoxia-inducible factor 2 suppresses chondrocyte autophagy. *Arthritis. Rheum.,* 2009; 60:1406–1415.

[59] Taniguchi N; Carames B; Ronfani L; Ulmer U; Komiya S; Bianchi ME, et al. Aging-related loss of the chromatin protein HMGB2 in articular cartilage is linked to reduced cellularity and osteoarthritis. *Proc. Natl. Acad. Sci. USA*, 2009; 106:1181–1186.

[60] Buckwalter JA; Roughley PJ; Rosenberg LC. Age-related changes in cartilage proteoglycans: quantitative electron microscopic studies. *Microsc. Res. Tech.*, 1994;28(5):398–408.

[61] Bayliss MT; Osborne D; Woodhouse S; Davidson C. Sulfation of chondroitin sulfate in human articular cartilage. The effect of age; topographical position; and zone of cartilage on tissue composition. *J. Biol. Chem.*, 1999;274(22):15892–15900.

[62] Wells T; Davidson C; Morgelin M; Bird JL; Bayliss MT; Dudhia J. Age-related changes in the composition; the molecular stoichiometry and the stability of proteoglycan aggregates extracted from human articular cartilage. *Biochem. J.*, 2003;370(Pt 1):69–79.

[63] Grushko G; Schneiderman R; Maroudas A. Some biochemical and biophysical parameters for the study of the pathogenesis of osteoarthritis: a comparison between the processes of ageing and degeneration in human hip cartilage. *Connect Tissue Res.*, 1989;19(2-4):149–176.

[64] Verzijl N; Bank RA; TeKoppele JM; DeGroot J. AGEing and osteoarthritis: a different perspective. *Curr. Opin. Rheumatol.*, 2003;15(5):616–622.

[65] DeGroot J; Verzijl N; Wenting-van Wijk MJ; Jacobs KM; Van El B; Van Roermund PM, et al. Accumulation of advanced glycation end products as a molecular mechanism for aging as a risk factor in osteoarthritis. *Arthritis. Rheum.*, 2004;50(4):1207–1215.

[66] Hollander AP; Pidoux I; Reiner A; Rorabeck C; Bourne R; Poole AR. Damage to type II collagen in aging and osteoarthritis starts at the articular surface; originates around chondrocytes; and extends into the cartilage with progressive degeneration. *J. Clin. Invest.*, 1995;96:2859– 69.

[67] Wu W; Billinghurst RC; Pidoux I; Antoniou J; Zukor D; Tanzer M, et al. Sites of collagenase cleavage and denaturation of type II collagen in aging and osteoarthritic articular cartilage and their relationship to the distribution of matrix metalloproteinase 1 and matrix metalloproteinase 13. *Arthritis. Rheum.*, 2002;46:2087-94.

[68] Burr DB; Radin EL. Microfractures and microcracks in subchondral bone: are they relevant to osteoarthrosis? *Rheum. Dis. Clin. North Am.*, 2003;29(4):675–685.

[69] Burr DB. The importance of subchondral bone in the progression of osteoarthritis. *J. Rheumatol. Suppl.*, 2004;70:77–80.

[70] Sanchez C; Deberg MA; Bellahcene A; Castronovo V; Msika P; Delcour JP, et al. Phenotypic characterization of osteoblasts from the sclerotic zones of osteoarthritic subchondral bone. *Arthritis. Rheum.*, 2008;58(2):442–455.

[71] Felson DT; Chaisson CE; Hill CL; Totterman SM; Gale ME; Skinner KM, et al. The Association of Bone Marrow Lesions with Pain in Knee Osteoarthritis. *Ann. Intern. Med.*, 2001;134(7):541–549.

[72] Baranyay FJ; Wang Y; Wluka AE; English DR; Giles GG; Sullivan RO, et al. Association of bone marrow lesions with knee structures and risk factors for bone marrow lesions in the knees of clinically healthy; community-based adults. *Semin. Arthritis. Rheum.*, 2007;37(2):112 118.

[73] Haywood L; McWilliams DF; Pearson CI; Gill SE; Ganesan A; Wilson D, et al. Inflammation and angiogenesis in osteoarthritis. *Arthritis. Rheum.*, 2003;48(8):2173–2177.

[74] Spector TD; Hart DJ; Nandra D; Doyle DV; Mackillop N; Gallimore JR, et al. Low-level increases in serum C-reactive protein are present in early osteoarthritis of the knee and predict progressive disease. *Arthritis. Rheum.*, 1997;40(4): 723–727.

[75] Livshits G; Zhai G; Hart DJ; Kato BS; Wang H; Williams FM, et al. Interleukin-6 is a significant predictor of radiographic knee osteoarthritis: The Chingford study. *Arthritis. Rheum.*, 2009;60(7):2037–2045.

[76] van Beuningen HM; van der Kraan PM; Arntz OJ; van den Berg WB. Transforming growth factor-beta 1 stimulates articular chondrocyte proteoglycan synthesis and induces osteophyte formation in the murine knee joint. *Lab. Invest.*, 1994;71(2):279–290.

[77] Olmez N; Schumacher HR Jr. Crystal deposition and osteoarthritis. *Curr. Rheumatol. Rep.*, 1999 Dec;1(2):107-11.

[78] Doherty M; Dieppe P. Clinical aspects of calcium pyrophosphate dihydrate crystal deposition. *Rheum. Dis. Clin. North. Am.*, 1988;14(2):395–414.

[79] Srikanth VK; Fryer JL; Zhai G; Winzenberg TM; Hosmer D; Jones G. A meta-analysis of sex differences prevalence; incidence and severity of osteoarthritis. *Osteoarthritis Cartilage,* 2005;13(9):769–81.

[80] Wluka AE; Cicuttini FM; Spector TD. Menopause; oestrogens and arthritis. *Maturitas,* 2000;35(3): 183–99.

[81] Hannan MT; Felson DT; Anderson JJ; Naimark A; Kannel WB. Estrogen use and radiographic osteoarthritis of the knee in women. The Framingham Osteoarthritis Study. *Arthritis. Rheum.*, 1990;33(4):525–32.

[82] Nevitt MC; Cummings SR; Lane NE; Hochberg MC; Scott JC; Pressman AR, et al. Association of estrogen replacement therapy with the risk of osteoarthritis of the hip in elderly white women. Study of Osteoporotic Fractures Research Group. *Arch. Intern. Med.,* 1996;156(18):2073–80.

[83] Zhang Y; McAlindon TE; Hannan MT; Chaisson CE; Klein R; Wilson PW, et al. Estrogen replacement and worsening of radiographic knee osteoarthritis: the Framingham Study. *Arthritis. Rheum.,* 1998;41:1867-73.

[84] Golightly YM; Dominick KL. Racial variations in self-reported osteoarthritis symptom severity among veterans. *Aging Clin. Exp. Res.,* 2005;17:264–269.

[85] Ang DC; Ibrahim SA; Burant CJ; Kwoh CK. Is there a difference in the perception of symptoms between African Americans and whites with osteoarthritis. *J. Rheumatol.,* 2003;30(6): 1305–1310.

[86] Allen KD. Racial and ethnic disparities in osteoarthritis phenotypes. *Curr. Opin. Rheumatol.,* 2010;22(5):528-32.

[87] Allen KD; Helmick CG; Schwartz TA; DeVellis RF; Renner JB; Jordan JM. Racial differences in self-reported pain and function among individuals with radiographic hip and knee osteoarthritis: The Johnston County Osteoarthritis Project. *Osteoarthritis Cartilage,* 2009;17(9): 1132–6.

[88] Clark AG; Jordan JM; Vilim VV; Renner JB; Dragomir AD; Luta G, et al. Serum cartilage oligomeric matrix protein reflects osteoarthritis presence and severity: the Johnston County Osteoarthritis Project. *Arthritis. Rheum.*, 1999;42: 2356-64.

[89] Spector TD; Cicuttini F; Baker J; Loughlin J; Hart D. Genetic influences on osteoarthritis in women: a twin study. *BMJ,* 1996;312(7036):940–3.

[90] Palotie A; Vaisanen P; Ott J; Ryhänen L; Elima K; Vikkula M, et al. Predisposition to familial osteoarthrosis linked to type II collagen gene. *Lancet,* 1989;1(8644):924–7.

[91] Felson DT; Couropmitree NN; Chaisson CE; Hannan MT; Zhang Y; McAlindon TE, et al. Evidence for a Mendelian gene in a segregation analysis of generalized radiographic osteoarthritis: the Framingham Study. *Arthritis. Rheum.*, 1998;41(6):1064–71.

[92] Ishimori ML; Altman RD; Cohen MJ; Cui J; Guo X; Rotter JI, et al. Heritability patterns in hand osteoarthritis: the role of osteophytes. *Arthritis. Res. Ther,* 2010;12(5):R180.

[93] Felson DT; Niu J; Clancy M; Aliabadi P; Sack B; Guermazi A, et al. Low levels of vitamin D and worsening of knee osteoarthritis: results of two longitudinal studies. *Arthritis. Rheum.*, 2007;56(1):129–36.

[94] McAlindon TE; Jacques P; Zhang Y; Hannan MT; Aliabadi P; Weissman B, et al. Do antioxidant micronutrients protect against the development and progression of knee osteoarthritis? *Arthritis. Rheum.,* 1996;39(4):648–56.

[95] Wluka AE; Stuckey S; Brand C; Cicuttini FM. Supplementary vitamin E does not affect the loss of cartilage volume in knee osteoarthritis: a 2 year double blind randomized placebo controlled study. *J. Rheumatol.,* 2002;29(12):2585–91.

[96] Fang W; Wu P; Hu R; Huang Z. Environmental Se-Mo-B deficiency and its possible effects on crops and Keshan-Beck disease (KBD) in the Chousang area; Yao County; Shaanxi Province; China. *Environ Geochem Health*, 2003;25(2):267–80.

[97] Neogi T; Booth SL; Zhang YQ; Jacques PF; Terkeltaub R; Aliabadi P, et al. Low vitamin K status is associated with osteoarthritis in the hand and knee. *Arthritis. Rheum.*, 2006;54(4):1255–61.

[98] Sowers M; Lachance L; Jamadar D; Hochberg MC; Hollis B; Crutchfield M, et al. The associations of bone mineral density and bone turnover markers with osteoarthritis of the hand and knee in pre- and perimenopausal women. Arthritis Rheum, 1999;42:483-9.

[99] Zhang Y; Hannan MT; Chaisson CE; McAlindon TE; Evans SR; Aliabadi P, et al. Bone mineral density and risk of incident and progressive radiographic knee osteoarthritis in women: the Framingham Study. *J. Rheumatol.,* 2000;27:1032-7.

[100] Dougados M; Gueguen A; Nguyen M; Tiesce A; Listrat VV; Jacob L, et al. Longitudinal radiologic evaluation of osteoarthritis of the knee. *J. Rheumatol.*, 1992;19:378-83.

[101] Schouten JS; van den Ouweland F; Valkenburg HA. A 12 year follow up study in the general population on prognostic factors of cartilage loss in osteoarthritis of the knee. Ann. *Rheum. Dis.,* 1992;51:932-7.

[102] Felson DT; Zhang Y; Anthony JM; Naimark A; Anderson JJ. Weight loss reduces the risk for symptomatic knee osteoarthritis in women. The Framingham Study. *Ann. Intern. Med.*, 1992;116(7): 535–9.

[103] Messier SP; Loeser RF; Miller GD; Morgan TM; Rejeski WJ; Sevick MA, et al. Exercise and dietary weight loss in overweight and obese older adults with knee osteoarthritis: the Arthritis, Diet, and Activity Promotion Trial. *Arthritis. Rheum.*, 2004;50(5):1501–10.

[104] Christensen R; Bartels EM; Astrup A; Bliddal H. Effect of weight reduction in obese patients diagnosed with knee osteoarthritis: a systematic review and meta-analysis. *Ann. Rheum. Dis.*, 2007;66(4):433–9.

[105] Tepper S; Hochberg MC. Factors associated with hip osteoarthritis: data from the First National Health and Nutrition Examination Survey (NHANES-I). *Am. J. Epidemiol.*, 1993;137(10):1081–8.

[106] van Saase JL; Vandenbroucke JP; van Romunde LK; Valkenburg HA. Osteoarthritis and obesity in the general population. A relationship calling for an explanation. *J. Rheumatol.*, 1988;15(7):1152–8.

[107] Sharma L; Lou C; Felson DT; Kirwan-Mellis G; Dunlop DD; Hayes KW, et al. Laxity in healthy and osteoarthritic knees. *Arthritis. Rheum.*, 1999;42:861-70.

[108] Sharma L; Pai YC; Holtkamp K; Rymer WZ. Is knee joint proprioception worse in the arthritic knee versus the unaffected knee in unilateral knee osteoarthritis? *Arthritis. Rheum.,* 1997;40:1518-25.

[109] Sharma L; Hurwitz DE; Thonar EJ; Sum JA; Lenz ME; Dunlop DD, et al. Knee adduction moment; serum hyaluronan level; and disease severity in medial tibiofemoral osteoarthritis. *Arthritis. Rheum.,* 1998;41:1233-40.

[110] Golightly YM; Allen KD; Renner JB; Helmick CG; Salazar A; Jordan JM. Relationship of limb length inequality with radiographic knee and hip osteoarthritis. *Osteoarthritis Cartilage,* 2007;15(7):824–9.

[111] Murray RO. The aetiology of primary osteoarthritis of the hip. *Br. J. Radiol.,* 1965;38(455):810–24.

[112] Stulberg SD; Cooperman DR; Wallensten R. The natural history of Legg-Calve-Perthes disease. *J. Bone Joint Surg. Am.,* 1981;63(7):1095–108.

[113] Harris WH. Etiology of osteoarthritis of the hip. *Clin. Orthop. Relat. Res.,* 1986;213:20–33.

[114] Lane NE; Lin P; Christiansen L; Gore LR; Williams EN; Hochberg MC, et al. Association of mild acetabular dysplasia with an increased risk of incident hip osteoarthritis in elderly white women: the study of osteoporotic fractures. *Arthritis. Rheum.,* 2000;43(2):400–4.

[115] Lohmander LS; Ostenberg A; Englund M; Roos H. High prevalence of knee osteoarthritis; pain; and functional limitations in female soccer players twelve years after anterior cruciate ligament injury. *Arthritis. Rheum.,* 2004;50(10):3145–52.

[116] Roos EM; Ostenberg A; Roos H; Ekdahl C; Lohmander LS. Long-term outcome of meniscectomy: symptoms; function; and performance tests in patients with or without radiographic osteoarthritis compared to matched controls. *Osteoarthritis Cartilage,* 2001;9(4):316–24.

[117] Englund M; Guermazi A; Gale D; Hunter DJ; Aliabadi P; Clancy M, et al. Incidental meniscal findings on knee MRI in middle-aged and elderly persons. *N. Engl. J. Med.,* 2008;359(11):1108–1115.

[118] Englund M; Guermazi A; Roemer FW; Aliabadi P; Yang M; Lewis CE, et al. Meniscal tear in knees without surgery and the development of radiographic osteoarthritis among middle-aged and elderly persons: The Multicenter Osteoarthritis Study. *Arthritis. Rheum.,* 2009;60(3):831–839.

[119] Hill CL; Seo GS; Gale D; Totterman S; Gale ME; Felson DT. Cruciate ligament integrity in osteoarthritis of the knee. *Arthritis. Rheum.,* 2005;52(3):794–799.

[120] Croft P; Cooper C; Wickham C; Coggon D. Osteoarthritis of the hip and occupational activity. Scand. *J. Work Environ. Health,* 1992;18(1):59–63.

[121] Lawrence JS. Rheumatism in cotton opertatives. Br J Industr Med, 1961;18:270–276.

[122] Hadler NM; Gillings DB; Imbus HR; ; Levitin PM; Makuc D; Utsinger PD, et al. Hand structure and function in an industrial setting. *Arthritis. Rheum.,* 1978;21(2):210–20.

[123] Felson DT; Hannan MT; Naimark A; Berkeley J; Gordon G; Wilson PW, et al. Occupational physical demands; knee bending; and knee osteoarthritis: results from the Framingham Study. *J. Rheumatol.,* 1991;18(10):1587–92.

[124] Buckwalter JA; Lane LE. Athletics and osteoarthritis. *Am. J. Sports Med.,* 1997;25:873-81.

[125] Kujala UM; Kettunen J; Paananen H; Aalto T; Battie MC; Impivaara O, et al. Knee osteoarthritis in former runners; soccer players; weight lifters; and shooters. *Arthritis. Rheum.,* 1995;38:539-46.

[126] Tveit M; Rosengren BE; Nilsson JK; Karlsson MK. Former Male Elite Athletes Have a Higher Prevalence of Osteoarthritis and Arthroplasty in the Hip and Knee Than Expected. *Am. J. Sports Med.,* 2012;40(3):527-33.

[127] Spector TD; Harris PA; Hart DJ; Cicuttini FM; Nandra D; Etherington J, et al. Risk of osteoarthritis associated with long-term weightbearing sports: a radiologic survey of the hips and knees in female ex-athletes and population controls. *Arthritis. Rheum.,* 1996;39(6):988–95.

[128] Lane NE; Michel B; Bjorkengren A; Oehlert J; Shi H; Bloch DA, et al. The risk of osteoarthritis with running and aging: a 5-year longitudinal study. *J. Rheumatol.,* 1993;20(3):461–8.

[129] Newton PM; Mow VC; Gardner TR; Buckwalter JA; Albright JP. Winner of the 1996 Cabaud Award. The effect of lifelong exercise on canine articular cartilage. *Am. J. Sports Med,* 1997;25(3): 282–7.

[130] Neogi T; Felson D; Niu J; Nevitt M; Lewis CE; Aliabadi P, et al. Association between radiographic features of knee osteoarthritis and pain: results from two cohort studies. *BMJ,* 2009:21;339:b2844.

[131] Slemenda C; Heilman DK; Brandt KD; Katz BP; Mazzuca SA; Braunstein EM, et al. Reduced quadriceps strength relative to body weight: a risk factor for knee osteoarthritis in women? *Arthritis. Rheum.,* 1998;41:1951-9.

[132] Sharma L; Dunlop DD; Cahue S; Song J; Hayes KW. Quadriceps strength and osteoarthritis progression in malaligned and lax knees. *Ann. Intern. Med.,* 2003;138(8):613–9.

[133] Altman R; Alarcon G; Appelrouth D; Bloch D; Borenstein D; Brandt K, et al. The American College of Rheumatology criteria for the classification and reporting of osteoarthritis of the hip. *Arthritis. Rheum.,* 1991;34:505-14.

[134] Altman R; Asch E; Bloch D; Bole D; Borenstein K; Brandt K, et al. Development of criteria for the classification and reporting of osteoarthritis. Classification of osteoarthritis of the knee. *Arthritis. Rheum.,* 1986;29:1039-49.

[135] Altman R; Alarcon G; Appelrouth D; Bloch D; Borenstein K; Brandt K, et al. The American College of Rheumatology criteria for the classification and reporting of osteoarthritis of the hand. *Arthritis. Rheum.,* 1990;33:1601 10.

[136] Zhang W; Doherty M; Leeb BF; Alekseeva L; Arden NK; Bijlsma JW, et al; ESCISIT. EULAR evidence-based recommendations for the diagnosis of hand osteoarthritis: report of a task force of ESCISIT. *Ann. Rheum. Dis,* 2009;68(1):8-17.

[137] Kerkhof HJ; Meulenbelt I; Akune T; Arden NK; Aromaa A; Bierma-Zeinstra SM, et al. Recommendations for standardization and phenotype definitions in genetic studies of osteoarthritis: the TREAT-OA consortium. *Osteoarthritis Cartilage,* 2011;19: 254-264.

[138] Dougados M. Clinical features of osteoarthritis. In: Haris ED, Budd RC, Firestein GS, Genovese MC, Sergent JS, Ruddy S, Sledge CB (Eds). Kelley's Textbook of Rheumatology. Philadelphia: *Elsevier Saunders*; 2005;1514-1527.

[139] Altman R; Asch E; Bloch D; Bole G; Borenstein D; Brandt K, et al. Development of citeria for the classification of osteoarthritis of the knee. *Arthritis. Rheum.,* 1986;29:1039-1049.

[140] Seed SM; Dunican KC; Lynch AM. Treatment options for osteoarthritis: considerations for older adults. Hosp. Pract. (Minneap), 2011;39(1):62-73.

[141] Altman RD; Dean D. Pain in osteoarthritis. Semin. *Arthritis. Rheum.,* 1989;18(4 Suppl 2)1-3.

[142] Kellgren JH; Moore R: Generalized osteoarthritis and Heberden's nodes. *Br. Med. J.,* 1952 Jan 26;1(4751):181-7.

[143] Dougados M; Nakache JP; Gueguen A. Criteria for generalized and focal osteoarthritis. *Rev. Rhum. Engl. Ed, 1996*;63(9):569-75.

[144] Spector TD; Cicuttini F; Baker J; Loughlin J; Hart D. Genetic influences on osteoarthritis in women: a twin study. *BMJ,* 1996;312:940-3.

[145] Resnick D. Patterns of migration of the femoral head in osteoarthritis of the hip. Roentgenographic-pathologic correlation and comparison with rheumatoid arthritis. *Am. J. Roentgenol. Radium. Ther. Nucl. Med.,* 1975;124(1):62– 74.

[146] Typpö T. Osteoarthritis of the hip. Radiologic findings and etiology. *Ann. Chir. Gynaecol. Suppl.,* 1985;201:1-38.

[147] Auleley GR; Duche A; Drape JL; Dougados M; Ravaud P. Measurement of joint space width in hip osteoarthritis: influence of joint positioning and radiographic procedure. *Rheumatology* (Oxford), 2001;40(4):414-9.

[148] Hochberg MC; Altman RD; Brandt KD; Clark BM; Dieppe PA; Griffin MR, et al. Guidelines for the medical management of osteoarthritis. Part I. Osteoarthritis of the hip. American College of Rheumatology. *Arthritis. Rheum.,* 1995;38(11):1535– 40.

[149] Ledingham J; Regan M; Jones A; Doherty M. Radiographic patterns and associations of osteoarthritis of the knee in patients referred to hospital. *Ann. Rheum. Dis.,* 1993;52:520-6.

[150] Vignon E; Piperno M; Le Graverand MP; Mazzuca SA; Brandt KD; Mathieu P, et al. Measurement of radiographic joint space width in the tibiofemoral compartment of the osteoarthritic knee: comparison of standing anteroposterior and Lyon schuss views. *Arthritis. Rheum.,* 2003;48(2):378-84.

[151] Chaisson CE; Zhang Y; McAlindon TE; Hannan MT; Aliabadi P; Naimark A, et al. Radiographic hand osteoarthritis: incidence; patterns; and influence of pre-existing disease in a population based sample. *J. Rheumatol.,* 1997;24(7):1337– 43.

[152] Alexander CJ. Heberden's and Bouchard's nodes. *Ann. Rheum. Dis.,* 1999;58(11): 675 –8.

[153] Campion G; Dieppe P; Watt I. Heberden's nodes in osteoarthritis and rheumatoid arthritis. *Br. Med. J.* (Clin Res Ed), 1983;287(6404):1512.

[154] Haugen IK; Bøyesen P. Imaging modalities in hand osteoarthritis - status and perspectives of conventional radiography; magnetic resonance imaging; and ultrasonography. *Arthritis. Res. Ther.,* 2011 Dec 13;13(6):248.

[155] Cobby M; Cushnaghan J; Creamer P; Dieppe P; Watt I. Erosive osteoarthritis: is it a separate disease entity? *Clin. Radiol.,* 1990;42(4):258-63.

[156] Moskowitz RW. Clinical and laboratory findings in osteoarthritis. In: McCarty DJ, Koopman WJ (Eds). Arthritis and Allied Conditions. Philadelphia: Lippincott Williams and Wilkins; 1993;1735-1760.

[157] Resnick D; Niwayama G. Radiographic and pathologic features of spinal involvement in diffuse idiopathic skeletal hyperostosis (DISH). *Radiology,* 1976;119(3):559-68.

[158] Mitchell NS; Cruess RL. Classification of degenerative arthritis. *Can. Med. Assoc. J.* 1977; 117: 763-5.

[159] Group for the Respect of Ethics and Excelllence in Science (GREES): Osteoarthritis section: Recommendations for the registrations of drugs used in the treatment of osteoarthritis. *Ann. Rheum. Dis.,* 1996; 55:552-557.

[160] Hunter DJ; Felson DT. Osteoarthritis. BMJ, 2006;18;332(7542):639–42.

[161] Dougados M: Synovial fluid cell analysis. *Bailliere's Clin. Rheumatol.*, 1996;10:519-534.

[162] Nalbant S; Martinez JA; Kitumnuaypong T; Clayburne G; Sieck M; Schumacher HR Jr. Synovial fluid features and their relations to osteoarthritis severity: new findings from sequential studies. *Osteoarthritis Cartilage,* 2003;11(1):50-4.

[163] Kraus VB. Osteoarthritis year 2010 in review: biochemical markers. *Osteoarthritis Cartilage,* 2011; 19: 346-353.

[164] Deberg M; Dubuc JE; Labasse A; Sanchez C; Quettier E; Bosseloir A, et al. One-year follow-up of Coll2-1; Coll2-1NO2 and myeloperoxydase serum levels in osteoarthritis patients after hip or knee replacement. *Ann. Rheum. Dis.*, 2008;67(2):168-74.

[165] Gangl M; Serteyn D; Lejeune JP; Schneider N; Grulke S; Peters F, et al. A type II-collagen derived peptide and its nitrated form as new markers of inflammation and cartilage degradation in equine osteochondral lesions. *Res. Vet. Sci.,* 2007;82(1):68-75.

[166] Henrotin Y; Deberg M; Dubuc JE; Quettier E; Christgau S; Reginster JY. Type II collagen peptides for measuring cartilage degradation. *Biorheology,* 2004;41(3-4): 543-7.

[167] Golightly Y; Marshall S; Kraus V; Renner J; Villaveces A; Casteel C, et al. Serum cartilage oligomeric matrix protein; hyaluronan; high-sensitivity C-reactive protein; and keratan sulfate as predictors of incident radiographic knee osteoarthritis: differences by chronic knee symptoms. *Osteoarthritis Cartilage,* 2010;18:62-3.

[168] Chua SD Jr; Messier SP; Legault C; Lenz ME; Thonar EJ; Loeser RF. Effect of an exercise and dietary intervention on serum biomarkers in overweight and obese adults with osteoarthritis of the knee. *Osteoarthritis Cartilage*, 2008;16(9):1047-53.

[169] Gordon CD; Stabler TV; Kraus VB. Variation in osteoarthritis biomarkers from activity not food consumption. *Clin. Chim. Acta,* 2008;398(1-2):21-6.

[170] Hayashi D; Guermazi A; Hunter DJ. Osteoarthritis year 2010 in review: imaging. *Osteoarthritis Cartilage*, 2011;19(4):354-60.

[171] Roemer FW; Crema MD; Trattnig S; Guermazi A. Advances in imaging of osteoarthritis and cartilage. *Radiology,* 2011;260(2):332-54.

[172] Kellgren J; Lawrence J. Radiological assessment of osteo-arthrosis. *Ann. Rheum. Dis.*, 1957;16:494–501.

[173] Guermazi A; Roemer FW; Burstein D; Hayashi D. Why radiography should no longer be considered a surrogate outcome measure for longitudinal assessment of cartilage in knee osteoarthritis. *Arthritis. Res. Ther.*, 2011 Nov 24;13(6):247.

[174] Peterfy CG; Guermazi A; Zaim S; Tirman PF; Miaux Y; White D, et al. Whole-Organ Magnetic Resonance Imaging Score (WORMS) of the knee in osteoarthritis. *Osteoarthritis Cartilage,* 2004;12:177–90.

[175] Kornaat PR; Ceulemans RY; Kroon HM; Riyazi N; Kloppenburg M; Carter WO, et al. MRI assessment of knee osteoarthritis: Knee Osteoarthritis Scoring System (KOSS)– inter-observer and intraobserver reproducibility of a compartment-based scoring system. *Skeletal. Radiol.,* 2005;34:95–102.

[176] Hunter DJ; Lo GH; Gale D; Grainger AJ; Guermazi A; Conaghan PG. The reliability of a new scoring system for knee osteoarthritis MRI and the validity of bone marrow lesion assessment: BLOKS(Boston Leeds Osteoarthritis Knee Score). *Ann. Rheum. Dis.*, 2008;67:206–11.

[177] Roemer FW; Eckstein F; Guermazi A. Magnetic resonance imaging-based semiquantitative and quantitative assessment in osteoarthritis. *Rheum. Dis. Clin. North* Am, 2009;35(3):521-55.

[178] Eckstein F; Ateshian G; Burgkart R; Burstein D; Cicuttini F; Dardzinski B, et al. Proposal for a nomenclature for magnetic resonance imaging based measures of articular cartilage in osteoarthritis. *Osteoarthritis Cartilage,* 2006; 14 (10): 974-983.

[179] Eckstein F; Burstein D; Link TM. Quantitative MRI of cartilage and bone: degenerative changes in osteoarthritis. *NMR Biomed.*, 2006;19:822–54.

[180] Gray ML; Eckstein F; Peterfy C; Dahlberg L; Kim YJ; Sorensen AG. Toward imaging biomarkers for osteoarthritis. *Clin. Orthop. Relat. Res.*, 2004;(427 Suppl):S175–81.

[181] Eckstein F; Cicuttini F; Raynauld JP; Waterton JC; Peterfy C. Magnetic resonance imaging (MRI) of articular cartilage in knee osteoarthritis (OA): morphological assessment. *Osteoarthritis Cartilage,* 2006;14(Suppl A):A46–75.

[182] Mosher TJ. Musculoskeletal imaging at 3T: current techniques and future applications. *Magn. Reson. Imaging Clin. N. Am.*, 2006;14:63–76.

[183] Burstein D; Bashir A; Gray ML. MRI techniques in early stages of cartilage disease. *Invest. Radiol.,* 2000;35:622–38.

[184] Burstein D; Velyvis J; Scott KT; Stock KW; Kim YJ; Jaramillo D, et al. Protocol issues for delayed Gd(DTPA) (2-)-enhanced MRI (dGEMRIC) for clinical evaluation of articular cartilage. *Magn. Reson. Med.*, 2001;45:36–41.

[185] Kimelman T; Vu A; Storey P; McKenzie C; Burstein D; Prasad P. Three-dimensional T1 mapping for dGEMRIC at 3.0 T using the Look Locker method. *Invest. Radiol.*, 2006;41:198–203.

[186] Mosher TJ; Dardzinski BJ. Cartilage MRI T2 relaxation time mapping: overview and applications. *Semin. Musculoskelet. Radiol.,* 2004; 8(4): 355-368 .

[187] Hunter DJ; Arden N; Conaghan PG; Eckstein F; Gold G; Grainger A, et al; OARSI OA Imaging Working Group. Definition of osteoarthritis on MRI: results of a Delphi exercise. *Osteoarthritis Cartilage*, 2011;19(8):963-9.

[188] Bansal PN; Joshi NS; Entezari V; Grinstaff MW; Snyder BD. Contrast enhanced computed tomography can predict the glycosaminoglycan content and biomechanical properties of articular cartilage. *Osteoarthritis Cartilage*, 2010;18:184-91.

[189] Aula AS; Jurvelin JS; Töyras J. Simultaneous computed tomography of articular cartilage and subchondral bone. *Osteoarthritis Cartilage*, 2009;17:1583-8.

[190] Alvarez C; Chicheportiche V; Lequesne M; Vicaut E; Laredo JD. Contribution of helical computed tomography to the evaluation of early hip OA: a study in 18 patients. *Joint Bone Spine,* 2005;72:578-84.

[191] Qvistgaard E; Kristoffersen H; Terslev L; Danneskiold-Samsøe B; Torp-Pedersen S; Bliddal H. Guidance by ultrasound of intraarticular injections in the knee and hip joints. *Osteoarthritis Cartilage,* 2001; 9(6): 512 –517.

[192] Monteforte P; Rovetta G. Sonographic assessment of soft tissue alterations in osteoarthritis of the knee. *Int. J. Tissue React,* 1999; 21(1):19-23.

[193] Iagnocco A; Coari G. Usefulness of high resolution US in the evaluation of effusion in osteoarthritic first carpometacarpal joint. *Scand. J. Rheumatol.*, 2000; 29(3):170-173.

[194] Keen HI; Wakefi eld RJ; Conaghan PG. A systematic review of ultrasonography in osteoarthritis. Ann Rheum Dis, 2009; 68 (5):611–619.

[195] Lim AY; Doherty M. What of guidelines for osteoarthritis? *Int. J. Rheum. Dis.*, 2011;14(2):136-44.

[196] Summers MN; Haley WE; Reveille JD; Alarcon GS. Radiographic assessment and psychologic variables as predictors of pain and functional impairment in osteoarthritis of the knee or hip. *Arthritis. Rheum.*, 1988;31; 204–9.

[197] Weinberger M; Tierney WM; Booher P; Hiner SL. Social support; stress and functional status in patients with osteoarthritis. *Soc. Sci. Med.*, 1990;30:503–8.

[198] Hannan MT; Anderson JJ; Pincus T; Felson DT. Educational attainment and osteoarthritis: differential associations with radiographic changes and symptom reporting. *J. Clin. Epidemiol.*, 1992;45:139–47.

[199] Wise BL; Niu J; Zhang Y; Wang N; Jordan JM; Choy E et al. Psychological factors and their relation to osteoarthritis pain. *Osteoarthritis Cartilage*, 2010;18: 883–7.

[200] Lugtenberg M; Burgers JS; Clancy C; Westert GP; Schneider EC. Current guidelines have limited applicability to patients with comorbid conditions: a systematic analysis of evidence-based guidelines. *PLoS One,* 2011;6(10):e25987.

[201] Hoffman C; Rice D; Sung HY. Persons with chronic conditions: their prevalence and costs. *JAMA,* 1996;276:1473–1479.

[202] Schoen C; Osborn R; Doty M; Bishop M; Peugh J; Murukutla N. Toward higher-performance health systems: adults' health care experiences in seven countries. *Health Aff*, 2007;26: w717–734.

[203] Brand C; Cox S. Systems for implementing best practice for a chronic disease: management of osteoarthritis of the hip and knee. *Intern. Med. J.*, 2006;36:170–9.

[204] Chevalier X; Marre JP; de Butler J; Hercek A. Questionnaire survey of management and prescription of general practitioners in knee osteoarthritis: a comparison with 2000 EULAR recommendations. *Clin. Exp. Rheumatol.*, 2004;22:205–12.

[205] DeHaan MN; Guzman J; Bayley MT; Bell MJ. Knee osteoarthritis clinical practice guidelines – how are we doing? *J. Rheumatol.*, 2007;34; 2099 105.

[206] Kirkley A; Webster-Bogaert S; Litchfield R; Amendola A; MacDonald S; McCalden R, et al. The effect of bracing on varus gonarthrosis. *J. Bone Joint Surg. Am.*, 1999;81(4): 539–548.

[207] Hinman RS; Crossley KM; McConnell J; Bennell KL. Efficacy of knee tape in the management of osteoarthritis of the knee: blinded randomised controlled trial. *BMJ*, 2003;19;327(7407):135.

[208] Brosseau L; Yonge KA; Robinson V; Marchand S; Judd M; Wells G, et al. Thermotherapy for treatment of osteoarthritis. *Cochrane Database Syst. Rev.*, 2003;(4):CD004522.

[209] Yurtkuran M; Kocagil T. TENS; electroacupuncture and ice massage: comparison of treatment for osteoarthritis of the knee. *Am. J. Acupunct.*, 1999;27:133-40.

[210] Clarke RG; Willis LA; Stenner L; Nichols PJR. Evaluation of physiotherapy in the treatment of osteoarthritis of the knee. Rheumatol. Rehabil., 1974;13:190-7.

[211] Rutjes AW; Nuesch E; Sterchi R; Juni P. Therapeutic Ultrasound for Osteoarthritis of the Knee or Hip. *Cochrane Database Syst. Rev.*, 2010 Jan 20;(1): (CD003132).

[212] Loyola-Sanchez A; Richardson J; Macintyre NJ. Efficacy of Ultrasound Therapy for the management of knee osteoarthritis: a systematic review with meta-analysis. *Osteoarthritis Cartilage*, 2010;18(9):1117-29.

[213] Huang MH; Lin YS; Lee CL; Yang RC. Use of ultrasound to increase the effectiveness of isokinetic exercise for knee osteoarthritis. *Arch. Phys. Med. Rehabil.*, 2005 Aug;86(8):1545-51.

[214] Zhang W; Moskowitz RW; Nuki G; Abramson S; Altman RD; Arden N, et al. OARSI recommendations for the management of hip and knee osteoarthritis; Part I: Critical appraisal of existing treatment guidelines and systematic review of current research evidence. *Osteoarthritis Cartilage*, 2007;15:981-1000.

[215] Osiri M; Welch V; Brosseau L; Shea B; McGowan J; Tugwell P, et al. Transcutaneous electrical nerve stimulation for knee osteoarthritis. *Cochrane Database Syst. Rev.*, 2000; (4): CD002823.

[216] Brosseau L. Efficacy of transcutaneous electrical nerve stimulation for osteoarthritis of the lower extremities: a meta-analysis. *Phys. Ther. Rev.,* 2004;9:213-33.

[217] Bjordal JM; Johnson MI; Lopes-Martins RAB; Bogen B; Chow R; Llunggren AE. Short-term efficacy of physical interventions in osteoarthritic knee pain. A systematic review and meta-analysis of randomised placebo-controlled trials. *BMC Musculoskelet Disord,* 2007;8:51.

[218] Rutjes AW; Nuesch E; Sterchi R; Kalichman L; Hendriks E; Osiri M, et al. Transcutaneous electrostimulation for osteoarthritis of the knee. *Cochrane Database Syst. Rev.*, 2009 Oct 7;(4):(CD002823).

[219] Ezzo J; Hadhazy V; Birch S; Lixing L; Kaplan G; Hochberg M, et al. Acupuncture for osteoarthritis of the knee: a systematic review. *Arthritis. Rheum.,* 2001;44:819-25.

[220] Manheimer E; Cheng K; Linde K; Lao L; Yoo J; Wieland S, et al. Acupuncture for peripheral joint osteoarthritis. *Cochrane Database Syst. Rev.,* 2010 Jan 20;(1): (CD001977).

[221] Roddy E; Zhang W; Doherty M. Aerobic walking or strengthening exercise for osteoarthritis of the knee? A systematic review. *Ann. Rheum. Dis.*, 2005;64:544-8.

[222] Thomas KS; Muir KR; Doherty M; Jones AC; O'Reilly SC; Bassey EJ. Home based exercise programme for knee pain and knee osteoarthritis: randomised controlled trial. *BMJ,* 2002;325:752.

[223] Roddy E; Zhang W; Doherty M; Arden NK; Barlow J; Birrell F, et al. Evidence-based recommendations for the role of exercise in the management of osteoarthritis of the hip or knee the MOVE consensus. *Rheumatolog*y (Oxford), 2005;44:67-73.

[224] Bartels EM; Lund H; Hagen KB; Dagfinrud H; Christensen R; Danneskiold-Samsoe B. Aquatic exercise for the treatment of knee and hip osteoarthritis. *Cochrane Database Syst. Rev.,* 2007 Oct 17;(4): (CD005523).

[225] American Geriatrics Society Panel on Exercise and Osteoarthritis. Exercise prescription for older adults with osteoarthritis pain: consensus practice recommendations. A supplement to the AGS Clinical Practice Guidelines on the management of chronic pain in older adults. *J. Am. Geriatr. Soc.,* 2001;49(6):808-23.

[226] Fisher NM; Kame VD; Rouse L; Pendergast DR. Quantitative evaluation of a home exercise program on muscle and functional capacity of patients with osteoarthritis. *Am. J. Phys. Med. Rehabil.*, 1994;73:413–420.

[227] O'Reilly SC; Muir KR; Doherty M. Effectiveness of home exercise on pain and disability from osteoarthritis of the knee: a randomized controlled trial. *Ann. Rheum.* Dis., 1999;58:15–19.

[228] Papaleontiou M; Henderson CR Jr; Turner BJ; Moore AA; Olkhovskaya Y; Amanfo L, et al. Outcomes associated with opioid use in the treatment of chronic noncancer pain in older adults: a systematic review and meta-analysis. *J. Am. Geriatr. Soc.*, 2010;58(7):1353–1369.

[229] Nüesch E; Rutjes AW; Husni E; Welch V; Jüni P. Oral or transdermal opioids for osteoarthritis of the knee or hip. *Cochrane Database Syst. Rev.*, 2009;(4):CD003115.

[230] AGS Panel on Persistent Pain in Older Persons. The management of persistent pain in older persons. *J. Am. Geriatr. Soc.*, 2002;50(6 Suppl):205-24.

[231] Zhang W; Nuki G; Moskowitz RW; Abramson S; Altman RD; Arden NK, et al. OARSI recommendations for the management of hip and knee osteoarthritis: part III: changes in evidence following systematic cumulative update of research published through January 2009. *Osteoarthritis Cartilage,* 2010;18(4):476–499.

[232] Kuffner EK; Temple AR; Cooper KM; Baggish JS; Parenti DL. Retrospective analysis of transient elevations in alanine aminotransferase during long-term treatment with acetaminophen in osteoarthritis clinical trials. *Curr. Med. Res. Opin.*, 2006;22(11): 2137–2148.

[233] Tramer MR; Moore RA; Reynolds DJ; McQuay HJ. Quantitative estimation of rare adverse events which follow a biological progression: a new model applied to chronic NSAID use. Pain 2000;85:169-82.

[234] Stucki G; Johannesson M; Liang MH. Use of misoprostol in the elderly: is the expense justified? *Drugs Aging*, 1996;8:84-88.

[235] Schnitzer TJ; Burmester GR; Mysler E; Hochberg MC; Doherty M; Ehrsam E, et al. TARGET Study Group. Comparison of lumiracoxib with naproxen and ibuprofen in the Therapeutic Arthritis Research and Gastrointestinal Event Trial (TARGET); reduction in ulcer complications: randomised controlled trial. *Lancet,* 2004;364:665-74.

[236] Bombardier C; Laine L; Reicin A; Shapiro D; Burgos-Vargas R; Davis B, et al. Comparison of upper gastrointestinal toxicity of rofecoxib and naproxen in patients with rheumatoid arthritis. The VIGOR Study Group. *N. Engl. J. Med.*, 2000;343:1520-1528.

[237] Silverstein FE; Faich G; Goldstein JL; Simon LS; Pincus T; Whelton A, et al. Gastrointestinal toxicity with celecoxib vs. nonsteroidal anti-inflammatory drugs for osteoarthritis and rheumatoid arthritis. The CLASS study: a randomized controlled trial. Celecoxib Long-term Arthritis Safety Study. *JAMA*, 2000;284:1247-1255.

[238] Kearney PM; Baigent C; Godwin J; Halls H; Emberson JR; Patrono P. Do selective cyclo-oxygenase inhibitors and traditional non-steroidal anti-inflammatory drugs increase the risk of atherothrombosis? Meta-analysis of randomised trials. *BMJ,* 2006;332:1302-8.

[239] Li Wan Po A; Zhang WY. Systemic overview of co-proxamol to assess analgesic effects of addition of dextropropoxyphene to paracetamol. BMJ, 1997;315:1565-1571.

[240] Kroenke K; Krebs EE; Bair MJ. Pharmacotherapy of chronic pain: a synthesis of recommendations from systematic reviews. Gen Hosp Psychiatry, 2009;31(3):206–219.

[241] Rosenberg MT. The role of tramadol ER in the treatment of chronic pain. *Int. J. Clin. Pract.,* 2009;63(10):1531–1543.

[242] Avouac J; Gossec L; Dougados M. Efficacy and safety of opioids for osteoarthritis: a meta-analysis of randomized controlled trials. *Osteoarthritis Cartilage*, 2007;15:957-65.

[243] Choquette D; McCarthy TG; Rodrigues JF; Kelly AJ; Camacho F; Horbay GL, et al. Transdermal fentanyl improves pain control and functionality in patients with osteoarthritis: an open-label Canadian trial. *Clin. Rheumatol.,* 2008;27(5):587–595.

[244] Langford R; McKenna F; Ratcliffe S; Vojtassák J; Richarz U. Transdermal fentanyl for improvement of pain and functioning in osteoarthritis: a randomized; placebo-controlled trial. *Arthritis. Rheum.,* 2006;54(6):1829–1837.

[245] Lin J; Zhang W; Jones A; Doherty M. Efficacy of topical NSAIDs in the treatment of osteoarthritis: a meta-analysis of randomized controlled trials. *Chin. J. Evid. Based Med.*, 2005;5(9):667-74.

[246] Zhang WY; Li Wan Po A. The effectiveness of topically applied capsaicin. A meta-analysis. *Eur. J. Clin. Pharmacol.*, 1994;46:517-22.

[247] Gammaitoni AR; Galer BS; Onawola R; Jensen MP; Argoff CE. Lidocaine patch 5% and its positive impact on pain qualities in osteoarthritis: results of a pilot 2-week; open-label study using the Neuropathic Pain Scale. *Curr. Med. Res. Opin.*, 2004;20(suppl 2):13–19.

[248] Kivitz A; Fairfax M; Sheldon EA; Xiang Q; Jones BA; Gammaitoni AR, et al. Comparison of the effectiveness and tolerability of lidocaine patch 5% versus celecoxib for osteoarthritis-related knee pain: post hoc analysis of a 12 week; prospective; randomized; active-controlled; open-label; parallel-group trial in adults. *Clin. Ther.* 2008;30(12):2366–2377.

[249] Verbruggen G. Chondroprotective drugs in degenerative joint diseases. *Rheumatology* (Oxford), 2006; 45; 129–138.

[250] Hunter; DJ; Hellio Le Graverand- Gastineau MP. How close are we to having structure-modifying drugs available? *Rheum. Dis. Clin North Am.*, 2008; 34; 789–802.

[251] Le Graverand-Gastineau MP. Disease modifying osteoarthritis drugs: facing development challenges and choosing molecular targets. *Curr. Drug. Targets*, 2010;11;528–535.

[252] Abramson SB; Attur M; Yazici Y. Prospects for disease modification in osteoarthritis. *Nat. Clin. Pract. Rheumatol.,* 2006; 2; 304–312.

[253] Schett G. Erosive arthritis. *Arthritis. Res. Ther.*, 2007; 9 (Suppl 1): S2.

[254] Salminen-Mankonen HJ; Morko J; Vuorio E. Role of cathepsin K in normal joints and in the development of arthritis. *Curr. Drug Targets*, 2007;8:315–323.

[255] Jones; AR; Gleghorn JP; Hughes CE; Fitz LJ; Zollner R; Wainwright SD, et al. Binding and localization of recombinant lubricin to articular cartilage surfaces. *J. Orthop. Res.*, 2007;25:283–292.

[256] Kashiwagi; M; Tortorella M; Nagase H; Brew K. TIMP-3 is a potent inhibitor of aggrecanase 1 (ADAM-TS4) and aggrecanase 2 (ADAM-TS5). *J. Biol. Chem.*, 2001;276:12501–12504.

[257] Glasson SS; Askew R; Sheppard B; Carito B; Blanchet T; Ma HL, et al. Deletion of active ADAMTS5 prevents cartilage degradation in a murine model of osteoarthritis. *Nature,* 2005;434: 644–648.

[258] Hunter DJ; Losina E; Guermazi A; Burstein D; Lassere MN; Kraus V. A pathway and approach to biomarker validation and qualification for osteoarthritis clinical trials. *Curr. Drug Targets*, 2010;11:536–545.

[259] Hunter DJ. Pharmacologic therapy for osteoarthritis--the era of disease modification. *Nat. Rev. Rheumatol.,* 2011 ;7(1):13-22.

[260] Clegg DO; Reda DJ; Harris CL; Klein MA; O'Dell JR; Hooper MM, et al. Glucosamine; chondroitin sulfate; and the two in combination for painful knee osteoarthritis. *N. Engl. J. Med.*, 2006;354(8):795–808.

[261] Sawitzke AD; Shi H; Finco MF; Dunlop DD; Bingham CO 3rd; Harris CL, et al. The effect of glucosamine and/or chondroitin sulfate on the progression of knee osteoarthritis: a report from the glucosamine/chondroitin arthritis intervention trial. *Arthritis. Rheum.*, 2008;58(10):3183–3191.

[262] Towheed TE; Maxwell L; Anastassiades TP; Shea B; Houpt J; Robinson V, et al. Glucosamine therapy for treating osteoarthritis. *Cochrane Database Syst. Rev.*, 2005;(2):CD002946.

[263] McAlindon TE; LaValley MP; Gulin JP; Felson DT. Glucosamine and chondroitin for treatment of osteoarthritis: a systematic quality assessment and meta-analysis. *JAMA,* 2000;283(11):1469–1475.

[264] Wandel S; Jüni P; Tendal B; Nüesch E; Villiger PM; Welton NJ, et al. Effects of glucosamine; chondroitin; or placebo in patients with osteoarthritis of hip or knee: network meta-analysis. *BMJ*, 2010;341:c4675.

[265] Danao-Camara T. Potential side effects of treatment with glucosamine and chondroitin. *Arthritis. Rheum.*, 2000;43(12):2853.

[266] Reginster JY; Deroisy R; Rovati LC. Long-term effects of glucosamine sulphate on osteoarthritis progression: a randomized; placebo controlled clinical trial. *Lancet*, 2001;357:251-6.

[267] Richy F; Bruyere O; Ethgen O; Cucherat M; Henrotin Y; Reginster J-Y. Structural and symptomatic efficacy of glucosamine and chondroitin in knee osteoarthritis: a comprehensive meta-analysis. *Arch. Intern. Med.,* 2003;163:1514-22.

[268] Leeb BF; Schweizer M; Montag K; Smolen J. A meta-analysis of chondroitin sulphate in the treatment of osteoarthritis. *J. Rheumatol.,* 2000; 27:205-11.

[269] Reichenbach S; Sterchi R; Scherer M; Trelle S; Burgi E; Burgi U, et al. Meta-analysis: chondroitin for osteoarthritis of the knee or hip. *Ann. Intern. Med.*, 2007;146:580-90.

[270] Dougados M; Nguyen M; Berdah L; Maziéres B; Vignon E; Lequesne M; ECHODIAH Investigators Study Group. Evaluation of the structure-modifying effects of diacerein in hip osteoarthritis: ECHODIAH; a three-year; placebo-controlled trial. Evaluation of the Chondromodulating Effect of Diacerein in OA of the Hip. *Arthritis. Rheum.*, 2001;44(11):2539–2547.

[271] Fidelix TS; Soares BG; Treviani VF. Diacerein for osteoarthritis. *Cochrane Database Syst. Rev.,* 2006 Jan 25;(1):CD005117.

[272] Brandt KD; Mazzuca SA; Katz BP; Lane KA; Buckwalter KA; Yocum DE, et al. Effects of doxycycline on progression of osteoarthritis: results of a randomized; placebo-controlled; double-blind trial. *Arthritis. Rheum.*, 2005;52(7):2015–2025.

[273] Nüesch E; Rutjes AW; Trelle S; Reichenbach S; Jüni P. Doxycycline for osteoarthritis of the knee or hip. *Cochrane Database Syst. Rev.,* 2009;(4):CD007323.

[274] Lane NE; Schnitzer TJ; Birbara CA; Mokhtarani M; Shelton DL; Smith MD, et al. Tanezumab for the treatment of pain from osteoarthritis of the knee. *N. Engl. J. Med.*, 2010;363(16):1521–1531.

[275] Malemud CJ. Anticytokine therapy for osteoarthritis: evidence to date. *Drugs Aging*, 2010;27(2):95–115.

[276] Bellamy N; Campbell J; Robinson V; Gee T; Bourne R; Wells G. Intraarticular corticosteroid for treatment of osteoarthritis of the knee. *Cochrane Database Syst. Rev.*, 2006;(2):CD005328.

[277] Shimizu M; Higuchi H; Takagishi K; Shinozaki T; Kobayashi T. Clinical and biochemical characteristics after intra-articular injection for the treatment of osteoarthritis of the knee: prospective randomized study of sodium hyaluronate and corticosteroid. *J. Orthop. Sci.*, 2010;15(1):51–56.

[278] Robinson P; Keenan AM; Conaghan PG. Clinical effectiveness and dose response of image-guided intra-articular corticosteroid injection for hip osteoarthritis. *Rheumatology* (Oxford), 2007;46(2):285–291.

[279] Lambert RGW; Hutchings EJ; Grace MG; Jhangri GS; Conner-Spady B; Maksymowych WP . Steroid injection for osteoarthritis of the hip. A randomized; double-blind; placebo-controlled trial. *Arthritis. Rheum.*, 2007;56:2278–87.

[280] Jones A; Regan M; Ledingham J; Pattrick M; Manhire A; Doherty M. Importance of placement of intra-articular steroid injections. BMJ, 1993;307:1329-30.

[281] Day B. The indications for arthroscopic debridement for osteoarthritis of the knee. *Orthop. Clin. North Am.*, 2005;36:413-7.

[282] Hubbard MJ. Articular debridement versus washout for degeneration of the medial femoral condyle. *J. Bone Joint Surg. Br.*, 1996;78:217-9.

[283] Moseley JB; O'Malley K; Petersen NJ; Menke TJ; Brody BA; Kuykenall DH, et al. A controlled trial of arthroscopic surgery for osteoarthritis of the knee. *N. Engl. J. Med.*, 2002;347:81-8.

[284] Chambers K; Schulzer M; Sobelov B. A controlled trial of arthroscopic surgery for osteoarthritis of the knee. *Arthroscopy,* 2002;18:683-7.

[285] Harris WH; Sledge CB. Total hip and total knee replacement (1). *N. Engl. J. Med.*, 1990;323:725-31.

[286] Harris WH; Sledge CB. Total hip and total knee replacement (2). *N. Engl. J. Med.*, 1990;323:801-7.

[287] Ethgen O; Bruyere O; Richy F; Dardennes C; Reginster J-Y. Health related quality of life in total hip and total knee arthroplasty: a qualitative and systematic review of the literature. *J. Bone Joint Surg. Am.*, 2004;86:963-74.

[288] Nilsdotter AK; Petersson IF; Roos EM; Lohmander LS. Predictors of patient-relevant outcome after total hip replacement for osteoarthritis: a prospective study. *Ann. Rheum. Dis.,* 2003;62:923-30.

[289] Lingard EA; Katz JN; Wright EA; Sledge CB; Kinemax Outcomes Group. Predicting the outcome of total knee arthroplasty. *J. Bone Joint Surg. Am.*, 2004;86:2179-86.

[290] Quintana JM; Arostegui I; Azkarate J; Goenaga JI; Elexpe X; Letona J, et al. Evaluation of explicit criteria for total hip replacement. *J. Clin. Epidemiol.*, 2000;53:1200-8.

[291] Escobar A; Quintana JM; Arostegui I; Azkarate J; Guenaga JI; Arenaza JC, et al. Development of explicit criteria for total knee replacement. *Int. J. Technol. Assess Health Care,* 2003;19:57-70.
[292] Quintana JM; Escobar A; Arostegui I; Bilbao A; Azkarate J; Goenaga JI, et al. Health-related quality of life and appropriateness of knee or hip joint replacement. *Arch. Intern. Med.,* 2006;166:220-6.
[293] Fortin PR; Clarke AE; Joseph L; Liang MH; Tanzer M; Ferland D, et al. Outcomes of total hip and knee replacement: preoperative functional status predicts outcomes at six months after surgery. *Arthritis. Rheum.,* 1999;42(8):1722–1728.
[294] Griffin T; Rowden L; Morgan D; Atkinson R; Woodruff P; Maddern G. Unicompartmental knee arthroplasty for the treatment of unicompartmental osteoarthritis: a systematic study. *ANZ J. Surg.*, 2007;77:214-21.
[295] Brand RA. Hip osteotomies: a biomechanical consideration. *J. Am. Acad. Orthop. Surg.* 1997;5:282-91.
[296] Millis MB; Kim YJ. Rationale for osteotomy and related procedures for hip preservation: a review. *Clin. Orthop. Relat. Res.,* 2002;405:108-21.
[297] Jackson JP; Waugh W. Tibial osteotomy for osteoarthritis of the knee. *J. Bone Joint Surg. Br.,* 1961;43:746-51.
[298] Harris WR; Kostiuk JP. High tibial osteotomy for osteoarthritis of the knee. *J. Bone Joint Surg. Am.,* 1970;52:330-6.
[299] Virolainen P; Aro HT. High tibial osteotomy for the treatment of osteoarthritis of the knee: a review of the literature and a meta-analysis of follow-up studies. *Arch. Orthop. Trauma Surg.,* 2004;124:258-61.
[300] Insall JN; Dorr D; Scott RD; Scott WN. Rationale of the knee society clinical rating system. *Clin Orthop,* 1999;248:13-4.
[301] Conway JD; Mont MA; Bezwada HP. Arthrodesis of the knee. *J. Bone Joint Surg. Am.,* 2004;86:835-48.
[302] Damron TA; McBeath AA. Arthrodesis following failed total knee arthroplasty: comprehensive review and meta-analysis of recent literature. *Orthopedics,* 1995;18:361-8.
[303] Bellamy N; Kirwan J; Boers M; Brooks P; Strand V; Tugwell P, et al. J Rheumatol. Recommendations for a core set of outcome measures for future phase III clinical trials in knee; hip; and hand osteoarthritis. Consensus development at OMERACT III. *J. Rheumatol.,* 1997;24(4):799-802.
[304] Bellamy N; Buchanan WW; Goldsmith CH; Campbell J; Stitt LW. Validation study of WOMAC: a health status instrument for measuring clinically important patient relevant outcomes to antirheumatic drug therapy in patients with osteoarthritis of the hip or knee. *J. Rheumatol.,* 1988;15:1833-40.
[305] Bellamy N; BuchananWW; Goldsmith C H; Campbell J; Stitt L. Validation study of WOMAC: a health status instrument for measuring clinicallyimportant patient-relevant outcomes following total hip or knee arthroplasty in osteoarthritis. *J. Orthop.* Rheumatol., 1988; 1: 95-108.
[306] Lequesne M G; Mery C; Samson M; Gerard P. Indexes of severity for osteoarthritis of the hip and knee: Validation-value in comparison with other assessment tests. *Scand. J. Rheumatol.*, 1987;(suppl 65): 85-9.

[307] Guccione AA; Felson DT; Anderson JJ; Anthony JM; Zhang Y; Wilson PW, et al. The effects of specific medical conditions on the functional limitations of elders in the Framingham Study. *Am. J. Public Health*, 1994 ;84(3):351-8.

[308] Gabriel SE; Crowson CS; O'Fallon WM. Costs of osteoarthritis: estimates from a geographically defined population. *J. Rheumatol. Suppl.,* 1995;43:23–5.

[309] Buckwalter JA; Saltzman C; Brown T. The impact of osteoarthritis: implications for research. *Clin. Orthop. Relat. Res.,* 2004;(427 Suppl):6-15.

[310] Ettinger WH; Davis MA; Neuhaus JM; Mallon KP. Long-term physical functioning in persons with knee osteoarthritis from NHANES I: effects of comorbid medical conditions. *J. Clin. Epidemiol.,* 1994;47:809–15.

[311] Kaplan RM; Alcaraz JE; Anderson JP; Weisman M. Quality adjusted life years lost to arthritis: effects of gender; race; and social class. Arthritis. Care Res., 1996;9:473–82.

[312] Lapsley HM; March LM; Tribe KL; Cross MJ; Brooks PM. Living with osteoarthritis: patient expenditures; health status; and social impact. *Arthritis. Rheum.*, 2001;45: 301–6.

[313] Blais R. Variations in the use of healthcare services: why are more studies needed? Can. Med. Assoc. J., 1994;151:1701–3.

[314] Rao JK; Callahan LF; Helmick CG. Characteristics of persons with self-reported arthritis and other rheumatic conditions who do not see a doctor. *J. Rheumatol.,* 1997;24:169–73.

[315] Hawker GA; Wright JG; Coyte PC; Williams JI; Harvey B; Glazier R, et al. Differences between men and women in the rate of use of hip and knee arthroplasty. *N. Engl. J. Med.*, 2000;342:1016–22.

[316] Katz JN; Wright EA; Guadagnoli E; Liang MH; Karlson EW; Cleary PD. Differences between men and women undergoing major orthopedic surgery for degenerative arthritis. *Arthritis. Rheum.,* 1994;37:687–94.

[317] Dominick KL; Ahern FM; Gold CH; Heller DA. Health-related quality of life and health service use among older adults with osteoarthritis. *Arthritis. Rheum.*, 2004 Jun 15;51(3):326-31.

In: New Horizons in Geriatric Medicine. Volume 1
Editors: Ahmet Turan Isik, M. Refik Mas et al.
ISBN: 978-1-62808-972-1

Chapter 14

URINARY TRACT INFECTIONS

Omer Coskun[1] and Hakan Erdem[2]
[1]Gulhane Medical Academy,
Department of Infectious Diseases and Clinical Microbiology, Ankara, Turkey
[2]Kasımpasa Hospital, Department of Infectious Diseases and Clinical Microbiology,
Istanbul/Turkey

ABSTRACT

An elder patient with a urinary tract infection (UTI) is not an infrequent applicant in the emergency department and poor outcome in this patient population admitted to emergency room with UTI has been known. UTIs have been classified as complicated or uncomplicated to emphasize the underlying urinary comorbid conditions, upper or lower to point anatomic localization, catheter-associated symptomatic or asymptomatic to delineate the catheterization status of a given patient. Contributing factors specific to gender include prostate enlargement in men, the increase of vaginal pH, vaginal atrophy due to postmenopausal estrogen depletion, and incomplete emptying of the bladder in elder women. Since classic clinical manifestations of UTIs such as dysuria, fever, urinary frequency and suprapubic tenderness may be absent or masked in the elderly, treating these infections in this group of patients is a special challenge for physicians. Vague symptoms such as nausea, vomiting and decreased urinary output must be distinguished from symptoms of other common illnesses. Thus, infections often present in subtle fashion in the elderly. Physicians must be aware of unique predispositions to infection among elder adults and must seek early recognition and diagnosis of disease and early initiation of therapy.

INTRODUCTION

Infection has a marked impact on mortality and morbidity in older adults, exacerbating underlying illnesses and initiating functional decline. Infections have been known to cause death primarily in one-third of the population over the age of 65 and contribute to mortality due to other medical reasons [1]. Urinary tract infections (UTI), in particular, may have either a mild clinical course or may progress to sepsis and death in patients with advanced age. They make up one-fourth of all infections in the elderly population and are the important causes of bacteremias [2-4]. In fact, genitourinary system has been found to be the source of bloodstream invasion in one-third to one-fifth of the elders with bacteremia [5-7]. It is reported that mortality due to bacteremic UTIs was found to be 10-30 % in the elderly population [8-11]. Furthermore, UTIs frequently have serious consequences such as delirium and dehydration other than urosepsis in the vulnerable elders [12]. Thus, an elder patient with a UTI is not an infrequent applicant in the emergency department and poor outcome in elderly patients admitted with any infection was derived and validated in the emergency rooms [13].

Caljouw et al. [14] reported that the incidence of UTI was 11.2 per 100 person years for individiuals over 86 years of age. This may be an overestimation due to the frequent presence of bacteriuria. Further, it is known that long-term catheterization is a strong risk factor for UTI and bacteriuria in institutionalized older persons [12]. In one nationwide study in the United States, 10.3% of hospital admissions due to infections were attributed to kidney, urinary tract, or bladder infections [15]. Hospitalization was more common in women than in men, and patients over 80 years of age had the highest admission rate. UTIs increase morbidity but not mortality in the elderly population [16].

Clinical Definitions

A UTI may involve the lower or upper urinary tract. Lower UTIs include cystitis and upper UTIs involve the kidneys (pyelonephritis). Acute cystitis is the most common type of UTI and is often referred to as a bladder infection. On the other hand, pyelonephritis is a potentially more serious disease [17, 18]. In this context, UTIs have been classified as complicated or uncomplicated to emphasize the underlying urinary comorbid conditions, upper or lower to point anatomic localization, catheter-associated symptomatic or asymptomatic to delineate the catheterization status of a given patient.

a) *Asymptomatic bacteriuria* (ASB) in women is defined as two consecutive clean-catch midstream urine samples growing $\geq 10^5$ CFU/mL of the same uropathogen (no more than two species) in a patient without symptoms of a UTI and no indwelling urinary catheter within seven days of the first urine culture. In men, a single clean-catch midstream sample growing $\geq 10^5$ CFU/mL without symptoms is consistent with the presence of an asymptomatic UTI [19]. ASB occurs in more than 10% of men over 65 years of age, 30% of female patients over 65 residing at home or within residential homes, and in up to 55% of women and between 15% and 40% of men residing within long-term care facilities (LTCFs) [20].
b) *Symptomatic UTI (cystitis)* is defined as a clean-catch urine culture growing $\geq 10^5$ CFU/mL of no more than 2 species of a uropathogen in a patient with UTI symptoms [21]. An alternative definition proposed on clinical grounds includes two of the following: Fever (>38°C [fever is not seen in uncomplicated cystitis]), dysuria, frequency, urgency, or suprapubic pain, and at least one of the following: Positive Gram stain, pyuria ≥ 10 white blood cells [WBCs]/mL^3), positive leucocyte esterase and/or nitrite by dipstick method, or two positive urine cultures with the same

uropathogen ($\geq10^2$) in a nonvoided sample. Another sign of UTI include foul-smelling urine and the urine that appears cloudy. The Infectious Diseases Society of America's (IDSA) 1999 consensus statement, however, recommends using $\geq10^2$ CFU/mL of a uropathogen for diagnosis of uncomplicated cystitis [22]. A consensus on the minimum CFU/mL value that is associated with a UTI has yet to be reached.

c) *Complicated UTIs* can affect the lower or upper urinary tract and occur in situations in which there are functional or structural abnormalities of the urinary tract that interfere with the normal flow of urine or defense mechanisms. These may result from the following: stone formation, indwelling catheters, prostatic hypertrophy, obstruction, cancer, or neurologic conditions [23]. UTIs in elderly men are generally considered complicated due to a potential prostate source [24].

d) *Uncomplicated UTIs* affect patients without functional or structural abnormalities of the urinary tract that interfere with the flow of urine or normal voiding mechanisms. The patient most commonly presents with urinary frequency, urgency, or dysuria with or without suprapubic pain. Patients with bacterial cystitis commonly have bacteriuria and pyuria, in conjunction with symptoms. Almost 15% of adult women and 3% of adult men are diagnosed with a UTI or cystitis each year [25]. Additionally, this patient population may be more prone to display neurological changes, including alterations in mental status from their baseline, with the onset of cystitis [26]. This finding is especially true in the elderly population residing in LTCFs. These unique features of disease presentation in the elderly population make the diagnosis of cystitis or pyelonephritis difficult, and there is a tendency to over treat with antibiotics in this patient population [27].

e) *Acute Pyelonephritis:* Acute pyelonephritis is a serious, potentially life threatening infection of the kidneys. The incidence in women was 12 to 13 cases per 10.000 population and three to four cases per 10.000 populations for outpatients and inpatients, respectively [28]. In men, the incidence was two to three cases per 10.000 outpatient population and one to two cases per 10.000 inpatient populations. The rates in men treated as outpatients or inpatients were generally lower than in women at almost all age groups, but discrepancy diminished at the older ages. When considering renal or infectious disease as a cause of death, overall mortality in hospitalized patients was 0.5/1000 for females and 0.6/1000 for males.

f) *Catheter-Associated (CA) Bacteriuria (Asymptomatic)/Catheter-Associated Symptomatic UTI*: CA-bacteriuria (indwelling urethral, suprapubic, freshly applied condom catheter in a male or intermittent catheterization) is defined as an asymptomatic presence of bacteria in the urine at a level $\geq10^5$ CFU/mL of ≥1 uropathogen. A CA-UTI is defined as a correctly obtained urine sample that grows $\geq10^3$ CFU/mL of ≥1 uropathogen in a patient with symptoms of a UTI with no other source of infection identified. The same criteria are applied to clean-catch midstream urine samples obtained from patients who have had a catheter removed 48 hours before obtaining a sample for culture. For a newly placed urinary catheter, a count $\geq10^2$ CFU/mL is sufficient for diagnosis of a UTI. There is no consensus on what constitutes a quantitative bacteria count for men with a condom catheter and a symptomatic UTI. CA-bacteriuria occurs at a rate of 3% to 8% per day and after about 30 days, virtually all patients will have bacteriuria [29]. Bacteriuria in patients who undergo short-term catheterization typically grow a single organism.

PREDISPOSING FACTORS TO UTI IN THE ELDERLY

Factors that predispose older adults to UTIs include the use of urethral or condom catheters, and neurogenic bladders with increased residual urine. Contributing factors specific to gender include prostate enlargement in men, the increase of vaginal pH, vaginal atrophy due to postmenopausal estrogen depletion, and incomplete emptying of the bladder in women. These aforementioned factors provide the opportunity for bacterial colonization and are likely to contribute to the higher rates of asymptomatic bacteriuria and UTIs in the elderly [30].

Multiple age-related changes contribute to decreased protection from infection in older adults. Due to the lessening quality of skin, respiratory, and gastrointestinal barriers with advanced age, microorganisms find easier ways of invasion, thus leading to infections. [31]. In addition, changes in cellular and humoral immunity including decreases in specific cell populations, losses of the proliferative capacity of immune cells, and decreased production of specific cytokines like IL-2 may lead to increased risk for intracellular pathogens [32, 33]. Impaired signal transduction after cytokine binding is also associated with impaired defense against fungal and viral pathogens. Decreased antibody response to vaccines, related to reductions in toll-like receptors and senescence of CD8+ T cells along with the reductions in immunoglobulin production and naive B-cells facilitate the development of infectious diseases in the elderly [34, 35].

THE CAUSATIVE AGENTS OF UTI IN THE ELDER POPULATION

The incidence rate approaches 10 % in women and 5.3 % in men over the age of 80 [36]. Gram-negative bacilli (e.g., *Escherichia coli, Enterobacter spp., Klebsiella spp., Proteus spp.*) are most common, but there is a shift to more resistant isolates in the elders towards *Pseudomonas aeruginosa*, and gram-positive organisms including enterococci, coagulase-negative staphylococci and *Streptococcus agalactiae*, when compared to young adults [37]. Elderly patients, particularly with chronic urological devices, often have polymicrobial bacteriuria [20].

In CA-bacteriuria, *E. coli* is the most common gram-negative organism isolated (incidence of 12%-29%). Gram-positive organisms include but are not limited to *Enterococcus species* (19%-20%), *coagulase-negative staphylococci* (21%-26%), and *S. aureus* (2.9%-4%). From the literature, fungi (mostly *Candida species*) have been isolated in 2.9% to 32% of cultures in this patient population. Unlike short-term catheterization, bacteriuria in patients with long-term catheter insertion is often polymicrobial, and organisms found in a sample may not persist in subsequent cultures [38, 39].

CLINICAL MANIFESTATIONS

Physicians must be aware of these unique predispositions to infection among elder adults and must seek early recognition and diagnosis of disease and early initiation of therapy. A challenge of early diagnosis is the often subtle and unique presentation of infections among elderly adults. For example, the basal body temperature of older adults may be lower than the standardized mean temperature of 37^{0}C (or 98.6^{0}F) [40]. In one study evaluating the elderly nursing home residents, the sensitivity of a single temperature of 38.3^{0}C (or 101^{0}F) was observed only 40 % among elderly residents with infection. Besides, UTIs are less likely to present with characteristically documented appearances like dysuria, and they more commonly present with changes in cognitive function like confusion or in physical functions like the inability to carry out daily activities [41]. This altered presentation is facilitated by underlying sensory deficits like impairments of hearing and vision, and dementia in the elderly host. The impaired vasopressin responses that occur in association with age lead to dehydration, hypernatremia, and azotemia when infection develops, and they also contribute to cognitive and functional decline. The subtle presentation of infection in older adults can have adverse consequences for both the underrecognition of disease and the overuse of empirical antibiotics. Because it is often difficult to distinguish true infection, overuse of antibiotics is common, particularly among individuals who reside in long-term care facilities, for whom 25 %-75 % of antibiotic use has been found to be "inappropriate" and for whom strict adherence to the minimum criteria for initiation of antibiotics should be practiced [42].

Since classic clinical manifestations of UTIs such as dysuria, fever, urinary frequency and suprapubic tenderness may be absent or masked in the elderly, treating these infections in this group is a special challenge for physicians. Vague symptoms such as nausea, vomiting and decreased urinary output must be distinguished from symptoms of other common illnesses [43]. Thus, infections often present in subtle fashion in the elderly. The clinical dilemma that the clinicians face is to determine what defines "symptomatic" in frail and often cognitively impaired seniors. Older adults with UTIs and comorbidities and those who are at risk for dehydration due to fever, nausea or vomiting should be strongly considered for hospitalization.

Patients with pyelonephritis typically present with fever, nausea, vomiting, and chills, with or without costovertebral angle pain or tenderness. Less commonly, patients may complain of pain in the right or left abdominal quadrants or in the epigastric region. Symptoms attributed to the bladder include urgency, frequency, dysuria, nocturia, and suprapubic discomfort. Hematuria may or may not be present. The fever response to serious infection may be blunted or absent in 20% to 30% of the elderly population. The IDSA defines a fever in the elderly population living in LTCFs as a single oral temperature >100°F (>37.8°C), or repeated oral temperatures >99°F (37.2°C), an increase in baseline temperature >2°F (>1.1°C), or a rectal temperature >99.5°F (>37.5°C) [44]. A patient's current medications should be reviewed for the presence of antipyretic or anti-inflammatory agents because these may blunt a fever response. Classic signs and symptoms of infection are more common in the independent elderly population [45]. The institutionalized patient may also demonstrate classic signs and symptoms; however, these elderly subjects may exhibit atypical presentations of infection like changes in mental status, lethargy, increased weakness, and complaints of abdominal pain. In addition, the inability to communicate with health care providers by more debilitated patients as in stroke or dementia, and the presence of multiple comorbidities adds to the diagnostic challenge in this population [45, 46].

CA-UTI's signs and symptoms may include new onset of fever or increase in body temperature, rigors, hypotension, altered mental status, costovertebral angle pain, malaise or lethargy, pelvic discomfort, and acute hematuria. Patients with recent catheter removal may experience frequency, urgency, suprapubic pain, and dysuria. Patients with spinal cord injury may experience an increased sense of restlessness, dysreflexia, and increase in spasticity.

Patients with short-term catheters can experience all of these signs and symptoms as well. In addition to the aforementioned findings, patients using intermittent catheterization or in whom the catheter has been removed, can complain of urgency, dysuria, and frequency [29].

Diagnosis

Physicians distinguish UTIs from other diseases that have similar clinical presentations with use of a small number of tests, none of which, if used individually, have adequate sensitivity and specificity. Among the diagnostic tests, urinalysis is useful mainly for excluding bacteriuria. Urine culture may not be necessary as part of the evaluation of outpatients with uncomplicated UTIs, but it is necessary for outpatients who have recurrent UTIs, experience treatment failures, or have complicated UTIs, as well as for inpatients who develop UTIs. Diagnosis of an UTI in an elderly patient relies on clinical signs and symptoms, supported by laboratory data. Urine cultures in infected elderly patients may have lower colony counts (10^2 to 10^3) compared to 10^5 in younger patients [47].

However, it is known that symptomatic UTI is over-diagnosed in the elderly population given the high prevalence of asymptomatic bacteriuria [48], for which the prevalence in residents of homes for the elderly is 25 % to 50 %, even rising to 100 % in catheterized patients. Asymptomatic bacteriuria in men is more common in the elder age compared to women [49, 50]. The detection of asymptomatic bacteriuria was higher when three specimens were obtained: 11 % of men had bacteriuria on at least one specimen. However, the bacteriuria was generally transient as persistence of the same organism in all three cultures occurred in only 1.3 % of men. Asymptomatic bacteriuria in young healthy men is rare [20].

The detection of signs and symptoms attributed to uncomplicated cystitis, the evaluation of the urine is an important step in making a diagnosis. A workup should include a microscopic evaluation for WBCs or a dipstick test for the presence of nitrite and leucocyte esterase. The presence of nitrites in the urine is indicative that gram-negative bacteria and nitrate reductase are present (specificity, 92%-100%; sensitivity, 25%). A positive urine leucocyte esterase test result may also aid in the diagnosis of a UTI, with the specificity ranging from 94% to 98% and the sensitivity ranging from 75% to 96% [51, 52].

A urine culture is not always indicated in elderly women with signs and symptoms of uncomplicated cystitis. The independent elderly woman should have a urine culture and sensitivity obtained if she does not respond to initial therapy, experiences a relapse, or has a history of recurrent UTIs. In elderly women and men residing in an LTCF or with a suspected hospital acquired infection, with signs and symptoms compatible with uncomplicated cystitis, a urine culture with sensitivity should be obtained if pyuria, that is more than 10 leucocytes per high power field, and the dipstick test is positive for leucocyte esterase or nitrite due to the risk of antimicrobial-resistant organism in these settings [48, 53].

Patients should be questioned about underlying conditions that may suggest the presence of complicated pyelonephritis. The physical examination should include vital signs and assessment for signs and symptoms of AP. A urine analysis including a microscopic examination should be obtained. Although the presence of pyruia is not sufficient to diagnose a urinary source of infection, a lack of WBCs in the urine essentially rules out a urinary infection unless there is complete obstruction of the affected kidney [54]. A positive result on the nitrite test, changes in urine odor, color, or turbidity are not sufficient by themselves to diagnose a urinary source of infection [55]. A urine culture and antimicrobial sensitivity should be obtained in all patients in whom pyelonephritis is suspected. This step is especially important due to the increasing prevalence of resistant uropathogens, including *E. coli* [56]. Knowledge of the causative organism and antibiotic susceptibility will assist in the choice of the antimicrobial agent. Generally, a clean-catch urine is ideal for obtaining a sample for culture, although an uncleansed first void urine may be sufficient in men [57]. In the frail elderly population or institutionalized individuals, obtaining clean-catch urine may be difficult. If a condom catheter is being used, a newly applied unit with prior cleansing of the glans penis can be used to collect urine. If the patient has an indwelling catheter, a sample can be obtained from the catheter port. Symptomatic patients with an indwelling urethral catheter placed for over two weeks should have the catheter replaced and the urine collected from the new catheter [29].

In patients of both sexes who are unable to provide a suitable urine sample for culture, an in-and-out catheterization can be performed. The urine culture should be obtained before initiating antibiotic treatment, and efforts should be made to determine whether the patient is currently receiving antibiotics. A gram stain of the urine can assist in directing initial therapy. A complete blood count, including a peripheral WBC with differential, should be obtained on all patients.

Additional blood work should include a serum chemistry panel and a serum creatinine to determine if antibiotic therapy will need to be adjusted due to altered kidney function. Blood cultures are commonly obtained in patients suspected of having AP; however, some have questioned their value when paired with a urine culture in the management of women with uncomplicated or complicated pyelonephritis. Others recommend that paired urine and blood cultures should be obtained in all patients suspected of having complicated pyelonephritis. Renal ultrasound and/or computerized axial tomography, urography and urodynamic tests are used to delineate complicated from uncomplicated AP. In the patient with uncomplicated disease, these tests add little to management if the patient responds to therapy within 72 hours [58, 59].

In the catheterized elders, neither dip sticks nor urine culture is useful in confirming the clinical diagnosis of UTI. Only a negative urine culture can exclude an infection [19]. In noncatheterized bacteriuric elderly institutionalized patients with fever and no localizing signs or symptoms, bacteriuria has only a 10 % positive predictive value for a urinary source of fever [60]. In addition, difficulties in communication, chronic genitourinary symptoms, and the high frequency of positive urine cultures make detection of symptomatic UTI problematic for the functionally impaired elderly [61].

Also urine cultures are often contaminated and the lack of existence of specific markers of infectious bladder inflammation makes it difficult to diagnose UTI in impaired elderly. Clinical guidelines from the Infectious Diseases Society of America (IDSA) for evaluation of infection in older residents of LTCFs advise that urinalysis and urine cultures should not be ordered for asymptomatic individuals. Clinical findings and a urinalysis are usually sufficient for diagnosis in older adults; however, a urine Gram stain and culture should be considered to direct therapy [62].

Because CA-bacteriuria is ubiquitous in patients with long-term catheterization and symptoms may be difficult to solicit in the elderly population, the presence of a CA-UTI is by necessity a diagnosis of exclusion. The urinalysis and quantitative urine culture are not helpful in differentiating CA-bacteriuria from CA-UTI. In the symptomatic patients with a short-term catheter, urine samples for culture should be obtained using sterile technique through the catheter port or by puncturing the catheter. Symptomatic patients with a catheter in place for two weeks should have the catheter removed and replaced by a new catheter if the catheter use is still indicated.

The urine sample for culture should be obtained using sterile technique from the new catheter and before the initiation of antimicrobial therapy. If the catheter can be discontinued, a midstream clean-catch urine specimen should be obtained for culture and sensitivity before the initiation of antimicrobial treatment [29, 63].

TREATMENT

Treatment for UTIs should be directed at the organism identified by Gram stain and culture. Unfortunately, polymicrobial infections occur in about 30 % of patients and more often if the UTI is related to the use of a catheter. In these patients, the use of a broad-spectrum antibiotic may be necessary. In general, seven days is an adequate duration of therapy in older women and 14 days in older men. The duration of therapy is routinely doubled for infections considered to be serious.

Lower Tract UTI

When true UTI is documented in an older woman, therapy is based on the location of infection and likely causative agent. Lower tract UTIs (cystitis) are often treated with short courses of antibiotics for three to five days in young women. A systematic review comparing antibiotic course duration as single-day, three to six days, or seven to 14 days for uncomplicated symptomatic lower UTI in elderly women found that three to six day courses were sufficient for treatment [64].

Asymptomatic Bacteriuria

Asymptomatic bacteriuria is not infrequent in the elderly, and with the use of chronic catheters the rates are even higher. Persistent bacteriuria does not appear to impair renal function or cause hypertension.

Numerous studies suggest that there is no clinical benefit when asymptomatic bacteriuria is treated, but treatment can lead to significant side effects, expense and potential for selection of resistant organisms. Thus, treatment is not recommended, even in the presence of white blood cells in the urine. Exceptions to treatment of asymptomatic bacteriuria are patients scheduled for a genitourinary procedure who have obstructive uropathy, stones or a history of recurrent symptomatic infections. Because of the usual presence of anatomic abnormalities or prostatitis, bacteriuria in men is typically difficult to eradicate with antibiotic therapy [49]. Thus, most authorities advocate withholding antibiotics in patients who are completely asymptomatic [30].

Upper Tract UTI

Upper tract infections require longer courses of therapy than lower tract infection. Because of the excellent bioavailability of many antibiotics, particularly the fluoroquinolones, intravenous therapy is not essential if the patient can tolerate oral medications, is not septic, and the infecting organism is sensitive to oral agents.

The location of therapy in the elderly population with AP will depend on the severity of illness, living conditions, existing comorbidities, and the ability of the patient to comply with therapy and to seek assistance should conditions not improve. The choice of antibiotic therapy will depend on local resistance patterns of likely organisms, the severity of the infection, and patient factors [18].

Currently, there are few guidelines specifically for the management of the elderly population with AP. Patient therapy recommendations will be based on the severity of illness like mild, moderate, or severe. Patients with mild disease are defined as those patients with signs and symptoms that would not require admission to the hospital like low-grade fever, normal or slightly elevated peripheral WBC, absence of nausea or vomiting, and stable hemodynamics. Empiric therapy with an oral fluoroquinolone (ciprofloxacin 500 mg orally BID or levofloxacin 750 mg orally once daily) with or without an initial intravenous dose is appropriate when the resistance rate of suspected organisms to the fluorquinolone is less than 10% and the patient does not have risk factors for quinolone resistance [65-67]. If local fluoroquinolone resistance is over 10%, an initial dose of ceftriaxone or an aminoglycoside can be administered. Adjustments to therapy should be made once culture and sensitivity results are available. Although co-trimoxazole would not be a first-choice agent for AP due to high initial resistance, it can be used for susceptible organisms once sensitivity is known. In patients with moderate disease, that is more ill than patients with mild disease but without severe sepsis, an oral fluoroquinolone can be used assuming the aforementioned resistance issues are not present and the patient can take oral medication. If the patient cannot tolerate oral medication due to gastrointestinal intolerance, a fluoroquinolone can be administered intravenously and switched to oral therapy once the patient can tolerate it. In cases of suspected resistance or intolerance to a fluoroquinolone, consideration should be given to the use of ceftriaxone, cefotaxime, cefepime, an aminoglycoside with or without ampicillin, a carbapenem, or piperacillin/tazobactam with or without an aminoglycoside. Aminoglycoside antibiotics should be used cautiously in the elderly population with decreased kidney function. Intravenous therapy should be switched to an appropriate oral antibiotic as soon as the patient improves, within 48-72 hours in particular, and can tolerate oral administration of therapy [68-70]. Patients with severe disease as in severe sepsis. diastolic blood pressure less than 60 mm Hg, altered mental status, need of vasopressors, and presence of at least three of the following parameters like temperature over 38.3°C, chills, nausea or vomiting, WBC more than 15,000/mm^3, moderate to severe flank pain will require hospitalization and parenteral therapy [71]. Choice of regimen should be based on expected antibiotic susceptibility. A fluoroquinolone, ceftriaxone, cefotaxime, ceftazidime, cefepime, an aminoglycoside with or without ampicillin, piperacillin/tazobactam with or without an aminoglycoside, or a carbapenem can be considered [68]. The carbapenem antibiotics have activity against organisms that produce extended-spectrum beta-lactamases and AmpC beta-lactamases [72]. Ertapenem should not be used as initial therapy if *P. aeruginosa* is suspected because it has no activity against the organism. In general, the length of antibiotic therapy should be between 10 and 14 days for women and 14 days for men. Levofloxacin 750 mg once daily can be administered for 5 days. Failure to respond to appropriate therapy within 72 hours warrants a search for complicating factors such as obstruction or intrarenal abscess. Length of therapy will need to be individualized in patients with complicated AP, which is approximately two to three weeks. In patients with complicated AP, efforts should be carried out to correct the underlying defect if possible. All doses and interval designations for the antibiotics mentioned here are based on patients with normal kidney function [73].

Catheter-Associated Bacteriuria (Asymptomatic)/Catheter-Associated Symptomatic UTI

Current guidelines do not recommend treatment of CA-bacteriuria [29]. Because health care associated CAUTI are often polymicrobial and caused by multidrugresistant organisms, the choice of initial antibiotic therapy will depend on local resistance patterns [18]. Initial therapy should be revised if indicated by culture and sensitivity results. A urine Gram stain can be used to guide initial therapy. Patients who respond quickly to therapy can be treated for seven days, whereas patients with delayed response should be treated for 10 to 14 days, regardless of whether the catheter is removed. Levofloxacin may be effective in select patients when administered for five days [29, 38, 74]. If the indwelling catheter is removed, a three-day regimen may be tried in women 65 years of age without signs or symptoms of pyelonephritis. Overall length of therapy depends on response to therapy and severity of infection. If possible, the catheter should be removed. Guidelines have been published to assist in reducing the incidence of CA-UTI, including the following: Use indwelling catheters only when indicated and discontinue as soon as clinically indicated; catheters should be placed by skilled personnel using aseptic techniques in placement and maintenance; use the smallest catheter caliber possible; and use condom catheters or other methods like intermittent catheterization, suprapubic catheter where appropriate [29, 75, 76]. Antimicrobial and silver-coated urethral catheters have been shown to provide short-term delay or reduction in CA-bacteriuria [29, 77]. Measures that have not been shown to be helpful in preventing CA-bacteriuria/CA-UTI include meatal cleansing, systemic prophylactic antibiotics, bladder irrigation, and use of antibacterial agents in the urine bag. Prophylactic antibiotics have resulted in selection of resistant organisms. The IDSA guidelines for CA-UTIs in adults do not recommend the use of prophylactic antimicrobial agents at the time of catheter removal or replacement [29, 78]. Methenamine (mandelate or hippurate) products have demonstrated inconsistent effects in patients with indwelling urinary or intermittent catheterization and are not currently recommended for suppression or prophylaxis to prevent bacteriuria [29, 78, 79]. Cranberry supplements have generally failed to demonstrate a benefit in catheterized patients with a neurogenic bladder [80]. More research will be needed to determine the validity of these approaches.

Prevention

Several strategies to prevent UTI have been developed, such as treatment of those at high risk with low-dose, long-term antibiotics [81, 82], oestrogens [83] and cranberry products [81,

84]. These strategies have been shown to be effective in preventing UTI in younger women with recurrent UTI, but not yet in vulnerable older people. Preventive strategies are best applied to those at risk; however, factors associated with UTI in ambulatory older patients in the community setting have not been described. Several studies have shown that increasing age [85], diabetes mellitus [86], stroke [87], urine incontinence [88], prior history of UTI, urogenital surgery, and impaired functional and cognitive status predict the development of UTI among older individuals [89]. To target preventive strategies against UTIs in older individuals, those with highest risk to develop UTI have to be identified.

CONCLUSION

Physician awareness of UTI, which often present in subtle fashion in the elderly, is imperative in routine medical practice. Physicians must be prepared for unique predispositions to UTI among elder adults and must seek early recognition and diagnosis of disease and early initiation of therapy.

REFERENCES

[1] Mouton CP, Bazaldua OV, Pierce B, et al. Common infections in older adults. *American family physician*. 2001 Jan 15;63(2):257-68.

[2] Foxman B, Brown P. Epidemiology of urinary tract infections: transmission and risk factors, incidence, and costs. *Infectious disease clinics of North America*. 2003 Jun;17 (2):227-41.

[3] Ruben FL, Dearwater SR, Norden CW, et al. Clinical infections in the noninstitutionalized geriatric age group: methods utilized and incidence of infections. The Pittsburgh Good Health Study. *Am. J. Epidemiol.* 1995 Jan 15;141(2):145-57.

[4] Foxman B. Epidemiology of urinary tract infections: incidence, morbidity, and economic costs. *The American journal of medicine*. 2002 Jul 8;113 Suppl 1A:5S-13S.

[5] Payeras A, Garcia-Gasalla M, Garau M, et al. [Bacteremia in very elderly patients: risk factors, clinical characteristics and mortality]. *Enferm. Infecc. Microbiol. Clin.* 2007 Dec;25(10):612-8.

[6] Esposito AL, Gleckman RA, Cram S, et al. Community-acquired bacteremia in the elderly: analysis of one hundred consecutive episodes. *Journal of the American Geriatrics Society*. 1980 Jul;28(7):315-9.

[7] Greenberg BM, Atmar RL, Stager CE, et al. Bacteraemia in the elderly: predictors of outcome in an urban teaching hospital. *J. Infect.* 2005 May;50(4):288-95.

[8] Meyers BR, Sherman E, Mendelson MH, et al. Bloodstream infections in the elderly. *Am. J. Med.* 1989 Apr;86(4):379-84.

[9] Chin BS, Kim MS, Han SH, et al. Risk factors of all-cause in-hospital mortality among Korean elderly bacteremic urinary tract infection (UTI) patients. *Arch. Gerontol. Geriatr.* Jan-Feb;52(1):e50-5.

[10] Ackermann RJ, Monroe PW. Bacteremic urinary tract infection in older people. *Journal of the American Geriatrics Society*. 1996 Aug;44(8):927-33.

[11] Ackermann RJ, Monroe PW. Bacteremic urinary tract infection in older people. *J. Am. Geriatr. Soc.* 1996 Aug;44(8):927-33.

[12] Engelhart ST, Hanses-Derendorf L, Exner M, et al. Prospective surveillance for healthcare-associated infections in German nursing home residents. *J. Hosp. Infect.* 2005 May;60(1):46-50.

[13] Caterino JM, Kulchycki LK, Fischer CM, et al. Risk factors for death in elderly emergency department patients with suspected infection. *Journal of the American Geriatrics Society.* 2009 Jul;57(7):1184-90.

[14] Caljouw MA, den Elzen WP, Cools HJ, et al. Predictive factors of urinary tract infections among the oldest old in the general population. A population-based prospective follow-up study. *BMC Med.* 2011;9:57.

[15] Christensen KL, Holman RC, Steiner CA, et al. Infectious disease hospitalizations in the United States. *Clin. Infect. Dis.* 2009 Oct 1;49(7):1025-35.

[16] Tal S, Guller V, Levi S, et al. Profile and prognosis of febrile elderly patients with bacteremic urinary tract infection. *J. Infect.* 2005 May;50(4):296-305.

[17] Zalmanovici Trestioreanu A, Green H, Paul M, et al. Antimicrobial agents for treating uncomplicated urinary tract infection in women. *Cochrane database of systematic reviews (Online).* (10):CD007182.

[18] Coskun O, Erdem H, Avcı A. Management of community-acquired acute bacterial cystitis in Turkey *Turkish Journal of Medical Sciences.* 2011;41(1):149-57.

[19] Schmiemann G, Kniehl E, Gebhardt K, et al. The diagnosis of urinary tract infection: a systematic review. *Dtsch. Arztebl. Int.* 2010 May;107(21):361-7.

[20] Nicolle LE. Asymptomatic bacteriuria in the elderly. *Infect. Dis. Clin. North Am.* 1997 Sep;11(3):647-62.

[21] Matthews SJ, Lancaster JW. Urinary Tract Infections in the Elderly Population. *Am. J. Geriatr Pharmacother.* 2011 Aug 11.

[22] Warren JW, Abrutyn E, Hebel JR, et al. Guidelines for antimicrobial treatment of uncomplicated acute bacterial cystitis and acute pyelonephritis in women. Infectious Diseases Society of America (IDSA). *Clin. Infect. Dis.* 1999 Oct;29(4):745-58.

[23] Abrahamian FM, Moran GJ, Talan DA. Urinary tract infections in the emergency department. *Infect. Dis. Clin. North Am.* 2008 Mar;22(1):73-87, vi.

[24] Lipsky BA. Urinary tract infections in men. Epidemiology, pathophysiology, diagnosis, and treatment. *Ann. Intern. Med.* 1989 Jan 15;110(2):138-50.

[25] Kidney and Urologic Diseases Statistics for the United States. In: US Department of Health and Human Services PHS, National Institutes of Health, National Institute of Diabetes and Digestive and Kidney Diseases., ed. Washington DC: US Government Printing Office, NIH Publication No. 10-3895. 2010.

[26] Sobel JD, Kaye D. Urinary tract infections. In: Mandell GL, Bennett JE, Dolin R, eds. *Principles and Practice of Infectious Diseases.* 7th ed. Philadelphia: PA: Churchill Livingstone 2010:957–85.

[27] Rotjanapan P, Dosa D, Thomas KS. Potentially inappropriate treatment of urinary tract infections in two Rhode Island nursing homes. *Arch. Intern. Med.* 2011 Mar 14;171(5):438-43.

[28] Czaja CA, Scholes D, Hooton TM, et al. Population-based epidemiologic analysis of acute pyelonephritis. *Clin. Infect. Dis.* 2007 Aug 1;45(3):273-80.

[29] Hooton TM, Bradley SF, Cardenas DD, et al. Diagnosis, prevention, and treatment of catheter-associated urinary tract infection in adults: 2009 International Clinical Practice Guidelines from the Infectious Diseases Society of America. *Clinical infectious diseases : an official publication of the Infectious Diseases Society of America*. 2010 Mar 1;50(5):625-63.

[30] Zhanel GG, Harding GK, Guay DR. Asymptomatic bacteriuria. Which patients should be treated? *Archives of internal medicine*. 1990 Jul;150(7):1389-96.

[31] Gomez CR, Boehmer ED, Kovacs EJ. The aging innate immune system. *Current opinion in immunology*. 2005 Oct;17(5):457-62.

[32] Castle SC, Uyemura K, Fulop T, et al. Host resistance and immune responses in advanced age. *Clinics in geriatric medicine*. 2007 Aug;23(3):463-79, v.

[33] Weiskopf D, Weinberger B, Grubeck-Loebenstein B. The aging of the immune system. *Transplant international : official journal of the European Society for Organ Transplantation*. 2009 Nov;22(11):1041-50.

[34] Goronzy JJ, Fulbright JW, Crowson CS, et al. Value of immunological markers in predicting responsiveness to influenza vaccination in elderly individuals. *Journal of virology*. 2001 Dec;75(24):12182-7.

[35] Listi F, Candore G, Modica MA, et al. A study of serum immunoglobulin levels in elderly persons that provides new insights into B cell immunosenescence. *Annals of the New York Academy of Sciences*. 2006 Nov;1089:487-95.

[36] Foxman B, Brown P. Epidemiology of urinary tract infections: transmission and risk factors, incidence, and costs. *Infect. Dis. Clin. North Am*. 2003 Jun;17(2):227-41.

[37] Gavazzi G, Mallaret MR, Couturier P, et al. Bloodstream infection: differences between young-old, old, and old-old patients. *Journal of the American Geriatrics Society*. 2002 Oct;50(10):1667-73.

[38] Nicolle LE. Catheter-related urinary tract infection. *Drugs Aging*. 2005;22(8):627-39.

[39] Cohen A. A microbiological comparison of a povidone-iodine lubricating gel and a control as catheter lubricants. *J. Hosp. Infect*. 1985 Mar;6 Suppl A:155-61.

[40] Roghmann MC, Warner J, Mackowiak PA. The relationship between age and fever magnitude. *Am. J. Med. Sci*. 2001 Aug;322(2):68-70.

[41] Berman P, Hogan DB, Fox RA. The atypical presentation of infection in old age. *Age Ageing*. 1987 Jul;16(4):201-7.

[42] Loeb M, Bentley DW, Bradley S, et al. Development of minimum criteria for the initiation of antibiotics in residents of long-term-care facilities: results of a consensus conference. *Infection control and hospital epidemiology: the official journal of the Society of Hospital Epidemiologists of America*. 2001 Feb;22(2):120-4.

[43] McCue JD. Antibiotic use in the elderly: issues and nonissues. *Clinical infectious diseases: an official publication of the Infectious Diseases Society of America*. 1999 Apr;28(4):750-2.

[44] High KP, Bradley SF, Gravenstein S, et al. Clinical practice guideline for the evaluation of fever and infection in older adult residents of long-term care facilities: 2008 update by the Infectious Diseases Society of America. *Clin. Infect. Dis*. 2009 Jan 15;48(2): 149-71.

[45] Jarrett PG, Rockwood K, Carver D, et al. Illness presentation in elderly patients. *Arch. Intern. Med*. 1995 May 22;155(10):1060-4.

[46] Stott DJ, Falconer A, Miller H, et al. Urinary tract infection after stroke. *QJM*. 2009 Apr;102(4):243-9.

[47] Wilson ML, Gaido L. Laboratory diagnosis of urinary tract infections in adult patients. *Clinical infectious diseases : an official publication of the Infectious Diseases Society of America*. 2004 Apr 15;38(8):1150-8.

[48] Nicolle LE. Urinary tract infections in the elderly. *Clinics in geriatric medicine*. 2009 Aug;25(3):423-36.

[49] Nicolle LE, Bradley S, Colgan R, et al. Infectious Diseases Society of America guidelines for the diagnosis and treatment of asymptomatic bacteriuria in adults. *Clinical infectious diseases : an official publication of the Infectious Diseases Society of America*. 2005 Mar 1;40(5):643-54.

[50] Boscia JA, Kobasa WD, Knight RA, et al. Epidemiology of bacteriuria in an elderly ambulatory population. *The American journal of medicine*. 1986 Feb;80(2):208-14.

[51] Wilson ML, Gaido L. Laboratory diagnosis of urinary tract infections in adult patients. *Clin. Infect. Dis*. 2004 Apr 15;38(8):1150-8.

[52] Rahn DD, Boreham MK, Allen KE, et al. Predicting bacteriuria in urogynecology patients. *Am. J. Obstet. Gynecol*. 2005 May;192(5):1376-8.

[53] High KP, Bradley SF, Gravenstein S, et al. Clinical practice guideline for the evaluation of fever and infection in older adult residents of long-term care facilities: 2008 update by the Infectious Diseases Society of America. *Clinical infectious diseases : an official publication of the Infectious Diseases Society of America*. 2009 Jan 15;48(2):149-71.

[54] Juthani-Mehta M, Tinetti M, Perrelli E, et al. Role of dipstick testing in the evaluation of urinary tract infection in nursing home residents. *Infect. Control. Hosp. Epidemiol*. 2007 Jul;28(7):889-91.

[55] Arinzon Z, Peisakh A, Shuval I, et al. Detection of urinary tract infection (UTI) in long-term care setting: Is the multireagent strip an adequate diagnostic tool? *Arch. Gerontol. Geriatr*. 2009 Mar-Apr;48(2):227-31.

[56] Erdem H, Kilic S, Pahsa A, et al. Gram-negative bacterial resistance to cephalosporins in community-acquired infections in Turkey. *Journal of chemotherapy (Florence, Italy)*. 2005 Feb;17(1):61-5.

[57] Lipsky BA, Ireton RC, Fihn SD, et al. Diagnosis of bacteriuria in men: specimen collection and culture interpretation. *J. Infect. Dis*. 1987 May;155(5):847-54.

[58] Hsu CY, Fang HC, Chou KJ, et al. The clinical impact of bacteremia in complicated acute pyelonephritis. *Am. J. Med. Sci*. 2006 Oct;332(4):175-80.

[59] Demertzis J, Menias CO. State of the art: imaging of renal infections. *Emerg. Radiol*. 2007 Apr;14(1):13-22.

[60] Orr PH, Nicolle LE, Duckworth H, et al. Febrile urinary infection in the institutionalized elderly. *Am. J. Med*. 1996 Jan;100(1):71-7.

[61] Nicolle LE. Urinary infections in the elderly: symptomatic of asymptomatic? *International journal of antimicrobial agents*. 1999 May;11(3-4):265-8.

[62] Mouton CP, Bazaldua OV, Pierce B, et al. Common infections in older adults. *Am Fam Physician*. 2001 Jan 15;63(2):257-68.

[63] Steward DK, Wood GL, Cohen RL, et al. Failure of the urinalysis and quantitative urine culture in diagnosing symptomatic urinary tract infections in patients with long-term urinary catheters. *Am. J. Infect. Control*. 1985 Aug;13(4):154-60.

[64] Lutters M, Vogt-Ferrier NB. Antibiotic duration for treating uncomplicated, symptomatic lower urinary tract infections in elderly women. *Cochrane database of systematic reviews*. 2008(3):CD001535.

[65] Rattanaumpawan P, Tolomeo P, Bilker WB, et al. Risk factors for fluoroquinolone resistance in Gram-negative bacilli causing healthcare-acquired urinary tract infections. *J. Hosp. Infect*. 2010 Dec;76(4):324-7.

[66] van der Starre WE, van Nieuwkoop C, Paltansing S, et al. Risk factors for fluoroquinolone-resistant Escherichia coli in adults with community-onset febrile urinary tract infection. *J. Antimicrob. Chemother*. 2011 Mar;66(3):650-6.

[67] Peterson J, Kaul S, Khashab M, et al. A double-blind, randomized comparison of levofloxacin 750 mg once-daily for five days with ciprofloxacin 400/500 mg twice-daily for 10 days for the treatment of complicated urinary tract infections and acute pyelonephritis. *Urology*. 2008 Jan;71(1):17-22.

[68] Gupta K, Hooton TM, Naber KG, et al. International clinical practice guidelines for the treatment of acute uncomplicated cystitis and pyelonephritis in women: A 2010 update by the Infectious Diseases Society of America and the European Society for Microbiology and Infectious Diseases. *Clin. Infect. Dis*. 2011 Mar 1;52(5):e103-20.

[69] Mombelli G, Pezzoli R, Pinoja-Lutz G, et al. Oral vs intravenous ciprofloxacin in the initial empirical management of severe pyelonephritis or complicated urinary tract infections: a prospective randomized clinical trial. *Arch. Intern. Med*. 1999 Jan 11;159(1):53-8.

[70] Takahashi S, Kurimura Y, Takeyama K, et al. Efficacy of treatment with carbapenems and third-generation cephalosporins for patients with febrile complicated pyelonephritis. *J. Infect. Chemother*. 2009 Dec;15(6):390-5.

[71] Wells WG, Woods GL, Jiang Q, et al. Treatment of complicated urinary tract infection in adults: combined analysis of two randomized, double-blind, multicentre trials comparing ertapenem and ceftriaxone followed by appropriate oral therapy. *J. Antimicrob. Chemother*. 2004 Jun;53 Suppl 2:ii67-74.

[72] Baughman RP. The use of carbapenems in the treatment of serious infections. *J. Intensive Care Med*. 2009 Jul-Aug;24(4):230-41.

[73] Sperryville VA. The Sanford Guide to Antimicrobial Therapy In: Gilbert DN, Moellering RC, Eliopoulos GM, eds. *Antimicrobial Therapy*. 40th ed 2010:30.

[74] Dow G, Rao P, Harding G, et al. A prospective, randomized trial of 3 or 14 days of ciprofloxacin treatment for acute urinary tract infection in patients with spinal cord injury. *Clin. Infect. Dis*. 2004 Sep 1;39(5):658-64.

[75] Stamm WE, Hooton TM. Management of urinary tract infections in adults. *N. Engl. J. Med*. 1993 Oct 28;329(18):1328-34.

[76] Saint S, Kaufman SR, Rogers MA, et al. Condom versus indwelling urinary catheters: a randomized trial. *Journal of the American Geriatrics Society*. 2006 Jul;54(7):1055-61.

[77] Darouiche RO, Smith JA, Jr., Hanna H, et al. Efficacy of antimicrobial-impregnated bladder catheters in reducing catheter-associated bacteriuria: a prospective, randomized, multicenter clinical trial. *Urology*. 1999 Dec;54(6):976-81.

[78] Morton SC, Shekelle PG, Adams JL, et al. Antimicrobial prophylaxis for urinary tract infection in persons with spinal cord dysfunction. *Arch. Phys. Med. Rehabil*. 2002 Jan;83(1):129-38.

[79] Gould CV, Umscheid CA, Agarwal RK, et al. Guideline for prevention of catheter-associated urinary tract infections 2009. *Infect. Control. Hosp. Epidemiol.* 2010 Apr;31(4):319-26.

[80] Waites KB, Canupp KC, Armstrong S, et al. Effect of cranberry extract on bacteriuria and pyuria in persons with neurogenic bladder secondary to spinal cord injury. *J. Spinal. Cord. Med.* 2004;27(1):35-40.

[81] McMurdo ME, Argo I, Phillips G, et al. Cranberry or trimethoprim for the prevention of recurrent urinary tract infections? A randomized controlled trial in older women. *The Journal of antimicrobial chemotherapy*. 2009 Feb;63(2):389-95.

[82] Albert X, Huertas I, Pereiro, II, et al. Antibiotics for preventing recurrent urinary tract infection in non-pregnant women. *Cochrane database of systematic reviews*. 2004(3):CD001209.

[83] Perrotta C, Aznar M, Mejia R, et al. Oestrogens for preventing recurrent urinary tract infection in postmenopausal women. *Obstet. Gynecol.* 2008 Sep;112(3):689-90.

[84] Jepson RG, Craig JC. Cranberries for preventing urinary tract infections. *Cochrane database of systematic reviews*. 2008(1):CD001321.

[85] High KP, Bradley S, Loeb M, et al. A new paradigm for clinical investigation of infectious syndromes in older adults: assessment of functional status as a risk factor and outcome measure. *Clinical infectious diseases : an official publication of the Infectious Diseases Society of America*. 2005 Jan 1;40(1):114-22.

[86] Geerlings SE. Urinary tract infections in patients with diabetes mellitus: epidemiology, pathogenesis and treatment. *International journal of antimicrobial agents*. 2008 Feb;31 Suppl 1:S54-7.

[87] Powers JS, Billings FT, Behrendt D, et al. Antecedent factors in urinary tract infections among nursing home patients. *South. Med. J.* 1988 Jun;81(6):734-5.

[88] Moore EE, Jackson SL, Boyko EJ, et al. Urinary incontinence and urinary tract infection: temporal relationships in postmenopausal women. *Obstet. Gynecol.* 2008 Feb;111(2 Pt 1):317-23.

[89] Stamm WE, Raz R. Factors contributing to susceptibility of postmenopausal women to recurrent urinary tract infections. *Clinical infectious diseases : an official publication of the Infectious Diseases Society of America*. 1999 Apr;28(4):723-5.

EDITORS CONTACT INFORMATION

Ahmet Turan Isik, M.D., Associate Professor
Department of Geriatric Medicine,
Gulhane School of Medicine,
Ankara, TURKEY
atisik@yahoo.com

M. Refik Mas, M.D., Professor
Department of Geriatric Medicine,
Gulhane School of Medicine,
Ankara, TURKEY
masrefik@gmail.com

M. Akif Karan, M.D., Professor
Department of Geriatric Medicine,
University of Istanbul,
TURKEY
karanma@istanbul.edu.tr

George T. Grossberg, M.D., Professor
Department of Neurology & Psychiatry;
Department of Anatomy and Neurobiology;
Department of Internal Medicine,
Division of Geriatric Medicine.
1438 S. Grand Blvd., St. Louis, MO 63104
grossbgt@slu.edu

INDEX

#

A

B

D

E

F

G

H

I

J

K

N

Q

R

S

T

U

V

W

X

Y

Z